A Mortal Condition

A Mortal Condition

Martha Fay

Coward-McCann, Inc.
New York

Designed by Katy Fay Early & Mary Fay-Zenk

The text of this book is set in 11 point Palatino.

Library of Congress Cataloging in Publication Data

Fay, Martha.
A mortal condition.

1.Cancer—Patients—Biography.   2. Memorial
Sloan-Kettering Cancer Center.   I.Title.
RC265.5.F39 1983   362.1'96994'00924   83-7407
ISBN 0-698-11251-2

Printed in the United States of America

This book is dedicated with affection and gratitude to its eight subjects and their families, whom I feel lucky to count as friends: the Angells, the Finks, the Finkelsteins, the Giovias, the Johnsons, the Minduses, the O'Briens, and the Polacks.

Their faith in a perfect stranger, along with unstinting gifts of time and candor, are equally responsible for the book's completion and its strengths.

The cooperation and support of many other people helped sustain me in this project for close to three years. At Memorial, a long list of attending physicians, oncology fellows, nurses, social workers, and nonmedical staff with whom I came in periodic contact proved exceptionally openhanded in their assistance, but I would especially like to thank Jerry Delaney, Drs. Timothy Gee, Robert Golbey, Thomas Hakes, and Benjamin Koziner, and Mary Ann Barletta, Jean Campbell, Kathy Dietz and Claudia Delaquilla Higgins.

To my agent, Amanda Urban, I give exorbitant thanks for unending support and attention, and unparalleled judgment. To Linda Healy, who on scant evidence convinced both me and her bosses that I could write this book, I am affectionately and permanently indebted. And to Faith Sale, who adopted me and my book enthusiastically and without reservation, I am most grateful. Thanks also to Maura Walsh for her cheerful and meticulous attention, to Thelma Palmerio and Betsy Williams for reading and commenting on the early manuscript, and to my sisters Katy Fay Early and Mary Fay-Zenk for their respective calligraphic and design contributions.

To Loudon Wainwright, my best and truest friend, I give thanks for three years of confidence in and sympathy for this book, for advice particular, general, and even withheld, and especially for never losing sight of what is most important in life.

A Mortal Condition

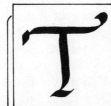
here is no inscription over the main entrance to Memorial Hospital. One enters beneath a broad steel canopy, past a uniformed doorman practiced at spotting who needs a cab on leaving, and how badly, and who would prefer to walk a while in the fresh air. Given the mixed promise and fearsomeness of the place, that small service is probably a more suitable notice to patients and the occasional passerby than any inspired phrase could ever be, for it is hard to imagine what words could be chiseled in stone without giving rise to either premature despair or an eventual sense of betrayal.

Few patients come to Memorial innocent. The full meaning of the diagnosis may still be in question, but the essential business that brings one there is known in advance. For all but a small number of patients with rare disorders who are treated at Memorial—the full and proper name, used in official accounts and obituaries, is Memorial Sloan-Kettering Cancer Center—that business is cancer. It may have been detected in a routine checkup, it may have been discovered one morning in a shockingly hard little lump that had not been there before, or it may confirm the source of a symptom of long standing. Between that moment and the time one arrives at Memorial, there will have been an interval of hours, days, months or years. For some, the reality of having cancer will have taken hold long ago; for others it will still be a fact beyond credibility, a piece of news so unwelcome that it simply cannot be let in.

Memorial is not a local hospital; people who live in New York City and have cancer are not routinely referred there, and virtually every patient at Memorial has been somewhere else first, at least for the original diagnosis; a large number live outside New York.

What brings them to Memorial (as it brings patients to Boston's Sidney Farber Institute, to M. D. Anderson in Houston, to Fred Hutchinson in Seattle) is a determination to spare nothing in the effort to beat the disease, and a judgment that this is where the experts are, the people who will know what to do, if anything can be done. What awaits a patient at Memorial depends on several things: the kind of cancer he has, how far it has progressed, which doctor he finds, the type of treatment available, how well he is able to tolerate it, and finally, whether it works.

The hospital itself will seem at times like a safe house to a man on the run; at others it will take on a repellent aspect, representative of all that is most intolerable and yet inescapable about the disease. An outpost of innovation, Memorial is also a solid, seemingly inimitable bastion of the established and self-congratulatory medical world, institutionally self-conscious and institutionally proud.

It is also a noticeably toney place, its immense respectability superficially mitigating the grim nature of its specialty. There is nothing shabby about Memorial; despite overcrowding and overuse, it retains a prosperous, well-cared-for look. The bathrooms are clean, the hardware intact; there are no thin patches in the carpeting, no broken chairs in the waiting rooms, no graffiti beside the phones. On the face of it, a patient need never feel that he has been shunted out of society's sight here; indeed, moneyed society takes a special interest in the place. Its donors and committee members are all big-time; the same names turn up on wall plaques at the Museum of Modern Art and the Metropolitan Opera, on the letterheads of the New York Public Library and Carnegie Hall. Roaming the halls, one soon learns to be alert for the careening carts of the gray ladies, a brigade of thin, middle-aged women whose winter tans and streaked blond hair seem as much a requirement of volunteerism as the trim blue lab coats they wear over their street clothes, tasteful knockoffs of the white coats worn by the medical staff. The gray ladies help out in the clinics, staff the library and the solarium, and raise money for research and daily operations, but it is as flower girls, resolutely cheerful and artful, that they are most conspicuous. One never comes upon a bowl of daisies or anything so pedestrian as a vase of mums at Memorial. The gray ladies fill the place with long-stemmed spotted lilies, Oriental tableaux of floral arcana, exotic blooms with names as hard to pronounce as the polysyllabic cytotoxins measured out in the clinic pharmacy—*Alstroemeria, L-Aspariginase; orange euphorbia, Mithramycin; pittosporum, Adriamycin; dendrobium orchid, Hydroxyurea*—until the drabbest anteroom is fitted out with an arrangement worthy of the fur salon at Neiman-Marcus.

Such juxtapositions are common enough at Memorial; it is a closed universe in many ways, containing within its walls the richest, widest range of emotions and behavior—elation, despair, grief, hope, acceptance, giddiness, cruelty, indifference, tenderness, solicitude. Any feeling or attitude that can be imagined outside can be found inside, with one ultimately conclusive difference—that there is always something essential at stake here and that very little can be taken for granted.

It is, if not easy to forget what one is at Memorial for, a simple matter to begin to think of it as commonplace. This is both good and bad. Unlike the "real world," this world does not flinch from the words *cancer, malignancy, tumor, biopsy.* One does not have to explain everything slowly, one can speak in shorthand, leave sentences unfinished and be perfectly understood, make dreadful jokes and not give offense. The cancer patient is not singled out.

On the other hand, it takes only a couple of days for a cancer patient to begin to think that he has been at Memorial for months—or, for that matter, all his life—and to experience a stripping-away of the old contexts that can be excessively painful. The real world drops from sight along with street clothes, hard shoes, MacDonald's, Chinese food, and money that can be held in the hand. Patients with low platelets are asked to surrender their razors; usually the request is tactfully explained as a precaution against a nick that could precipitate unchecked bleeding, but one leukemic who did not receive this explanation was horrified to think the nurses imagined him a potential suicide.

Such lapses among the nursing staff are rare; patients may complain about the hospital, their private doctors, or the house staff, but rarely do they complain of the nurses, who tend to be young, intelligent and attractive, and who, as a rule, spare patients a lot of cheerfully unrealistic chatter. The unctuous "we" of the nursery is similarly absent; patients retain the right to be addressed in the second person singular. Memorial's nurses are better paid than average, but it is obvious that something else draws them to this work—a solidity and a realism that keep their compassion from turning maudlin and signal when it's time to transfer to a less punishing assignment. Memorial's nurses are known to leave after a few years and return again, and for most there is an ongoing tension between the inclination to stick with a specific floor and type of patient and the urge to transfer frequently to lessen the intensity of identification. The emotional reserve that a cancer nurse develops can be used up in a single bad day, and it takes more than a day to recover. And though their dealings with patients are more intimate than most of the doctors', though they are as a group more compassionate and more open-hearted, they commonly remain more anonymous, and their names are frequently forgotten. Even the patients who most truly value them can often do no better than "Donna on the fourth floor" or "Linda, who was on twelve my first stay." In part, this is due to the frequent shifting of staff among floors, but it also has to do with an imbalance of power untouched for decades; though nearly every patient will swear that the nurses make the hospital (and the smartest doctors will swear it as well), it is the appearance of one's doctor every morning or afternoon that counts. The nurses reassure, make comfortable, joke, commiserate, trade personal histories and reduce the mysteries of chemotherapy to human scale, but they do not pronounce one improved, cured, free to go.

It is harder to generalize about the doctors at Memorial. Their status allows them a more conspicuous individuality than the nurses, the upper-case title still works in their favor. There are 283 doctors on staff, about half of whom are involved in research as well, and they are held in greatly varying degrees of esteem by their patients and the hospital staff. A few are genuinely and deservedly loved, a good many more are not, and the majority fall in between. There are a lot of doctors who deserve to be labeled technicians, and not all of them are superior even at that task. To hear some fellows (postresidents planning to specialize in oncology) talk, the Memorial complex could be emptied of its current roster of physicians tomorrow and suffer no loss of stature. "The doctors here are all replaceable," one first-year fellow commented with perhaps predictable irreverence. "What makes the place great is the support staff, the equipment, the research."

What patients register of all this is necessarily fragmented, however. And though they speculate on the rankings of their own doctors, are curious about salaries and total income, wonder who runs the place and how the rules are set, in the end their imaginations turn back to their own difficulties. With occasional exceptions, a similar attitude toward other patients prevails. When they are at all compatible, inpatient roommates achieve an almost instantaneous intimacy, a closeness of the sort that many would shun on the outside. There is inevitable talk about life and death, or the hedging that sometimes substitutes for it, and there is sympathy offered between beds, as well as advice and confidences. One might think that such friendships would endure, if only in an occasional phone call or postcard, yet they rarely do.

It is not that the good will dissolves, only the contact, and there are many reasons for this. A reluctance to hear bad news is as common among people who already have cancer as it is among their anxious friends—no one wants to ask, "How are you?" when the stakes are so terribly high. There are also geographic barriers, inhibitions of age and social ranking that reassert themselves once a patient is again outside the hospital walls. But for the most part it is simply that once one has broken free, the last thing one wants is to be drawn back to the subject by seeking out another patient. With few exceptions, solidarity is no compensation for the comforts of distance and forgetfulness, while the ever-present temptation to retreat from the facts of one's own case is, of course, made easier with every mile the patient puts between himself and the hospital.

That it's all a mistake is an illusion that is easier to sustain on the bus or the plane en route to—or from—Memorial than it is when one is actually there. But it's an illusion that is especially hard to resist once the crisis of discovery, confirmation of the disease, and early treatment is past, when one is feeling well again. "Better than ever before" is the way many cancer patients who achieve remission put it, as if chemotherapy or radiation or even surgery, once its rough work is done, bestows some extra fillip of well-being on its subjects as compensation for the beating it has inflicted.

For many cancer patients, the idea of Memorial is almost as appalling as the disease that leads one there. Nevertheless, the beds—565 of them—are nearly always full, the clinics overflowing. Rich men arrive in their own ambulances, sometimes without advance notice, not knowing the name of a doctor, but expecting to be admitted and saved. Some time ago, a man arrived at Memorial in such bad shape that the doctors who met him and referred him elsewhere because there were no beds were afraid he would not live; he refused their recommendation of another hospital nearby and returned home as he came, dying en route. Such stories are not common, though neither are they apocryphal, but their meaning has less to do with Memorial than with their individual protagonists.

Which is equally true of the stories that might be more credibly described as typical. A patient arrives at Memorial with a disease and with the personal baggage of a lifetime. Every patient brings to the experience of having cancer all that he has been before, and all that he expects of life and his own possibilities. There is no special equipment issued cancer patients, just as there is no cancer personality, no certain marker that can warn of, or protect against, its arrival in one's life. No one knows ahead of time how, or how well, he will deal with it. And ahead of time, very few of us ever consider the question.

Indeed, the only defense that most people feel capable of mounting against cancer is to not think about it. Failing that—and it gets harder and harder all the time to block out information, correct or not, on the subject—one can at least insist on its being the sort of thing that happens to someone else, a tactic that we use every day to defend against all kinds of fears, and wisely. Only with cancer, the shock that one feels when that defense collapses can be stunning.

The fact is that only ordinary people get cancer; there is no other category of available targets. "That's what people should know," one teen-age patient said one day. "Mothers should read about people like me and say to their children, 'This kid's just like you. He's a fun guy, he clowns around. It could happen to anybody.'" And regularly does.

Still, the eight patients whose stories are presented here are not representatives of some cross section of cancer victims; they were not chosen for their typicality, or their symbolic value, nor because of their extreme unusualness. Though they were chosen with some thought of presenting a range of different diseases, greater reference was made to their willingness to let themselves be observed and to offer their own thoughts on what was happening to them.

Like most patients at Memorial, these eight (or their families) were protected by insurance at the time of their diagnosis, moderately to well educated or well connected, sufficiently realistic to get themselves to a specialty center, aggressive enough to push for what they believed to be the best care possible. Beyond these characteristics, and before they had in common the experience of being cancer patients, there would have been little to connect them. And, in that people who will get cancer in their lifetimes overwhelmingly outnumber redheads, or left-handers, or joggers in the general population (the figure is three in ten in the United States, with just under a million new cases diagnosed each year), there is virtually no way to define a subgroup of likely victims that protects the rest of us. Yet for a condition so nearly ubiquitous, the facts about cancer remain essentially obscure, understanding of it barred by a fear that has the simplest of causes. Cancer is believed still to be exactly the equivalent of death.

The association is undeniable, but it is not absolute. Survival statistics issued by the American Cancer Society and the National Cancer Institute project a five-year survival rate for 45 to 50 percent of all patients. The percentage is minutely disputed by reasonable people, but there is little argument among experts that over-all survival is inching up, and no argument that certain forms of cancer that were once nearly universally fatal are no longer so.

Indeed, of the eight patients whose stories are told here, only two have died. Three to four years after diagnosis the remaining six count as survivors, though with somewhat different long-term prospects. Surviving five years after diagnosis without a recurrence is considered evidence of a probable, though not certain, cure for most cancers; by that standard, five of the six still living are edging toward safety. For the one of these six whose cancer has returned after initial treatment, long-term survival is less likely, barring substantial new developments in treatment; but neither is death imminent or inevitable for her, except as it is to us all.

When things turn out well in a person's life, it is always possible to root around in the past and turn up the good news in embryo form—the Nobel Prize winner's fourth-grade report card, the Congressman's high-school valedictory address, neighborhood tales of the MVP's dominance of sandlot softball games. When catastrophe descends, a similar instinct takes over (though it is pursued more warily), and every aspect of the subject's life up to that moment is scrutinized for the early warning signs that must be there. Cancer patients are not immune from this inclination—if anything, they are more given to introspection and self-analysis at this time of their lives than at any other. And in the wake of recent psychological theories about "cancer types," self-sabotage and self-healing, some quite punishing reflections can turn up. To begin with, there is innate in most patients, as in most people everywhere, a wish to make sense of something that makes no sense at all. A patient can point his finger at the environment, at his own eating or smoking habits, at his family history, and yet recognize that others in similar circumstances did not get cancer. There must be something else, this line of reasoning goes, something that settles the question, "Why me?"

That the answer is most likely to be found deep in the intricate and still-not-understood workings of the immune system or cellular processes of the body is frequently overlooked in favor of unprovable theories involving the psyche. The idea that cancer can be thus explained, that its victims can be reasoned to have

17

arranged their own victimization may be a peculiarly American tendency, resonant of the puritanism that we commonly reserve for the poor, whose misfortunes many people would equally like to see laid to personal failings. It is understandably hard going for the cancer patient who intuitively shares this Calvinist view of affairs, for to swallow it whole leaves him not only with an enormous load of guilt but with the obligation to undo his sin as well and to make himself whole again.

In fact, working toward the return of health is the main business of most patients, however limited their personal contribution may, or must, be. But it is here that the most stubborn contradiction of the disease is displayed in sharpest relief: cancer treatment requires an essentially passive participation on the part of the patient; one submits—to the knife, to the machines, to the poisons—and one takes a beating. One does not *do,* one is *done to.* Yet the emotional and moral survival of the patient, including the wherewithal to keep showing up for such punishment, demands that he do whatever is possible to keep control of his life, to resist restrictions, to fight arbitrariness, to prevail. This struggle can be modest and private, or it can be monumentally troublesome and tangled. It can work for the patient, and it can sometimes prove disastrous.

In the end, the reaction of each patient to the experience of having cancer is singular, a reflection of all that he or she is and can handle. But of all the elements that combine to form each individual patient's attitude toward his disease, two—hope and denial—can be said to be universally essential to sanity and to making it through each day. Neither is easily maintained, and the capacity of the individual patient for each fluctuates continually. The first is critical to continuing treatment, because without the hope that one will recover—that the treatment will work—one simply would not submit. Hope is necessary also for sustaining a sense of oneself as a person with a future; without that expectation, the experience would be one of despair only. Denial—of death and of the immediate limits imposed by the disease—is necessary to the idea of oneself as someone who exists apart from the condition of illness, whose true self continues distinct throughout and emerges intact at the end.

To survive cancer altogether is not within the power of the patient alone, nor does it lie with his doctor or the treatment he is given. Identical treatments administered to different patients commonly yield different results, and optimistic—or pessimistic—early reports have a way of failing to prevail. What is within the power of the patient is the choice of how to live with what has

18

happened to him. That, rather than the question of survival alone, is what this book is about. The eight people who are its subjects have all been treated for cancer at Memorial, and the hospital has a special hold on their memories and their futures. But each of the eight also has a history that predates cancer, and a life he does not want to relinquish to a disease he did not ask for. Cancer patients do not enter some gray valley at diagnosis (though in their worst moments they do feel irreparably estranged from health and normal life); they are nowhere but here, ordinary people among us everywhere: mother, father, sister, brother, daughter, son, friend, self.

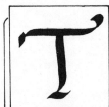heresa Sweeney O'Brien was born with a streak of red in her blond hair, what the Irish call Veronica's Veil and take for a sign of great good luck.

She often said, sometimes with a shudder and a look backward over her shoulder, "Oh, God's been good to me, God love me," and she said this very close to the end of her life, when her hair—which in turning darker with age and then beginning to gray, had kept its streak—had fallen out in patches as a result of chemotherapy, and she was debating whether to order a second wig, this time with a streak, to make her feel more like her old self again.

The good things in Terry O'Brien's life were seldom left unmentioned in any conversation that lasted more than a few minutes. It was sometimes hard to keep track of them all, impossible to scribble them all down in the time it took her to name them. But the most important to her were on her lips from moment to moment, and one did not have to list them in order to remember.

First there was her husband, Ray, about whom she was likely to say, while watching to see its effect, "Did I tell you that my husband is the Chairman of the Board of Emigrant Savings Bank? He is. Oh, he works very hard. He used to work for Chase. Do you want to hear about the time I christened a ship in Japan? It's quite a story."

There were also—and it was hard to trace the lines of her split allegiance, so fiercely was she devoted to him and them, and so visibly did she preside between him and them—six children: Susie, the oldest, was twenty-six the year her mother died, a first-year intern at a consortium of hospitals in New Jersey; Raymond was twenty-four, married less than a year and working in the loan division at Chase Manhattan Bank; Chris, twenty-two, a year out of college, had just started in a training program at Manufacturer's Hanover Trust, one of the few big New York banks—Chase was another—willing to hire an Irish Catholic Fordham graduate when his father started in banking; Sean was about to turn twenty near the end of his sophomore year at St. Mary's College in Maryland; Carol was seventeen, a senior at Red Bank Catholic, a private school for girls in New Jersey, and Nancy was fifteen and a sophomore at Red Bank Catholic.

There were a great many friends too, seemingly hundreds of them, enjoying varying degrees of intimacy with Terry O'Brien, and relatives, seen less frequently but recalled often, acidly or with affection, whenever an accomplishment or an offense proved spectacular enough to warrant repeating.

And there was the Bronx, where Terry Sweeney grew up, the third of four children, the second daughter, of James and Mary Sweeney. Both the senior Sweeneys were born in Ireland, which put them among the most recent arrivals in the parish but did not mark them as significantly different from their mainly Irish Catholic neighbors. James Sweeney was a supervisor for the New York City Sanitation Department. Mary Sweeney was handsome and straight-backed and gave the appearance of being taller than she was and possibly more prosperous, a talent certain women of her generation had. Her daughters remember that she could not be hurried out of the apartment; she would not budge until she looked the way a lady ought to look out of doors—which is to say, perfect.

One of Mary Sweeney's daughters was big-boned and tall and thriving—Kathleen, called Kak by the family; the other was small and given to childhood illnesses, though she made up for it in energy and stubbornness—Theresa, called Te-Te, or Te (pronounced *tee*) for short. Kak remembers herself as an often awkward child, gangly, too big, interested in athletics, and shy. Her younger sister she remembers as a curly-haired baby-contest winner whose appeal survived growing up into quite an ordinary physical attractiveness—not a beauty, skinny even, and flat-chested, but funny and friendly, and a great success with boys.

It took her little time to settle on one. She started going out with Ray O'Brien when she was seventeen and he was twenty-one. They were married four years later, on March 29, 1952, her twenty-first birthday. Ray had a degree from Fordham, had spent a year in Korea, and had just begun working toward a law degree from Fordham at night. He got a job at Chase and wound up staying for twenty-one years. Terry had worked since graduating from high school in June 1949, first for Blue Cross, then as a secretary on Wall Street, and she continued working until a few months before Susie was born, in October 1954, and she began the career that she had always planned on and knew she would be great at.

Meeting Terry O'Brien for the first time, one would never come away thinking of her as frail, though it was obvious that her strength was not physical. She was slightly built, five feet and a couple of inches tall and rarely weighing more than 115 pounds, though she liked to claim a high of 122 or 123 as her normal weight. She was more wired than wiry, slightly tense even when having a good time. In an athletic incarnation, she might have made a good runner, like her son, Chris, or like Sean, who of all her children most resembled her physically. But she was neither seriously athletic nor given to activities of the kind that fill the lives of women in similar circumstances.

She didn't cook fancy meals in her big kitchen, or sew except when she had to, do needlepoint, paint, or play great bridge at luncheon parties. She cooked for her family as simply and as infrequently as she could get away with, happy to order out a pizza on a moment's notice. She did the laundry, ironed Ray's handkerchiefs, and drove the kids to school.

In middle age, her face was like the rest of her—thin, though it was essentially a round Irish face, with faint traces of freckles under the powder she used to pick up her color when she was neither feeling nor looking well. She held her head high but with effort, and aimed her chin at whatever lay dead ahead, which gave her the appearance—correct, as it happened—of being alert and interested in everything going on around her. This impression was accentuated by the conspicuous if slight bucking of her front teeth, an imperfection that improved her small and otherwise regular-featured face and gave it a look of perpetual animation. On occasion, she withdrew this eager face in public, and certainly she did not maintain it in private. With lips drawn together tightly over those troublesome teeth, she could manage to look tranquil or even, for a minute of two, solemn. By letting the sides of her mouth drop, she could turn peckish and fierce as an angry nun. Her hazel-gray eyes, small behind large, tortoise-shell glasses, would go cold. This was her withering look, employed when necessary, and then quickly shaken off.

In pictures taken before she started chemotherapy, Terry O'Brien's thick hair is brushed back from her forehead, the better to show the just-visible streak. The wig she wears, though an impressive facsimile of that comb-defeating mass, is styled with the hair brushed forward at the hairline, to obscure its mounting, and she picks unfamiliarly at the strands above her eyebrows, unsure of where to place them. "You know," she would say from time to time, tugging at the base of the thing, "this is a very expensive wig." That was about the limit of her materialism, despite the material comforts of her life, which were considerable.

What she liked best was human company, her family and her friends. She loved going out to dinner, not to eat but to talk, and she liked parties and dances where people called to one another over the dance floor. She liked to hear secrets while sipping scotch, and she liked to smoke, which she started doing in high school, away from the house, where her mother couldn't catch her. She was a sociable woman, and her gifts and her pleasures were sociable ones.

In 1952, the year Terry and Ray O'Brien were married, Stuyvesant Town, a thirty-five–building apartment complex laid out among its own parks, playgrounds and patrolled walks along the East River in lower Manhattan, had been open for five years. It was planned as a place in which to raise children, a city-suburb, one of Robert Moses' grand ideas, and a perfect place for Terry O'Brien. There was always someone to talk to, everybody had kids, the apartments were big and inexpensive, the supermarkets were within walking distance, and everything else was at the end of a subway or bus ride.

The O'Briens might have stayed in Stuyvesant Town through the arrival of their sixth child, Nancy, if they had been able to get one of the coveted five-bedroom apartments for which there was a long wait list, or if Ray had not begun to long to live in the country. Just after their fifth child, Carol, was born, friends of the O'Briens' who had settled in New Jersey persuaded them to come look around, and in 1965 they bought a house in Matawan, forty miles down the Garden State Parkway from the Lincoln Tunnel. A few years later, they moved to the fancier township of Colts Neck, a few miles farther south, to a pleasant, two-story white house set on a slope at the back of a bowllike cul-de-sac. Susie, the oldest, was thirteen then; Nancy, the youngest, was two.

The O'Briens joined a country club, where Ray golfed and Terry played a little tennis and the kids swam in the summer. Most of their friends were prosperous, transplanted city people like themselves, Catholic, with kids, though not as many as the O'Briens. Ray traveled for Chase, and Terry went with him from time to time. And she eventually started taking the pill, on a medical dispensation from a Catholic priest, the sort of dispensation that became commoner than vocations in Catholic circles in the late 1960s.

Sometime in the middle of the night of February 11, 1974, Terry woke Ray to complain of a sharp pain that moved slowly down her right side, along her right arm, and down her right leg. They considered calling their doctor, but then the pain disappeared, and they went back to sleep.

The next afternoon, February 12, she had a second attack. Her son Sean, who was twelve at the time, remembers her coming into his room with a pile of laundry and suddenly "keeling over on the bed." Her right leg had collapsed, and she had blacked out. Sean remembers thinking that she was dead, and she remembered thinking that she was dying. It was a stroke, severe enough to leave her temporarily paralyzed along the right side, but one from which she made an essentially complete recovery. She was forty-two.

It is not clear what caused the stroke. For several years she had suffered from mild hypertension and had taken medication to control it. But Susie O'Brien, a sophomore at Mount Holyoke College at the time and now a doctor, says that she has since wondered whether it was set off by the birth-control pills that she had been taking.

Only an occasionally perceptible limp remained from that event, yet Susie believes that the stroke left her mother feeling very vulnerable. "She was always paranoid about it," Susie says in retrospect. "She would joke about it—she'd say something like, 'Don't walk so fast, I'll have another stroke,' and everyone would *pooh-pooh* it. But I guess if something hits you like that out of the blue when you're not expecting it, then all your life you're going to wonder if it's going to happen again."

Terry O'Brien never did have another stroke, but it was as if the first had started a jagged crack on the face of an enormous mirror, marking the onset of seven years of the worst sort of medical bad luck. Within a year of her stroke, she developed rheumatoid arthritis, and by the time she came to the attention of rheumatologist Arthur Brawer in October 1977 she had what he describes as "a bad case. A lot of swelling, a lot of pain in the joints, a lot of curtailment of motion. It was in the shoulders, the neck, the ankles, the wrists—you name it. She couldn't get out of bed in the morning."

Before going to Brawer, she had been treated with Cortisone and aspirin, but it was clear to him that she would make no improvement without escalating to a different class of drug. He started her on something called penicillamine, and within a year she was in remission, meaning that there was occasional discomfort still but little swelling in the morning and a good range of motion.

Despite the stroke and the arthritis, Susie O'Brien said, no one in the family ever really thought of their mother as sickly. "She had all these things wrong with her, it's true, but you never thought of her as being sick. She always seemed to do everything." Certainly there was no retreat from life, and no hint that it was to be foreshortened.

In fact, despite her history, she had no warning. Nothing related to what was coming. She had no cough, no shortness of breath, no pains in the chest, no blood on the pillow. It just turned up one day, on a routine X ray ordered by Brawer because penicillamine is known to cause inflammation of the lung. It was a small dot, on the lower right lung, and when Brawer did a repeat X ray, it was still there.

She spent one night in Riverview Hospital, where she had been treated after her stroke, and then Ray made arrangements for her to see Edward Beattie, at Memorial. Beattie is a thoracic surgeon, a man of reputation and self-assurance, and also something of a public figure, someone conspicuously suited for the front office. When Terry O'Brien came to him, he had been Chief Medical Officer at Memorial for thirteen years, and his specialty, surgery, was still the most effective treatment for lung cancer.

Terry's first appointment with Beattie was on March 19, 1979, a Monday. She checked into Memorial as a patient the following Sunday afternoon, March 25, four days short of her forty-eighth birthday and twenty-seventh wedding anniversary. The admitting form listed her occupation as "homemaker," named her father, mother, and husband, and also mentioned the fact of, but did not individually name, her six children. In the upper-right-hand corner of the form, in a small box indicating "reason for admission," was typed "lung lesion rule out ca." The following day, in a simple diagnostic procedure called a needle biopsy, "ca." was emphatically ruled in. The diagnosis was adenocarcinoma, one of the four major types of lung cancer.

On Tuesday, March 27, Terry signed a consent form authorizing Beattie to perform a "fiberoptic bronchial, thoracotomy, pulmonary resection"—a piece of surgery that would cut away the middle lobe of her right lung. The operation was scheduled for the twenty-ninth, which gave Terry something absurdly grisly to dwell on. "All I could think about," she would recall later on, mimicking the look and gestures of a starlet fantasizing her name in lights, "was the headline in the paper reading 'Terry O'Brien.

Born March 29. Married March 29. Died March 29.'"

As it happened, the surgery was postponed a day, which deflated the irony somewhat in Terry's opinion, but had the merit of giving her another twenty-four hours to smoke in the lounge at the end of the hall. The next morning, the thirtieth, Beattie removed the middle lobe of her right lung in a procedure nearly identical to one he described in a book completed about that time.

According to the pathologist's report completed later that day, the excised lobe, described as "reddish brown to purple" in color and with a "finely reticulated" surface, measured 12 x 6 x 3 centimeters and weighed 48 grams—roughly the size and weight of a soft pack of cigarettes. Beneath the surface, at the mid-portion of the lobe, was a little button of a tumor, a single nodule 1.8 centimeters in size—three-quarters of an inch of cancer.

The pathologist's report confirmed the earlier biopsy finding of adenocarcinoma for the tumor itself and ruled out malignancy for all nearby sites, which was very good news. Typically, lung cancer is not diagnosed until the original tumor has grown large enough to impinge on nearby vital organs or to interfere with the proper functioning of the body, with the result that more than 50 percent of all lung cancers prove inoperable. Terry O'Brien's cancer had been caught at what is called Stage I—no lymph node involvement, a single tumor in a single lobe, no evidence of metastases—giving her as good a statistical chance of survival as a lung-cancer patient is likely to get.

About half of all patients diagnosed with adenocarcinoma Stage I survive five years following successful surgery.* Twenty-four percent of all Stage I patients, however, will die within two years from recurrence within the lungs, or from distant metastases.

When Beattie told Terry that she was a very lucky woman, he was, for the moment, correct, and his reading matched her own view of how things would turn out. She was discharged on April 8, with a prescription for Percocet, a painkiller, and instructions from Beattie to "go home and have a happy life."

This last was supposed to be her specialty, and she worked hard in the next months to achieve it. Except for the pain following surgery, she did pretty well. But the pain was a problem. Despite her long experience with arthritis, she found it hard to function in the weeks after surgery. A month after being dis-

---

*Statistics vary by source. The figures used here are taken from *Lung Cancer, 1980*, a collection of papers presented at the Second World Congress on Lung Cancer, at Copenhagen. Editors Heine H. Hansen and Mikael Rørth. Excerpta Medica. Amsterdam-Oxford-Princeton.

charged, when she returned to Memorial for her first checkup, Beattie noted that she was "doing well except for pain." He renewed her prescription for Percocet and advised her to "take it freely."

It was not that simple for Terry, who was reluctant to take his advice flat out. It was not as if she intended to make herself feel wretched, just that she had her own rules about these things. Late in May, she and Ray flew to South Bend, Indiana, to attend Raymond's graduation from Notre Dame. On the way to the ceremony, Terry discovered that she had forgotten to transfer the Percocet when changing pocketbooks, and she insisted that they go back to the hotel to get it. She knew that she couldn't get through the whole day without it. Yet she would not take it "freely," and held religiously to the prescribed four-hour wait between pills. It was partly a suspicion of all drugs; "scotch is better," she would say, and it helped; partly a manifestation of her Catholicism—pain isn't all that bad, after all; and partly it was a matter of control—if you took a pill every time you hurt, then the pain ran you, and not the other way around. Terry always liked to be in control.

As the summer approached, she began to feel more like her old self. Her cancer surgery, just five years after her stroke, was similarly transformed into a good story. There were no more cigarettes for her, but at parties she would urge friends to "blow a little smoke my way."

In the middle of June, more than two months after her surgery, Terry was admitted to Riverview Hospital in New Jersey with severe chills and fever. Tests were run, the presumption being that she was suffering from a postoperative fever, but the cause of the fever was never pinpointed. In his report on her July 2 checkup, Beattie noted this "mysterious fever"—a phrase that turns up with some frequency in medical records—and raised a consideration that would recur later on in her illness: "I suppose it is always possible," he wrote, "that there might be an occult primary (a separate, unrelated cancer) elsewhere."

Though Beattie raised the question, and though it would be raised again, the evidence of all the tests ruled out a second primary cancer. And though Terry would have recurring problems with hypertension and arthritis through the remainder of the year and into the next spring, she had no more fevers and no symptoms relating to lung cancer. She came into Memorial again in November, for an X ray and a checkup, which were both clean. Her weight at the end of November was 123 lbs., quite good. (Although whoever typed up Beattie's report may have been somewhat distracted—the patient's name is given as Mrs. Margaret O'Brien.)

On March 7, 1980, almost a year after surgery, she came in again. Beattie noted that she was "getting along reasonably well as far as chest," although she "has been troubled a great deal with hypertension and arthritis some months ago, and developed rash from her medication."

In the spring there were two more graduations, Susie's from the College of Medicine and Dentistry of New Jersey and Chris's from Bucknell. Terry saw Beattie again on June 27. He reported that she had reached the fourteen-month mark "and is doing very well at this time."

Which is what she reported, and felt. The recovery period seemed well over, and she was more troubled by her prior conditions of hypertension and arthritis than by thoughts of a recurrence of the cancer. During the summer of 1980 she had something significant to look forward to: Raymond was going to be married in October, the first of the kids to take the plunge. It was a big, splashy, beautiful wedding, in Palm Beach, where the bride's parents lived. The ceremony was at a Catholic church where Jack Nicklaus is a parishioner, and the reception was at the Breakers. In the home movies taken by Terry's younger brother, Brian Sweeney, the camera bounces off one after another handsome Irish face—eight smiling O'Briens decked out in morning coats and bright dresses making their way past white stucco pillars and shocks of greenery.

Terry O'Brien is wearing a bright blue dress in the movie, and she charges the camera as she comes down some steps, her face lit, her mouth open. Ray is behind her, impeccably gray-haired and gray-striped. There is no sound, of course, but Terry is most emphatically saying something sassy to someone. Or maybe just, "Point the camera over here, Brian."

She especially liked weddings, and it was hard to imagine life offering her a better spectacle than a wedding that starred one of her own children, her boys picking at their collars, her girls tripping over their high heels, everyone dancing and drinking and having a wonderful time. She had a wonderful time certainly and later remembered that she looked and felt as healthy that October as she had in a long time.

The following spring she would look back on Raymond's wedding in some bewilderment, and with a degree of retrospective self-deception. Looking at the pictures from the wedding, she would seek confirmation of what she wanted to remember, that she really had been well. Yet the truth was that she had been conscious since the previous August of sensations of pain across her lower back. Because it was not crippling, it was easy enough to attribute to tension or to arthritis. And anything that did not stop her in her tracks did not slow her down.

Once the wedding was behind her, however, she began to pay more attention. In late October, in anticipation of her next appointment with Beattie, she had a series of X rays of her lower back taken by a radiologist in Red Bank.

Beattie's account of her November 3 visit is unalarmed. He notes that her X rays were "reported to show dense sclerotic areas throughout the lower and thoracic lumbar spine," and he recommended that she go for a bone scan, in order to "see whether there is anything in this. It may require further X rays of suspicious areas. If all is well," he concluded optimistically, "we will plan to see her again in three months."

The bone scan was done November 6, at Riverview Hospital in Red Bank. The radiologist who read the scan reported to Terry's rheumatologist in a letter dated November 25, 1980 (its essence had already been conveyed orally): ". . . evidence of blastic metastases involving the thoracic and lumbar spine. . . . Lytic metastases are also seen involving the pelvis . . . and in both femurs extending down to the midshaft. . . . there is involvement of lower rib cage. . . ."

There would be additional tests, X rays, bone-marrows, mammograms to ascertain whether this could be the result of a previously undetected breast cancer—but all the results would narrow down to one cause: the cancer had come back, with something of a vengeance, given the facts. It was in her bones, lots of them, and it hurt. She had not beat it out after all.

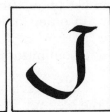immy Polack came in first, after a flight from Seattle with his grandparents and his aunt, who would settle into a too-expensive apartment a half hour's walk from the hospital and remain nearly six months. That was December 18, a Thursday, and Jimmy still felt fine. He was nineteen, and his only symptom was a swollen lymph node under his chin. But the bone-marrow test done the week before had confirmed that he had leukemia, and he had spent his last day in Seattle sorting through his possessions, with a mind to giving away things he thought he would never need again. The night before he left for New York, he parceled them out, with no explanations, to a group of close friends. He told them only that he was going away for a while and did not know when he'd be back. Then they stayed up most of the night drinking beer, and in the morning, numb as the battered bumper on his used Corvette, Jimmy boarded the plane to New York.

Sal Giovia was next. He came in on December 21, five days short of his seventeenth birthday and so sick that his parents didn't return home to Long Island for close to a week. They had been ferrying him back and forth to doctors for almost a year in an effort to find the cause of his recurrent fevers, strep throat, lassitude and, finally, bleeding gums, which their dentist suggested had been caused by pyorrhea. By the time leukemia cells were found in his blood, his platelet count was so low that he was in danger of bleeding to death. In his first ten days at Memorial he would receive 28 units of platelets and 2,000 cc's of whole blood. Over Christmas vacation, blood donors from his high school and others on Long Island were brought into New York by the hundreds; their extravagance made the local nightly news, and Sal's face, thin, bearded, excited and scared, was beamed to millions of viewers for a minute and a half. The exposure was not quite long enough to suit Sal, who hopes to become an entertainer, like his father; "But it's a start." And, although he would not admit it until long after he learned that it was not so, in those early days, Sal believed absolutely that "if you looked up the definition of leukemia in the dictionary, it would say 'Rest in Peace.'"

Karyn Angell came in on January 14, transferred from Norwalk Hospital in Fairfield County, Connecticut, less than two hours after hearing that she almost certainly had leukemia or, failing that, a lymphoma of some kind. The diagnosis would be confirmed within the day, but it would take a lot longer before Karyn or her family would begin to understand its enormous impact. It would be toughest, of course, on Karyn, a seventeen-year-old freshman at Mount Holyoke and the oldest of four sisters in a particularly close family, from which she had just begun to pull away. Encouraged by her parents, themselves not yet forty, Karyn had been rehearsing self-sufficiency for a long time. The summer before, as the Angells prepared to return to the United States after three years in Paris with IBM, Dave Angell's employer, Karyn had taken off on a tour of Europe with her backpack and only another teen-age girl for a companion. She went with her parents' blessing and a Eurailpass they had given her as a high-school-graduation present. She had a wonderful time and wound up staying so long that she had to go directly from Europe to college to get there on time. She didn't even see the house her parents had found in Westport until Thanksgiving, but that was very much what everyone expected. She was out of the nest, eager, accomplished, and expecting the best.

Jimmy Polack, Sal Giovia, and Karyn Angell are, or have all been at one time, patients of a man named Timothy Gee, a hematologist on the staff at Memorial who was born in Canton and raised in San Francisco. Gee's specialty is leukemia and when he is pressed to explain how he manages to sustain his balance in the everpresent face of death, he often answers, and not facetiously, "it helps to be Chinese."

Just about everybody comes to Gee recommended; that is, someone has said, "Don't go to anyone else," and then made the phone call that will guarantee the connection. The recommendations are made by hematologists around the country, by many of the more than one hundred former fellows (postresidents studying oncology) he has helped to train, by specialists and general practitioners with whom he keeps in touch by phone—and they are made not just because of his superb reputation as a clinician but because to land within the circle of Timothy Gee's practice is to land in one of the few places where having leukemia does not seem to be the end of everything else. Gee's relationship with his patients has an intimate, almost tribal quality, and his sense of what they need—from him, from their families, from other patients and, even more important, who they are as people—extends this connection well beyond the traditional one of doctor and patient.

A big, shaggy man, Gee roams the hospital coatless and at high speed, listing slightly to the right like a bear that's been nicked in the woods, the result of a bad back. If he is on his way to see a patient, a fellow (or two) usually trails behind, lab coat flapping in his wake. Gee's assistant, being nearly as tall as her boss and accustomed to the pace, keeps up easily, even when overtaken by a laughing fit. She is a young woman with shoulder-length blond hair and a freckled, sympathetic face; her name is Kathy Dietz, and she is indispensable equally to Gee and to his patients. She carries a clipboard on which are duplicated the vital facts on each patient that she and Gee carry in their heads, and manages to keep straight an incredible store of detail on the personal lives of Gee's patients as well. One of the rare criticisms one hears of Gee is that he has too many patients, that he might be spreading himself too thin. It may be true, if only at the theoretical level, but his patients do not complain of it. Kathy Dietz is one reason; Gee's manner is the other. Patients joke that everyone gets to see him for exactly twenty-six seconds—"the Minuteman," Sal Giovia calls him—and when you see him barreling down a corridor, it does seem as if he's always in a hurry. Once he and his entourage arrive at a patient's door, however, everyone, Gee included, slows down, and the patient is given the unshakable impression that this clutch of experts, smiling and joking and barking out optimistic news about blood counts, has all the time in the world to spend with him. This is something Gee learned long ago. "If you're in a hurry," Gee recalls being told by an old medical-school professor, "and a patient wants to talk, sit down. Don't stand there and shuffle your feet."

He is much more likely to shuffle patients, orchestrating and manipulating, arranging introductions (between Jimmy and Sal, between Karyn and an Iranian student down the hall), subtly interpreting for family members struck mute by disaster. All of this is accomplished amid reassurances that everything that can be done will be done, that his patients have landed in the best imaginable place, that the staff surrounding him, and them, is superb. And there are the difficult facts, too, laid out the first day, repeated if there is any doubt. Gee's open face is not to be doubted in one of these sessions. His big head bobs as he explains the disease, his eyebrows rise above the tops of his rimless glasses, indemnifying words spoken in a voice so soft and low it is like a murmur. The people who come to him haven't got many choices and he knows that. They can come to him or they can go to somebody else; either way, they have to trust somebody, and he works hard to earn their trust. He is careful, and precise, and truthful, so that even as he reassures a patient that his chances are good, or better than they were a month or a year earlier, no one is likely to suspect him of having dressed up the truth. And when the truth is particularly ugly, he is a good man to know. As Jimmy Polack would say when they had known each other for some time, "Dr. Gee could tell you you were going to die and that it was all right, and you'd believe him."

It is not a pose, though it may be in part the role a good doctor writes for himself and then tries to act. To attempt what Gee attempts in his practice requires, in addition to the obvious essentials of skill and energy and compassion, qualities of daring and confidence that come only with big, ambitious egos. Most doctors, Gee says, come so equipped, and he is no exception. Though in a private office he could earn more than the considerable amount he does now, he is not willing to give up what money can't buy and what only a place like Memorial can give him—the chance to excel in a business where success was, until recently, unknown. The bureaucratic in-fighting and political maneuvering at the hospital that he finds distasteful are made up for by the support staff, the facilities and the patients who come to him because he is there. And in the end, it is the patients who hold him. His unusual involvement with his patients takes him on occasion to their homes for dinner, to parties that celebrate a remission or a birth never really believed in ahead of time, and it inevitably places him at many painful scenes as well.

Gee is openly taken with the people who are his patients, curious about their lives outside the hospital, impressed by their qualities of nerve, endurance and adaptability. He says often that he gets back much more than he gives, and it is clear that that includes a sense of privilege at being allowed to see so much so close up because of the circumstances that bring them all together. The sheer variety of characters he is in contact with every day causes him to shake his head in amazement and fascination.

The winter Jimmy, Sal, and Karyn were diagnosed, one not

33

untypical Monday morning clinic began with Gee having a consultation with a sixty-eight-year-old foreign diplomat sailing home to begin his retirement. Because he was over sixty-five, the man needed a letter from Gee to the ship's doctor declaring him fit for sea travel. A few minutes later, Gee hurries to speak with a patient of six years, a housewife in her thirties who is terrified that she might be coming out of remission. In fact she is not, but because she has a bad case of herpes Gee wants her admitted to the hospital as a precaution and in hope of hurrying the normal herpes cycle with new drugs. He stays and talks with her for fifteen minutes, and the talk is largely about her fears for her marriage, which she is afraid would not survive a relapse. She dreads becoming a burden to her husband, who has just started a new job. "I feel like a plague or something," she says. "Sometimes I think I should just leave him so he'll be free. No one wants to be married to a sick person." She calls this latest hospitalization a bad omen. Gee says that he understands how she feels, that his wife often feels the same way, as do many women who have never been sick. Their husbands are caught up in exciting work and they feel left behind. He also reminds her that he knows her husband and children and knows how important she is to them. And she has a job, right? Yes, she says, for three years, and she is very proud of it. Then she returns to the bad-omen business, and Gee, who sits opposite her across a small desk, says, looking straight at her, "To the degree that you are scared, you are scaring me. Do you know that?" He lifts his eyebrows high above his glasses and gazes at her while this confession sinks in. He has granted to her the power of irrationality, of superstition, and admitted that he shares it. She nods, and they wordlessly agree that she will make it through.

Later in the morning he will get the name of a great Italian restaurant in Brooklyn from a patient who almost died last year and whose chief complaint now is charley horses in the middle of the night. Gee tells him to drink more milk for his charley horses and the man leaves in a buoyant mood.

A very edgy middle-aged nurse who has just had confirmation that she has leukemia waits to talk to Gee in another examining room. She tells him that she cannot take in the news, and it is obvious. She and Gee agree that they will meet when she is ready. Later in the day, she shows up in his office with a long list of questions to ask, mainly about available treatment and what she calls "quality of life," meaning, how much life can I have while on chemotherapy? Her final question is semirhetorical. She tells Gee that she worked as an X-ray technician, unshielded, for

34

about three years, twenty years ago. "What do you think?" she asks him. "Could that have caused this?" He nods his head once and says, "Very possibly."

Back in Examining Room 451, where Gee sees most of his patients, a young man from Indonesia and his uncle discuss his case with extreme politeness, in limited English. They would like Gee to review his situation; that's why they have come so far. If he agrees that the treatment the patient has been getting is proper, they will go home. If he has a better idea, they will stay. Gee sends them down the hall to prepare for a bone-marrow. He appears a few minutes later, loping into the room where the patient lies bare-chested on an examining table, his shoeless feet pointed at the door. Gee pulls on pale thin rubber gloves, the only sartorial evidence of his profession. A nurse hands him a swab, with which he wipes the dead center of the patient's pale yellow-brown chest. All the ribs show as the young man inhales. Gee warns him as he injects the anesthetic, "This will hurt," and the patient's feet slowly lift off the table in response, his toes curling toward the ceiling. He grips the nurse's hand fiercely, but neither grunts nor cries out. Gee takes a small metal plug resembling a pair of golf tees stacked one on top of the other, and twists it into the man's chest. He inserts another hypodermic needle into this plug, and slowly draws the marrow from the breastbone. The patient looks up at Gee, whose face is directly overhead, and asks, with understandable national pride, "Am I your first patient from Indonesia?" Gee smiles back, his hands still working to extract the marrow, and says gently, with a guarded shake of his head, "No."

If one hangs around Tim Gee long enough, the world itself seems to shrink in size and narrow in focus until it is possible to think of it as populated almost entirely by leukemics and the people who try to save them. In fact, leukemia remains rare among the general population, with an estimated 23,400 new cases in the United States in 1981, meaning that it occurs at an annual rate of about one in 10,000, as compared to the annual incidence of cancer generally, which is one in 300. Many leukemia patients are surprised to learn that their disease is rare, and this common distortion is of a piece with many misconceptions about this disease, a cancer with a singular and perversely contradictory reputation. Actually a broad category of related blood diseases, leukemia is perceived by some people as being something other than cancer—not as grisly, not as nasty, and yet as being irremediably fatal. Dr. Gee is at pains to correct as many of these misapprehensions as he can. When a patient at one of the monthly Monday-night discussion meetings that Gee holds for patients and their families suggested that life as a leukemia patient might be easier if the disease were not labeled a cancer, Gee responded quickly and emphatically by saying, "I don't think so. It *is* a cancer, and it's important to recognize that." He told the group about a patient who, on hearing that she had leukemia, said, "Whew, I'm glad it wasn't cancer." "But it is," Gee said, "and they are equally bad."

Still, in the popular mind, and therefore in the minds of virtually all his prospective patients, it is a cancer suitable for film treatments, for television specials, for love stories that end in the worst possible way. It is a disease that is obscured by myths, to which patients and even doctors remain susceptible. "In the old Memorial," one of the senior doctors there said one day, referring to the original hospital building that now houses offices, "all leukemics were grouped on the same floor, and the saying went that everyone on it was young and beautiful and that they all died. It wasn't true, of course, that they were all young and beautiful. It just seemed that way. But they did all die."

Now that is no longer true either. Many of Timothy Gee's patients will survive leukemia, and live to die of something else, to use the phrase that defines victory under these special circumstances. But most of his patients will die, usually within a few years after they come to him. It is a seemingly unbearable reality for someone who cares as much about his patients as Gee does, and it is a reality that everyone who works in hematology must to some degree block out of daily consciouness. Yet it is only in the context of such awful losses that Gee's work and attitude—and, to a certain extent, the attitudes of his patients—can be understood: so many more of the people who come to him now will live than did patients who came in when he first started working in hematology that, in talking about his practice, Gee inevitably sounds hopeful. This habit of optimism is more than a reflection of his confidence that the progress against leukemia made in the last fifteen to twenty years will continue apace; it is as well a necessary act of faith, deliberate and sober.

Much of Gee's warranted optimism has to do with the huge change that has taken place in the treatment of one form of the disease—acute lymphocytic, or lymphoblastic, leukemia (ALL)—the kind that Jimmy Polack, Sal Giovia, and Karyn Angell have. Often referred to as childhood leukemia because it most frequently occurs in children under ten, ALL is the most common form of cancer in children, cancer in turn being the second-biggest cause of death in children under fourteen. But ALL occurs in adults as well, accounting for 10 percent of all cases of leukemia in people over fifteen, the age at which patients are treated as adults at Memorial.

Tim Gee's is an adult practice. His oldest patient in 1982 was seventy-eight; his youngest was fifteen. Every year, he sees something like one hundred or so new cases of acute leukemia, perhaps twenty-five cases of chronic. About one third of the acutes are ALL, with the remainder a mixture of acute non-lymphoblastic leukemias, of which there are several distinct types. ANLL usually strikes after the age of forty and is the pre-eminent form of adult leukemia.

Though the two forms of acute leukemia differ in important respects, they are both fast-growing blood cancers that are invariably fatal if left untreated. In both, healthy white blood cells are displaced by rapidly proliferating immature or "precursor" white cells, with the result that the body's ability to fight harmful bacteria and infections is greatly reduced. The unchecked growth of cancerous white cells in the bone marrow (the point of origin for some leukemias, the primary site of active disease for all leukemia) eventually interferes as well with the production of red blood cells, used to transport oxygen throughout the body, and platelets, jagged-edged blood cells necessary to prevent abnormal bleeding. Acute leukemics are in greatest danger of dying from infection or hemorrhage. (Chronic leukemia manifests in two forms, chronic myelocytic—or granulocytic—leukemia, CML, typically a disease of young to middle-aged adults, and chronic lymphocytic leukemia, CLL, which mainly affects people in their sixties and older.)

Because leukemia is a blood disease, systemic rather than localized, historically it could not be treated the way other cancers were; it could neither be cut out by surgery, still the primary treatment for what are called solid tumor cancers, nor destroyed by radiation, since doses powerful enough to kill off cancerous cells in the bone marrow inevitably proved fatal. The logic of using drugs to treat leukemia was long apparent, but as one after another of the so-called miracle drugs developed during the 1930s and 1940s were tried against leukemia without result, it was not until several years after World War II and the emergence of what are called cytotoxic (poisonous to cells) drugs that hopes of chemical treatment appeared likely to be fulfilled. Still, as Tim Gee often tells his patients, few in the medical profession were willing to treat leukemia until recently. The high death rate, even after brief remissions began to be achieved, and the fact that most patients, in Gee's words, died "not easily," made it a field to shun.

Gee himself did not plan to enter it. He came to hematology sideways, in a self-improving move taken because he felt that he was weak in the subject during his residency. He planned to study with a "white-cell" specialist at Hammersmith Hospital in London for a year, but the summer before he was to leave for England, a professor suggested that he look into the fellow program at Memorial and perhaps apply there as well. Gee wrote to Memorial requesting an application, was sent an acceptance instead, and started working with Bayard D. Clarkson, chief of clinical hematology at Memorial and Gee's present boss, in February 1967.

His timing could not have been better. Since 1965, Memorial had been treating leukemia patients with a drug called 6-Mercaptopurine and obtaining what were, for the time, impressive results. Used alone, as all chemicals were at that stage, 6-Mercaptopurine was inducing remissions in some patients of up to six months' duration, a record.

6-Mercaptopurine is what is called an antimetabolite. It destroys cancer cells (as well as healthy cells) by interfering with the cell's ability to manufacture essential nucleic acids and proteins. It does this by imitating the functions of certain of the cell's natural components, with the result that the cell fails to complete functions necessary to its survival. It is in that sense a saboteur rather than an assassin and typical of most of the drugs used in chemotherapy, each class of which works against cell life in a distinct way (with the precise mechanism not known in every instance).

Because cancer cells as a rule reproduce themselves faster than do healthy cells, and because they are ingenious in adapting to circumstances, the early successes that resulted from treatment with 6-Mercaptopurine were from the start limited. While the lengths of some 6-Mercaptopurine-induced remissions were impressive, only 15 percent of the patients treated with it at Memorial actually achieved remission.

In early 1967, in an effort to identify additional drugs capable of bringing on remission, and just as Tim Gee arrived to start his fellowship in hematology, two new antimetabolites that are still being used in the treatment of ALL were introduced. These were Thioguanine (TGG) and Cytosine Arabinoside, or Ara-C.

TGG proved much more successful than 6-Mercaptopurine, bringing about remissions of varying lengths in 50 percent of the patients treated, and Ara-C showed equivalent promise. Over the next two years, Clarkson, Gee, and their colleagues conducted clinical tests of these and other newly available agents in alternation, laying the ground for Memorial's first combination-drug program, or "protocol," for the treatment of leukemia, called L-2, which was introduced in November 1969.

Aimed at both adults and children with acute leukemia of all kinds, L-2 represented the most important advance up to that time in Memorial's treatment of the disease. It was a two-phase program, induction and consolidation, and it included eight separate drugs that had come into use or existence since World War II.

In addition to Ara-C and TGG, a third antimetabolite, Methotrexate, was administered directly into the spinal canal, or intrathecally, to prevent stray leukemia cells from finding sanctuary there. A large percentage of relapses were believed to have resulted directly from this tendency, and injecting Methotrexate into the spinal canal was the first successful attempt to deal with it.

The five other drugs used in L-2 included one each from five different classes of drugs: Vincristine, a plant alkaloid; Daunomycin, an antitumor antibiotic; Prednisone, a steroid; L-Asparaginase, an enzyme; and, as an option, a nitrosurea called BCNU.* Each of the eight drugs threatened side effects that ranged in severity from minor weight gain to extreme nausea to stroke. Patients were forewarned of the risks involved and required to sign consent forms before beginning treatment. Given the alternative, the identified risks were universally judged tolerable by patients.

Twenty-two previously untreated adult patients and seventy-five children were started on the L-2 protocol in November 1969. As the results of the treatment began to be evaluated, it appeared that children were responding better than adults—that is, they were coming into remission with greater frequency, and those remissions were lasting longer than the adults'—and that adult ALL patients did better than patients with ANLL (all of whom were adult). From that point, separate lines of testing were pursued for each of the types of leukemia identified.

By January 1973, a new protocol aimed at prolonging remissions in adult ALL patients was ready for testing. Called L-10, the new treatment added four more drugs to the eight of L-2, altered the original sequence, and added a third phase, called maintenance, to the induction and consolidation phases of L-2. Of thirty-three previously untreated patients** enrolled in the L-10 program, fif-

---

*Many of these same drugs are used against other cancers as well, with varying degrees of efficacy.
**Only patients who have never been treated previously are included in Memorial's research data.

teen survive. Twenty-nine, or 88 percent, of the original thirty-three were successfully brought into remission; of that group, fourteen, or 48 percent, had not suffered relapses as of March 1983. Two patients died early in treatment, before coming into remission, a third after seven months, and a fourth after eleven months. (A fifth patient died in his fifth year of remission, in a construction accident, without ever relapsing.) Of the fourteen patients who suffered a relapse, only one survives.

Why some patients remain in remission while others on the same protocol relapse is still not known (although Dr. Gee believes that, as with the great variance between adult and childhood ALL, the consistent, but individually unpredictable, failure of roughly half the adult group to survive may actually reflect separate diseases that current classification and testing do not reveal). What is known is how monumental the cleavage between the two groups is. In leukemia, the first remission is everything, and its prolongation is the patient's only hope of survival. One never knows how long it will last, or whether it will. Patients who were treated in the early days of L-10 and whose remissions have held can reasonably begin to think of themselves as cured, though they can never be absolutely sure. But a relapse means death, certain, unquestioned, uncircumventible. One may be brought back into remission again, and one may live for several years, but one can never again reclaim the protection of an unbroken original remission. With relapse, all the rules are different.

In January 1977, a further modification of the adult ALL protocol was introduced, called L-10M, which achieved a remission and survival rate similar to L-10's. Of thirty-nine patients enrolled, thirty-three, or 85 percent, were brought into remission; thirteen, or 50 percent, have continued in remission through March 1983. L-10M was followed three years later by yet another protocol meant to boost remission and survival rates. Eight patients were started on this new program, called L-17, beginning in January 1980, but the protocol was dropped within three months because it proved too toxic. A milder version, L-17M, was substituted and had been in use for eight months when Jimmy Polack, Sal Giovia and Karyn Angell became patients of Tim Gee's.

By that time, L-17M gave every indication that it would turn out to be appreciably more effective than its predecessors. The odds on a patient's being brought into remission were close to 90 percent, while the odds on surviving leukemia altogether—and, in that peculiar, optimistic phrase, living to die of something else— were a flat 50–50. With every month in remission, those odds would sweeten: last a full year, and they would rise to 60 percent;

last two years, and they would soar, to 80 percent, or 90. At that rate, one could imagine a return to innocence at some point. Or at least to something that resembles it.

Of course, if you are not yet twenty, the idea that there are odds of any kind on your survival is close to impossible to credit, and disbelief and a somewhat fantastic air cling to young patients like the odor of rubbing alcohol. "It doesn't make any sense," is how Karyn Angell put it one day. She was trying to consider the statistical possibility that she could die of this disease before finishing college, but she could not get it to stand still. "Children never think of death for themselves," she said. And though there is no mistaking her for a child, she is certainly correct in pointing out that nothing in her short history has prepared her for the possibility of her own death at an early age. And her logic, if one suspends what one knows about how the world operates, is unassailable.

This is in the third week of her illness, in the middle of induction. Karyn has not yet gone into remission, so it is a bit premature to say she has begun her recovery, but she is confident that it will happen soon. Jimmy and Sal, whom she has met, had both come into remission well before a month was up, and she held to the idea that she would do as well.

On good days, or the halves of bad days that were okay, Karyn would sit up, cross-legged, on her big hospital bed and talk or write letters or fiddle with one of the small stuffed animals her family had brought to amuse her. Dozens of get-well cards stood open on shelves fitted into the corner of the room at the foot of the bed. More were stored in the drawer of her night table, along with writing paper, makeup, paperbacks, and a journal in which Karyn still found it too difficult to record her thoughts but in which she regularly entered the names of the drugs she was getting, the dates of bone-marrows done to check her progress and of spinals, daily blood counts, and assorted other facts about her medical situation that struck her as important. A few texts from college were shifted frequently from bed to floor to night table, out of sight some days, conspicuously open others.

Every morning, she gathered a little more hair from her pillow. It started coming out two weeks to the day after her inaugural dose of Vincristine, the first of thirteen drugs that she would receive on her "arm"—the long arm—of L-17M. For a few days, fine strands of pale hair hung like corn-row braids from the crown of her perfectly shaped balding head. This artful, if accidental, arrangement ends when Karyn asks her mother to snip off the remaining wisps, leaving her totally bald, but still so pretty that one of the hematology fellows assigned to her case later on will wonder what a head of hair could possibly do to improve her looks.

Karyn is small, five feet tall in a hospital gown and barefoot, but built so squarely and solidly, like her father, a member of the Lehigh University wrestling team twenty years before, that, heavy, as she was when she came into the hospital, or thin, as she became by midsummer, she seems as substantial as one of those painted wooden madonnas of the Black Forest. She has the same rosy cheeks, fuller now because of Prednisone, the round blue eyes and sweet, pleasing smile. She has her mother's heart-shaped face and a habit of smiling even when annoyed, having yet to develop the sense that her good luck in life up to this point does not disqualify her from legitimate complaint.

As diagnoses go, Karyn's was not especially hard-won. A month or so before she was hospitalized, she became aware that something was wrong with her, though as a first-semester freshman, she paid little attention.

"I couldn't put my finger on it," she recalled in February 1981, "but I knew I wasn't well. I had always been very healthy, always, and now I was tired. The first thing my mother said to me when she came to pick me up at school at Christmas was, 'You look horrible.' I had no symptoms. I just didn't feel well."

The night of December 29, Karyn woke from a sound sleep with symptoms. "I had these really bizarre hip pains," she recalls, "like spasms, or muscle cramps, in the groin area, right where the hip meets the leg. They were really, really painful, and I just didn't know what to do for them."

Her younger sister, Jennifer, had had a minor operation a few weeks earlier, and there was still some codeine in the house from her recovery. Karyn took it and managed to get through the night. In the morning, her mother took her to a local doctor, who took X rays and said she suspected tendonitis. The pain continued through the next day, made tolerable by a painkiller, then disappeared. Karyn felt better briefly and then, late on New Year's Eve, was hit with new spasms—"all up and down my back. I had trouble breathing. I felt like I was being squished. I was in a lot of pain. And I was scared. I was really frightened, because I didn't know what it was. I had no idea."

Because the Angells were new to Westport, they had no regular doctor to call, and there was some confusion as they tried to find one first on New Year's Eve and then the following day. Finally they located Dr. Paul Schulman, and the day after New Year's more tests were begun.

"For the next two weeks, I had the same thing on and off, with a fever sometimes, sometimes not." A CAT scan was done, and repeated X rays were taken in a search for possible tumors. A blurred optic nerve in her right eye led to her being treated by "about fifty-five neurologists," who made her "walk a straight line and follow their fingers," all of which Karyn did without blinking. Blood work had been extensive and had ruled out mononucleosis, hepatitis (considered seriously because her liver was inflamed), and several other possible diseases. The most significant clue that Schulman had to go on when almost every possibility had been ruled out was a general indicator of infection called the sed rate. A normal sed rate in a young woman is less than twelve; Karyn's was eighty. Schulman decided to take a sample of her bone marrow late on the one full day she spent at Norwalk Hospital, after the favorable neurological review was completed.

Karyn spent the night alone in a double room, and the next morning her parents returned to hear the results.

"They were called out of the room," Karyn recalls, the pace of her account slowing for dramatic effect, the pauses well-timed and wry, her voice a bit shallow. She takes a breath. "And there I was. And they were gone too long." She exhales for emphasis. "After a while, I just knew something was wrong. At that point I was so emotionally upset that no matter *what* they said, I knew I was going to break down.

"So they came into the room—the doctor, and my parents, and another woman I hadn't seen before, but who I later found out had had a lymphoma years ago; and she had been talking to my parents and was very helpful. And, of course, all I had to do was take one look at my mother—" Here Karyn suddenly laughs at the memory of her mother's face, and it is a laugh that holds in it the end of a thriller, the knowledge that the heroine survives— "and I knew I was in kind of tough shape."

The bone-marrow sample indicated leukemia or some type of lymphoma. Schulman thought the first more likely. Hearing this, Karyn says, "All I could feel at that point was, *I'm only seventeen.* But the other thing I remember is that I heard him say, 'We can cure this. You're not going to die in three months. It's going to be hard, it's going to be emotionally difficult, some of the treatments are going to be painful, but just remember this, we're trying to cure you. There's a possibility that we can. We're not just going to prolong anything.'

"So then I said to myself, Well, I *am* only seventeen, and I've got too many more things to do. I'll be sick for two years or whatever, and that's it. I made up my mind. That's what it was gonna be."

Schulman could have treated Karyn himself, but he told the Angells that he thought they should take her to Tim Gee to start her treatment, and he arranged by phone for Gee to take her as a patient. Dee and Dave Angell went back to Westport to pack a bag for Karyn and make arrangements for their other daughters, and Karyn sat down and waited for them to return. "I was getting ready to leave," Karyn remembers, "and I had had my initial cry, and I was numb, I still didn't understand, and I was just sitting there waiting, when another girl came in. She was with one of her friends and she went into the bathroom to get changed and her friend said to me, real quietly, 'She's having her tonsils out, and she's so scared.'"

Karyn breaks up telling this, and says, "I just looked at her, and than I said, 'Well, I had my tonsils out when I was six, and I made it. So I guess she'll be okay.'"

When he has all his hair it is black and glossy and thick as tar, slicked back and wavy now, where before chemotherapy it was halolike and wiry. In pictures taken before he got sick, it stands out from his face in an enormous bush, and with his full beard, he looks like one of the twelve Apostles, or his father's older brother. Five days short of his seventeenth birthday when he arrived at Memorial as a patient, Sal Giovia was a precocious, unformed high-school senior—smart, cocky, funny, and totally without motivation, as easily moved to anger by "jerks" and "morons" as to praise of his expanding list of heroes, a list that at that point included Sly Stallone, or more precisely the underdog heavy-weight he portrayed in *Rocky*, Robert de Niro, Frank Sinatra and Sal Richards, who also happened to be Sal Giovia, Sr.

At the time of his diagnosis, and for the first year and more of his illness, Sal was given to speaking of himself alternately as "just an ordinary guy," the sort people should realize can get something like leukemia, nobody special at all, and as someone unique and headed straight for stardom. The two versions are almost equally plausible. He seems at moments the embodiment of what it has meant to be a teen-ager in this country for the last twenty-five years, bearing traces of every decade since Buddy Holly in his "act." Most days he wears a tee shirt, blue jeans, and sneakers, a gold chain to fiddle with around his neck. It is the normal costume of a seventeen-year-old, and it fit the life he lived with his friends at the time he got sick, driving around, hanging out, moving from one club to another on "the strip" in Smithtown. Except as a place for meeting other kids, high school satisfied none of his desires. When leukemia interrupted his senior year, he appeared to care little. He never returned to regular classes, but, with only sporadic tutoring, he passed the exams he needed to graduate. At the time, he was adamant about how college would be useless to him. "If I can fight this battle without college," he said, "I can do whatever else I want without it."

The "whatever else" means becoming a professional entertainer like his father, a hard-working comic and singer who could retire the Al Pacino-Dustin Hoffman look-alike trophy. Sal senior finally made it to Las Vegas in the first year of his son's illness, after twenty years of playing the Catskills and clubs around New York. The prospect of a similar, but speedier, rise has shaped Sal's expectations of life. He has big dreams—of fame ("I think I'll be a household name in ten years"); of living in California, where he's never been, or Las Vegas, where he visited his father and had a date with the runner-up in the Our Ideal Miss contest; of becoming a producer, an actor, the guy who makes the whole country howl with laughter.

But the dreams are also a bit cloudy: they do not detail how to get from here to there. Some kids with such dreams are protected by their lack of talent, by their remove from a world where such a life seems possible, or by a shortage of self-perception. None of these defenses is available to Sal, who seems always to have seen through his own act and to have wondered, confusedly, at the contradiction between his aimless life in the suburbs and the world of glamour that he planned to join. It is the sort of muddle that is common among bright young people and is often sorted out by accident or time. Some kids go off to college, some join the Army, others find jobs. It is hard to say what Sal Giovia might have done had the end of high school arrived before leukemia did.

The confirmation that Sal had leukemia had come by phone, two days before he was admitted to Memorial. The doctor to whom the Giovias had taken him called the house to talk to Sal's parents. Sal answered the phone upstairs as his father answered downstairs, and he heard the news in a rawer form than anyone intended. He knew almost nothing about the disease except that people died from it and, sick as he was, he started running through the house screaming, "I'm gonna die, I'm gonna die." Later on, when he heard what Dr. Gee had to say, he would decide, like Karyn, that he was definitely going to be among the cured, and any reference to the opposite possibility made him angry.

Fear was the enemy, and Sal wasn't having any of it. A few days after he was released from Memorial the first time, he was asked to speak at a special teen-agers' Mass held every Saturday night at a Catholic church in Port Jefferson, a few miles from Smithtown. Many of the young people who attend regularly had donated blood for Sal in the previous weeks, and he wanted to thank them and show them how well he was doing.

"The only reason there isn't more love in the world, and why there is hate," Sal told his four hundred listeners, including his wet-eyed parents and brother, Guy, younger by a year, "is that people don't show love. They're afraid."

He went on to tell of his own experience, and of what lay ahead for him. His mood, or at least his language, was brave, accepting, pious, worthy of feature coverage in the local edition of the Sunday *New York Daily News.* "I know what I'll be going through the next couple of years of my life," he said, "and it's something I've got to do to live. But I asked God to help me, and believe me, I've been helped."

At home, the message was more urgent, the eloquence blunted. "He talks to himself in the mirror," his mother reported. "It's really something. He looks himself right in the eye and says, 'Okay, all you leukemia cells. Out!'"

On first hearing that he had leukemia, Jimmy Polack said to himself, "If they tell me I've got a month to live, that'll make it easy. If it gets painful, I'll just end it. No problem." So then he asked, "When am I going to die?" and he was given no answer, only the odds that meant he might or might not. It was 50–50, with no timetable. "That made it hard."

The possibility that he might die of leukemia was a very real prospect to Jimmy Polack in a way that it was not, at least consciously, to Karyn Angell and Sal Giovia, and in the first few months of his illness, he could not make the decision to place himself in the category of the saved as they had. He stuck hard on the awful either-or quality of the odds. Fifty–fifty has an all-or-nothing ring to it, as though everything has already been settled, as though the coin has already been tossed. In the first months of treatment, Jimmy seems to be waiting for official notification as to which side he has landed on, so that he will know what to do next. Beginning his second round of treatment, he is doing well medically, and for now, sojourns on the winning side of the tossup. But he doesn't feel like a winner. He looks awful, and he minds a lot.

In the course of a year, Jimmy will tolerate chemotherapy with less physical discomfort than either Sal, whose reactions to drugs are often severe, or Karyn, whose counts climb with exasperating slowness after each treatment. But from the beginning, he is the most changed in appearance, and he feels the sting of this transformation keenly. It is one more thing that separates him from the boy he used to be—a healthy, dark-haired boy accustomed to being outdoors half the day, slightly—and justly—vain about his body, serious about its care. At home, in Seattle, he fished, hiked, ran, biked. He lifted weights and poultry crates, ran a marathon for the hell of it, and once spent three days alone in the woods as part of a junior–high-school survival-training course.

Now his body is stiff from disuse after two months, his color poor from confinement. Prednisone has made his face round and his flesh puffy, like a fighter gone suddenly out of shape. He moves slowly, and even his facial expressions seem sluggish, as if his interior timing is off, or as if he is badly depressed. His baldness extends to his eyebrows and leaves his face without definition. Outside the hospital, he wears one of a collection of peaked caps pulled low over his eyes.

All of the physical changes that have overtaken him since he got leukemia are "disgusting" to him, but, safe from the gaze of his friends back home—for it is in their eyes that he imagines he would appear most frighteningly distorted—he reflects on what has happened to him with an almost abstract curiosity. Analyzing the breakdown of his sturdy body, he sounds like a biology teacher, or a football coach. He knows a lot about how the body works—about heartbeat, muscle development, stamina. Pairing that with what he has learned about his blood and its currently deranged functioning gives him plenty to think about when he is by himself. Which is seldom.

When he is not in the hospital, he is most often at the two-bedroom apartment off Madison Avenue that his grandfather rented soon after the family arrived in December. Morris Polack can afford the rent, and he would pay more if necessary to insure that Jimmy would not be alone, but $3,200 for an apartment that barely accommodates the four of them—Morris and his wife, their daughter Valerie, who is Jimmy's aunt, and Jimmy when he's there—seems a little steep, a little exaggerated, in keeping with the extraordinary circumstances that have brought them here.

None of the Polacks knows what to do with Jimmy, what to say to him. All they want is for him to get better, but no one knows how to make it happen. Mr. Polack has done the one thing it was in his power to do, which is to cart his heir, his grandson and, by adoption, also his son, clear across the country to be treated by the best doctor he could find. Never mind that other men might travel nearly that distance to bring a child to the town the Polacks had just left, which has a major cancer center with a fine reputation for treating leukemia particularly. Morris Polack had taken himself to the Mayo Clinic when he needed treatment, and he would have taken Jimmy to the Antarctic if he had thought it would help.

Mrs. Polack, after two months of mourning for the boy who is still alive, cannot shake her sorrow. Every time she looks at him, she is hit anew by the awfulness of it, and her frequent admonitions to him to bundle up, to rest, to take it easy, eat right and not talk about dying, fall on deaf ears. She has no capacity for recovery, it seems, and says, out of Jimmy's hearing, but often, "Life will never be the same."

Valerie Polack, in her thirties, often looks as sorrowful as her mother, but manages her voice and her conversation with Jimmy more skillfully. She is careful not to ride him and yet is torn between wanting to offer him a semblance of companionship and giving him the total privacy he sometimes seems to crave.

The four of them circle and talk and pull back, suspended, all four, from normal life. Jimmy calls the chemotherapy that knocks him flat and turns the veins in his thick arms to hard, useless crusts "abuse." It is a term appropriate to the entire business, but none of the other Polacks puts it so baldly, for fear of seeming to begrudge Jimmy a thing.

From experience, Tim Gee knows that a lot of what he tells patients the first time he meets with them will not register, and so he is careful to tell them this and to impress on them their right to come back and ask him what they most want to know over again. He is also careful to compensate for a patient's instinct to improve bad news as he takes it in. "I always paint a slightly more negative picture because people tend to remember only the positive things you say. And if it doesn't turn out well, they are unprepared."

Dee Angell remembers that the afternoon of Karyn's first day as his patient, Gee sat and talked with her "for a good hour. He came upstairs and sat and talked and answered all her questions. It was the setup for her whole stay. It gave her a mind-set in which to think about it and deal with it, and I think it was essential."

Karyn remembers that she asked first how he thought she would do. "I wanted to know my chances, first thing, obviously," and she recalls his giving what was in fact a quite cautious estimate. "He said 90 percent chance of remission, 40 to 50 percent chance of a cure." Reciting these figures three weeks after she first heard them, Karyn adds, "That to me means, I'm going to be cured. My age is a plus, the fact that I've always been healthy is a plus, and because I'm only seventeen, I haven't done anything yet. I just don't think it's time."

As it happened, Dave Angell was scheduled to leave for a three-week business conference in Belgium almost immediately after Karyn was diagnosed. His first thought was to cancel, but Karyn insisted that he go as planned, and for three weeks father and daughter carried on a transatlantic campaign of mutual support and sympathy. Their long-distance comfort of one another was not entirely telephonic. As a child, Karyn says, she used to read her parents' minds with considerable success. While Dave Angell was in Belgium, he several times experienced symptoms corresponding to reactions Karyn was having to drugs. One day in February he called to ask how she was feeling. When Karyn said she had a bad stomachache from Adriamycin, he said, "I know. I've had one for three days." The two of them shared headaches and fevers and, though separated by four thousand miles and living in different time zones, discovered they had fallen asleep at exactly the same time several days.

Before Dave Angell left for Belgium, he and Dee sat down with their three other daughters—Kim, then fifteen and a sophomore in high school, and Jennifer and Janet, fourteen-year-old twins, who were freshmen—and told them everything they knew about leukemia. "They made it so it wouldn't scare us," Kim said later that year, referring to the natural fear siblings have that they too will get terribly sick. What they could not explain was why Karyn should have gotten it. "When I first heard it," Kim said, "I stopped believing in God, because how could this happen to *her*. That it should happen to *her*," she repeated. "She was always so good." After a while, Kim changed her mind about God, and began making private appeals in Karyn's behalf during services at the church the Angells attend in Connecticut. "They ask you to speak out, like for the Pope [after he was wounded in an assassination attempt in May 1981]. I would pray, 'Please help Karyn to get well so I can stop being so angry.' I never do it when she's there."

While Dave Angell was out of the country, Dee's mother came from Florida to help out, and Dee became a daily commuter to New York. Most mornings she left Westport on a train that arrived at Grand Central sometime after eleven, then took a bus or cab to the hospital, getting there by noon, the start of visiting hours. Usually she stayed right through until the end of visiting hours, at eight, then retraced her route, arriving home each night around nine-thirty.

One is not acclimated to leukemia gradually. The experience is more like being plunged into a cold lake from a great height—one moment high above the water's surface, dry and ignorant, the next, deep beneath the water line, upside down, scrambling, out of breath. Everything looks different, nothing has its former weight; the words that matter are all new, numbers that one didn't know existed suddenly have exorbitant value. How many red cells, white cells and platelets one has in one's blood, or hatching in one's marrow, means everything. "Counts" are the mathematics of life for leukemics, and "my counts" is the most significant conversational opening.

The hospital is a sealed environment. Visitors come and go, but the patient's world is circumscribed by daily events that have no corollary elsewhere. Blood is drawn for testing, temperature and blood pressure are taken. For patients with leukemia, treatment is begun almost immediately, as soon as the necessary tests are completed. On L-17M that means five separate drugs in the first twenty days, as well as six spinals and two additional bone-marrows.

The effects of these drugs vary according to the patient. Nausea comes and goes. A severe siege of vomiting following a drug like Adriamycin can be followed by days of dulled appetite or by ravenous hunger. Karyn was invariably laid low by spinals. When Methotrexate is to be given intrathecally, a small amount of spinal fluid is first extracted in order to maintain the proper fluid balance in the spine: if the resulting balance is slightly off, the patient may wind up, as Karyn did several times, with a severe headache. The alternative is to lie still for several hours and hope that when you try to sit up enough time had passed.

Mouth sores are common, not just with leukemics but with all cancer patients whose counts have been lowered because of chemotherapy (or in some cases radiation). Jimmy and Sal had theirs; Karyn suffered a virtual plague. In the first month in the hospital, and, indeed, for the duration of nearly every stay, one's veins are the target of nearly continuous abuse. Several drugs are administered around the clock, others require repeated injections, but the effect of them all is to serially destroy the patient's veins: some collapse, some grow hard and useless, others are perforated by the I.V. needle in the middle of an infusion, so that blood or medication seeps into the surrounding tissue. Called infiltration, this last reaction is common and painful, raising a swollen bruise that can last for days or weeks, because the patient's platelet counts are usually so low. (Jimmy Polack, who liked to invite people to feel his ruined veins—wire-hard lengths beneath the skin—pointed out one of chemotherapy's unadvertised side effects over a bacon-and-eggs breakfast one morning. "Cancer patients don't have to worry about cholesterol," he said, smiling. "All that poison blasts it right out of the veins.")

In all these matters, one quickly becomes expert. Like Jimmy and Sal before her, Karyn has it all straight within days. She talks casually of her "polys" not coming up as fast as she'd like ("polys" being polymorphonuclear white cells, the most mature form of healthy white blood cells, whose return in number will signify that remission has been achieved) and what it's like to have a spinal or a bone-marrow. Jimmy Polack's approach to these subjects is technical and detailed, as if he's describing how he replaced a two-wheel-drive underbody with a four-wheel-drive one; Sal Giovia is offhand and elliptical when he describes hospital procedures, always eager to give the impression that they are of little consequence, yet he too can discuss the refinements of chemotherapy and its effects as convincingly as—and certainly more entertainingly than—a second-year resident. Karyn's tone in discussing these matters is curious, excited, cheerfully instructive, as if she has seized on a terrific subject for a term paper and is trying her ideas out.

She is aware of how she handles the material that could terrorize her. "When I talk about it, it's in an academic way," she says. "That's part of the way I operate. You can't be emotional all the time." Everybody uses tricks to get through the hard parts. Karyn's are intellectual, controlling, and, in retrospect if not in the actual moment, humorous. By her third week in the hospital, she had had a total of four bone-marrow extractions and four spinals, and she was able to talk about them freely, wincing occasionally as she remembered, but overlooking nothing important.

"I don't remember the one Dr. Gee did on my chest (at admittance), because I was crying and upset while they were doing that, but in the hips you feel a lot of pressure when they go in because they have to go right into the bone. You don't feel any pain, because they give you anesthesia. The novocaine stings, though, for about thirty seconds—it really stings. And then you just feel pressure going in. It feels funny. You can kind of hear it," she says, and makes a face. "It's the thought that's worse than anything else. It goes in and then they aspirate the fluid. And sometimes you can feel a sharp pull and you can feel it in the back of your legs, just as the fluid is being pulled out. Sometimes they have to take a biopsy, they have to take a piece of the bone to test that, and that again—you feel pressure, and you kind of hear them grinding away in there—" Karyn makes an odd noise from time to time, a sharp, cut-off laugh that suggests surprise at what she's saying, and she makes it now—"Really, the sounds are the worst, and it's the same with a spinal tap—that is, it's the thought of it, of a needle going in between [the vertebrae] and you're afraid it's going to hit something and you're waiting for it to hurt. But they are so skilled at this and they've done so many, that it's not going to hurt you. I just think—what it feels like is someone pressing a thumb into my back, and that's how I think of it—she's (most of Karyn's early spinals were done by Dr. Catherine Small, one of the fellows; bone-marrows were done by Dr. Gee) just sticking her thumb into my back. And then there's no problem. That's how I deal with it. Instead of thinking, Oh, my God, this needle is *driving* into my flesh."

Karyn gets most of her information about leukemia from Dr. Gee, Dr. Small, or Kathy Deitz, and Dee Angell is there to hear most of it, but she supplements their answers with reading. She has collected a shopping-bagful of pamphlets from the Cancer Information Service office down the street from Memorial, and she reads them while Karyn sleeps off the effects of treatment in midafternoon. Like her daughter, Dee Angell has always taken comfort in knowing what she is up against, although the more she reads on this subject the more she is forced to recognize the futility of her researches. "We were people who always had control over their lives," she said one day during Karyn's first month in the hospital. "We always felt we could make things happen. We can negotiate, we can manipulate, we can evaluate. But with this we can't. The way we can salvage the situation is by making something positive out of it. It doesn't make sense not to."

One of the few choices the Angells were free to make was where Karyn would be treated. Acting on Schulman's advice they had chosen Memorial and Gee, and they were glad of it in retrospect, not just for medical reasons but because in this hospital, as Dee bluntly puts it, "Karyn is not a freak. She is not unusual. If she were in our local hospital, people would be speaking in hushed tones, they'd be walking by with long faces—you know, this poor young girl, her whole life ahead of her. It's very different here. She's lucky—if you can conceive of someone who's just been diagnosed as having leukemia as being lucky in any way. The people who work here are simply better at helping people deal with things. They know what to say and how to behave."

In all of this, Karyn concurs and will, long after she has come to hate the place. It is true that the nurses, who are unstarched and wear bright shirts to work and are, most of them, only a few years older than Karyn, are wonderful to her. Also that Kathy Dietz and Dr. Small pay particular attention to her, attention that falls somewhere between sisterly and motherly. Everyone answers her questions, tells her that she is doing just great, that all is in order, that despite that fact that she is now bald as an egg she is still a beautiful girl. In the worst of situations, Karyn has landed in an almost ideal setting and at first that "luck," in her mother's tempered phrase, buoys her up. She and Memorial are a match; they share an attitude of energy and optimism, of conviction that obstacles can be overcome, that, given the best doctors, the best treatment, things will naturally work out for the best.

Yet, even while maintaining a personal hopefulness, as the weeks passed, Karyn could not help but become aware of how grim a place the hospital could be, once the newness had worn off. For a week or two, her roommate is a young married woman with acute nonlymphocytic leukemia who is in "for a fever," a common occurence during treatment. Regina* has already passed through many of the phases that lie ahead of Karyn, and she is generous with advice, about wigs and fever sores, headaches and nausea. Patients are always being cautioned not to compare themselves too pointedly with others, as everyone's response to treatment is different, but for most it is irresistible. It's important to be told in advance by one of the medical staff that Vincristine and Adriamycin will make your hair fall out, or that Prednisone may make you moody. It's quite another thing to hear it directly from someone who's already been there, to trace her collapsed veins with your fingers, to hear—from the bed across the room— how hard she shakes when her temperature is 104 degrees, to trade accounts of what you looked like before you lost your hair, of who you are in real life, and to hear that it is possible to pick up the thread of normal life again.

For Dee Angell, having Regina to talk to "was like having Dr. Spock. When the kids were little, whenever anything was wrong, I would look it up and see that so many children react this way, and so many come down with this in their first year. When you don't know what to expect, it can be very frightening, and we don't know what to expect with this. Regina was able to give us some idea of what's ahead of us."

---

*To protect the privacy of patients who figure incidentally in the narrative, pseudonyms have been substituted for real names. All major characters—patients, doctors and nurses, family members and friends—are identified by real names unless otherwise indicated.

Knowing something about Regina's case had other, more subtle effects on the Angells. Not only was Regina's long-term prognosis less favorable statistically than Karyn's, she had two small children at home, about whose future she was concerned, and for whom she had to care in the present. She wanted to spend as much time as she could with them between stays in the hospital, but exposure to them when her counts were down meant that she was always in danger of contracting an infection that could land her back in the hospital. It was a dilemma toward which the Angells were sympathetic, and it also worked to take some of the heat of sympathy off themselves. This sense of comparative well-being is one of the few true universals among cancer patients. Everyone takes comfort not from the suffering of another patient but from the perception (sometimes totally wrong, but that doesn't affect its power) that someone else is worse off in some way.

For Dee Angell, in whom openness and friendliness coexist with a fierce sense of her own individuality and personal autonomy, being privy by circumstance to Regina's private affairs was a very sensitive issue. One day, when the floor social worker was interviewing Regina, an educated middle-class woman with a husband who supported her, Dee found herself wishing that she could disappear, so acutely did she project her own sense of privacy onto Regina. When she in turn was approached by the social worker, who knew nothing of the Angell's circumstances, she realized that she was appalled by the implication that her family might need outside help.

"I wasn't defensive," she said in reflecting on it afterward, "but I wasn't ready to open up. It has to do mainly with control. And, very honestly, with pride." A similar situation had arisen at home, when a volunteer from the local welcome wagon appeared one day to ask if her group could help out by bringing in meals. "I found the hair standing up on my head," Dee said, telling about it now in full awareness of the many levels of irony contained in the scene and her reaction to it. Only in a town like Westport, Connecticut, could a volunteer from the welcome wagon be mistaken for an agent of the welfare state. Yet the hint of insufficiency that the offer implied set her off. It was as if by virtue of this one new fact in their lives, their status as independent people had been abruptly changed. And, of course, it had been, although it did not extend to getting meals on the table.

Nor was it just a matter of outsiders, Dee realized. An equivalent reluctance to become a burden on friends combined with the exhaustion that went with their changed lives and threatened to cut them off from people who wanted to stay in touch and help if they could. "You can isolate yourself unintentionally," she said. "Most people who call call at nine-thirty at night, when I've just gotten home and haven't eaten. But you can only say you're too tired to talk so many times before people stop calling. You have to be sensitive to other people trying to reach out to you."

A few friends and relatives were rendered mute by Karyn's illness—one distantly related couple surprised the Angells by showing up to visit Karyn at the hospital, but could not bring themselves to inquire about her. "They didn't say two words about the disease," Karyn says. "They just talked about what *they* were doing." But most of the people they cared about took their cue from the family. "All my college friends wanted to know everything," Karyn said, "about the disease and the treatment." Her four closest friends from school had driven down to see her and sent care packages. "They treat me exactly the same as before, which is good." Communication with other friends was less successful, giving Karyn the first hint that there would be people who would not treat her exactly as before. A boy she had known before the family moved to Paris called, and "was real quiet on the phone. I just went into my whole medical spiel, and told him I'm not going to die, these are my chances, this is what's going to happen, *blah blah blah,* and at the end of it, he said, 'I don't know what to say.' I said, 'Well, you think about it and get back to me when you think you can handle it.' And he called me back last week and said, 'I still don't know what to say.' I said, 'You don't have to say anything. I'm not different. I'm sick, but you don't have to feel differently toward me.' And he's really having a hard time with that."

Much later on, when Karyn was back in school and under the care of one of Gee's former fellows, Dr. Gee would look back on her first weeks in the hospital and confess that for a while he suspected that she might not really be taking in what had happened to her. "Her attitude was almost too good to believe," he said, "and in the beginning I thought, Is this getting through to her? And then I saw that it had, but that she was doing with it what she needed to do."

Karyn's own estimate of her strengths and limits was unusually shrewd, and not just for someone who was seventeen, about to turn eighteen. In trying to explain how she managed to be both optimistic and philosophical about her situation, she began by talking about the big changes that had taken place in her life before she got leukemia and how she believed those changes had consistently been for the best.

For the ten years before the Angells moved to Paris—an assignment they went after actively, believing that it would be good for the whole family—they lived on a farm in upstate New York, a short distance from the IBM Endicott plant, where Dave Angell worked. It was a quiet life, with horses and cows to tend, and days centered closely on family pursuits, school, sports, local events. Karyn and her sisters learned to ride, and she became a gymnast. Fall Sundays she spent watching football with her father, and in the summer the family usually rented or borrowed a sailboat to vacation on. Their life was comfortable, settled, idyllic in some respects, but also confining, and Dave and Dee Angell wanted to stretch themselves and their daughters with a big change. They succeeded.

Karyn was fourteen when they left Endicott. "We were zapped right into Paris," as she puts it, "and I loved it. I remember driving down the streets there the first day, on our way to the hotel. I didn't know there were that many people in the whole world."

The four girls were enrolled in the American School, with Karyn intent on finishing high school in three years, the term of her father's assignment. The American School was at once safe and familiar, exotic and revelatory. Virtually everyone in it knew, with the precision that only an American childhood can insure, just exactly how a hamburger with French fries and a Coke should smell, taste, and repeat within the hour, and there was in addition the assurance that no student of average ability would fall behind his counterparts at home. Yet included among the student body were kids who had lived everywhere in the world and had had experiences that would have been unimaginable in Endicott. There were lots of non-Americans too, so that when Karyn returned to the United States, the young Iranian whom she would meet while in the hospital would in some important ways seem more familiar to her than Jimmy or Sal.

Outside the school, the Angells leapt into French life. They lived in a rented house near the Bois de Boulogne, and Karyn remembers a parade of French acquaintances dragged home by her mother. "Every day we would come home from school and my mother would be sitting in the kitchen with another new face, talking away in French."

In the summers, the family traveled together, but the kids also went off on solo trips, with school groups or other families. One of Karyn's greatest triumphs was taking a train from Wales to London by herself when she was fourteen. Though she would eventually traipse all over Europe at a not much older age, faking

Italian and German and waving her arms, this first big trip alone occupies a huge place in her sense of herself as an independent person, and she cites it almost as if she is stroking a charm—it reminds her of what she's capable of.

"I know if I had lived on that farm until I got this disease, I would be thinking about it in a different way. It's because I've been through a lot of major changes that it doesn't affect me as hard, I don't get as uptight about things, little stupid things, as I used to. Something comes up, some crisis, some disaster, and I've learned to say, Okay, this is what's happening. Now what am I going to do about it? I know that has helped me."

Asked whether she feels angry at times, she replies quickly, as though she has been waiting for the question and knows that her answer is somewhat surprising. "That's one thing I've never felt. About this, that is. Dr. Gee said I would probably feel it at some point.

"I have felt—well, my first reaction was numbness, and just kind of a whole disbelief. It's the kind of thing that you see in movies and read in books, but it doesn't happen to you, and I don't know—but I've never been angry. I've been depressed. I've never thought, Oh, why me? I don't think it's a punishment. I'm not sure *what* I think. I'm having some thoughts about my belief in God and whether someone is up there calling the shots or whether we call the shots. I'm not sure about any of that, either. I think maybe it's just one of those things that are in store for me growing up."

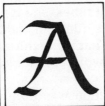 solid tumor cancer spreads in one of two ways: by direct, sometimes exponential, growth at the original site, leading to the involvement of nearby organs; or through metastasis, in which cancerous cells break away from the original tumor and make their way, by means of the blood or lymph systems, to a distant part of the body.

In lung cancer, the most common sites of distant metastases are the brain, the bones, the adrenal glands, and the liver, in that order of frequency. Because a cancer cell retains its original character regardless of its current host, however, cancers are treated according to their sites of origin, no matter where the metastases present. A lung cancer metastasized to bone is always treated as a lung cancer; a breast cancer metastasized to bone is treated as a breast cancer.

The problem with determining a course of treatment in Terry O'Brien's case was that she had already used up the most effective treatment available. When it works—as for the 50 percent of adenocarcinomas, Stage I, who *don't* suffer a recurrence within five years—surgery cannot be improved upon as a treatment for lung cancer. When it fails, there remains a scarily modest collection of treatments to turn to, essentially radiation and chemotherapy, with some experimental work being done in immunotherapy.

None of these is employed with great expectations in the treatment of metastatic lung cancer, and there is nothing that can be called a standard treatment for adenocarcinoma. There is no single drug or combination of drugs that is known to be consistently effective against lung cancer in the sense that such therapies exist for the treatment of Hodgkin's disease, testicular cancer, or breast cancer. The history of chemotherapeutic treatment of lung cancer consists rather of a series of drugs, tried over time, singly and in combination, and found wanting. Their effectiveness is spoken of cautiously, in terms of degree of response or level of activity, not survival, if the term can be circumvented, and never "cure."

Still, given Terry O'Brien's condition, and her resolution to pursue whatever treatment was offered, chemotherapy appeared to be her best chance, and in December 1980 her surgeon, Dr. Beattie, referred her for treatment to Robert B. Golbey, since 1967 the head of Memorial's Solid Tumor Service and one of its most senior clinical chemotherapists. Golbey had started working at Memorial in 1954, when chemotherapy was very much an embryonic science, and in the years since, he had seen it grow exponentially but unevenly, with truly spectacular results in the treatment of some cancers and virtual failure in others. Midway through his treatment of Terry O'Brien, Golbey would conclude a detailed explanation of the limits of his specialty with respect to lung cancer with the remark, "If we cure anybody, we are surprised."

At the time Terry O'Brien came to Golbey's attention, a drug called Vindesine—according to Golbey the "single most active agent" against lung cancer yet identified—was undergoing clinical trials in which it was being paired, one after another, with a series of other drugs known to have some activity against lung cancer. Used alone, Vindesine had demonstrated an average 30 percent response in lung patients—meaning that in 30 percent of the patients treated, some response, ranging from partial to full remission (with duration unknown) is obtained. It was hoped that, in combination, that response rate could be pushed higher, and in fact, when paired with a drug called cis-platinum, it climbed to 40 percent, with remissions of longer duration. The side effects of the combination, however, were much more severe than those of Vindesine alone, which meant that fewer patients could successfully tolerate the protocol, and for this reason, and in continued pursuit of more effective combinations, Vindesine was tested with yet additional drugs.

When Terry O'Brien appeared for her first appointment with Dr. Golbey on December 26 (she had not wanted to start treatment sooner, because of Christmas) a trial of Vindesine plus a drug called Methyl-GAG was underway, and it was this combination that Golbey recommended for her. He explained to her the value of the two drugs and the purpose and history of the trial and discussed with her the implications of treatment, which would be weekly. The consent form that Terry would sign a week later listed the following possible side effects: "lowering of the blood count, due to bone-marrow effect, which may cause increased susceptibility to infection or bleeding; muscle weakness, numbness and tingling and hair loss are also common. Other side effects seen are nausea, vomiting, fever, mouth soreness, laryngitis, skin rash, diarrhea, soreness of the esophagus or a low blood sugar." A final cautionary sentence warned that additional side effects could not be predicted, but that the patient would be "observed closely to minimize toxicity."

In exchange, there was a 30 percent chance (or better, if the hoped-for synergy between the two drugs materialized) that the treatment would slow the pace of her cancer, for an unspecified period of time.

Terry O'Brien spent no time reflecting on the mean nature of the bargain being offered her. She was afraid of chemotherapy, because, like everyone else, she had heard horror stories—not one person's real story so much as repeated fragments of a kind of floating tale of misery—hair loss, constant sickness, the cure worse than the disease, and futile, to boot. But that the medicine for something so terrible as lung cancer should be harsh seemed appropriate to her—the stronger the better, she would say more than once.

On December 29 Terry checked into Memorial for the second time in less than two years, and on New Year's Eve, she joked, "instead of drinking scotch I was drinking milk of magnesia." Over the next couple of days, she underwent a series of tests, and on January 3 she received her first dose of chemotherapy. The Vindesine, 4.8 milligrams, was given by I.V. push, the Methyl-GAG, 800 milligrams, by I.V. drip. Noting on her chart that "chemotherapy was well tolerated," Golbey discharged her the same day.

She received her second dose of chemotherapy, 3.0 mgs. of Vindesine, without Methyl-GAG, as an outpatient on the fourteenth. The following week, her white blood count was depressed and treatment was postponed. Her hair began to fall out in patches, and on her way home, she stopped to pick up a wig that she had ordered at a shop off Fifth Avenue.

On the twenty-eighth, her counts were up, and she received a full dose of Methyl-GAG, 800 mgs, but no Vindesine. On February 4, she got another combined dose of Vindesine and Methyl-GAG, at three-quarter strength.

After each treatment would come, within a few hours, a period of nausea, usually followed by vomiting. Most often, she was recovered by the next day, but as the treatment progressed, she began to be conscious of more general discomfort, and then a number of specific complaints.

On February 9, a Monday, Terry called Golbey from home to report that she had been suffering from chills all weekend, had a fever, a sore throat, pink eye, and a long list of other ailments, no two of which, Golbey later remarked, appeared to be related. He reserved a room on the twelfth floor and told her to come in as soon as possible.

She arrived in Bedholding, Memorial's equivalent of an emergency room, at two-thirty, "alert, oriented, and in good color." Her additional complaints included difficulty in swallowing, diarrhea and dehydration, a tender abdomen, burning on urination, one small lesion on the upper part of her right foot, and a second lesion on the inside of her mouth.

There were three more or less equally likely causes for her condition: drug toxicity, infection brought on by lowered resistance (the depressed white counts), or a combination of the two. Golbey started her on antibiotics and fluids for dehydration and ordered a series of tests to find out what was wrong.

I met Mrs. O'Brien for the first time in the middle of that hospital stay, by chance on the afternoon of February 11, 1981, the seventh anniversary of her stroke. She was, for the moment, not hooked up to anything and sat sideways on the high hospital bed, facing the window and the sunny view across midtown. This was a private room, the last one she would have, a simple accident of availability. A large hard-cover book, one of a series of best-sellers that she would recommend as interesting but would never finish herself, lay open on her lap. She wore a handsome blue-and-maroon robe that Ray had given her for Christmas, too long by a couple of inches in the hem and sleeves, but warm, and her new wig, an artifact so persuasively and lushly Celtic that I took it for her real hair. On her feet, which dangled halfway between the bottom of her robe and the floor, she wore cotton tennis socks, the kind with a fluff ball at each heel. She looked tired but not sick, and her greeting to Golbey was wry.

Terry O'Brien always seemed to be someone on the best of terms with herself—not at peace, but perfectly self-acquainted, and certain of exactly how much of that self she wanted to share, and with whom. She invited me to explain my project and listened with an attentiveness that was almost severe. Occasionally, she would utter an *"uh-huh"* from some locus of judgment far back in her throat. So composed and polite was she during the opening minutes of our interview that I was not conscious of being on trial until, with an abrupt change in the temperature, as we talked of our common origins in the Bronx, I realized I had passed.

The frequency of her comments increased, the *uh-huhs* and the nods gave way to questions, and what I had taken for a natural reserve collapsed and was replaced by a more truly characteristic engagement. Yet there were limits. Once she had agreed to let me trail her through her illness, she never changed her mind, but she could not resist pointing out, despite her agreement, that she was, after all, Irish. "And the Irish never tell you anything," she would say, with a perfectly straight face.

There was some truth in her claim, but it did not apply with precision to her. In the first place, her husband remarked more than once when he heard her speak of being Irish, they were "American-Irish. And there's a big difference." In the second place, Terry O'Brien happened to be an extremely blunt woman— "brutally honest" is how Ray put it, having seen her at the top of her form. She was likelier to tell you bad news about yourself than about her, and she was unquestionably tight-lipped about matters that she considered her business and no one else's, matters of pride and terror especially.

Her relations with the world, including those closest to her, skittered always between the antipodes of Irishness and Americanness, circumspection and openness. Much of the time, her habit of keeping her most serious thoughts to herself was obscured by the more immediately endearing and obvious side of her nature—gregarious, effusive, curious, sympathetic. Having cancer didn't radically change that balance, but it tipped Terry O'Brien's view of things a bit. Perhaps as significant is the fact, unmistakable as time went on, that Terry O'Brien believed that she deserved a biographer. She had few pretensions about herself in the worldly sense; she knew that she was a girl of a good family who had grown up in the Bronx. She hadn't gone to college, and she read best-sellers instead of Proust, but she knew she was someone special. When Golbey asked her whether she would like to speak to a writer interested in cancer patients, it seemed like the most natural development imaginable to her. Of course, someone would want to write about her before she died. And she was ready.

That first afternoon, honoring the intentions of her interviewer with great seriousness, she attempted to give an account of herself and her feelings about her illness with a deliberateness that she had clearly never before attempted. As she talked, she seemed to be struggling to reconcile several contradictory but equally instinctive reactions to her illness. Her tone was alternately formal, comic, outraged, sentimental. She frequently punctuated a sober statement with a one-liner, and easily half of what she said about anything was phrased parenthetically, with much of it having the quality of being spoken aloud for the first time. At moments she seemed surprised to learn—from her own busy mouth—just how she felt about certain matters or, indeed, how she had arranged things.

On the one hand were the facts and her long habit of facing them. She had always looked at life squarely. So had Ray; neither believed in fooling oneself. All the children had been told, she said, the three older ones as soon as it was known that the cancer had spread, the younger girls and Sean as soon as he returned for Christmas vacation. "They know it's serious," she said. "And they ask questions about the treatment. We talk about it," she said, and hesitated. "We don't talk about dying."

In that hedge was defined the limits of family realism for the present. Any suggestion that all was lost was intolerable. When her rheumatologist, on learning that her cancer had spread, asked her, "How are you going to handle it?" she was incensed. "He annoyed me," she said with a curl of her lip. "What did he think I was going to do? Grab a knife?"

Similarly, she had advised her friends of the limits of sympathy. "Have you ever been to a club—you know, a country club where you know everyone? Well, then you know that the minute something happens to a person, everybody knows. As soon as people heard I was in here, they descended on Ray. 'How's Terry? What's happening? How's she doing?' I tell my good friends, 'Listen, do me a favor. The man's there to have a drink, to relax. Ask him once how I am, and then leave him alone.'"

The phone rang several times during our first visit, her sister calling from Long Island, Raymond from the West Coast where he had gone on business, friends from Colts Neck. She told all callers that she was fine, just waiting to find out "what the hell is wrong with me. It's ridiculous. I've got them baffled." The tone was light—nothing serious is afoot.

And though she complained that the room was too cold and asked everyone who came in to check the thermostat, she was otherwise cavalier about the complaints that had brought her in. In fact, she was more comfortable now; her fever had abated, and her various lesions and sores had begun to heal. Her appetite was poor, but she was getting fluids and nourishment by I.V. and felt stronger. Her mood was good.

Indeed, her apparent turnaround and her attitude of calm were

63

very much at odds with both the overriding facts of her case and her own instinctive realism. Speculating on whether the current treatment would successfully stave off death, and for how long, she suddenly said, "I'd like to live to about sixty. But I don't have any control over the situation." Still, she said, she preferred to believe that she was going to make it, that the slim statistical chance that chemotherapy offered would swell for her into a future. Sixty was not quite a number picked from a hat—more a wish, half timid, half bold, midway between asking for a lot and very little at all. In another ten years, Nancy, her youngest, would be twenty-five, Ray would be sixty-four. She might get to see a few grandchildren, although the prospect did not excite her as much as rumor would suggest that such things do; she was a woman still engaged with her own children, and in the flesh, they were more important to her than the abstract idea of grandchildren.

And she knew that she did not want to live too long; she had no stomach for surviving into helpless senility the way her mother had. Mary Sweeney was now pushing eighty-three, still straight-backed and strong as an ox, but out of her head, speechless, needing to be clothed, fed, and bathed, living in a Catholic nursing home downtown; the three of her four children who lived near New York—Kak on Long Island, Brian in Connecticut and Terry in New Jersey, visited her regularly, but they disagreed on whether she knew them when they sat beside her chair. Terry was certain she did not. "You should see her," she said. "It's really pathetic. And if she knew—she would have died thinking she would end up like that. I'd rather go my way."

Hearing herself say such brave things out loud, Mrs. O'Brien felt obliged to acknowledge that she knew it was possible only because the exact date of her life's foreclosure was still unknown, and because she was still able to concentrate on lesser losses. She volunteers the absurdity that "I never cried when I heard I had cancer, but when my hair started to fall out, I cried for two hours. I thought it was the worst thing that could happen to me." Then she gets serious, and says, "I don't know how I'll feel if someone says, 'You have two weeks.'" She studies her hands a moment, then lifts her head again. "But I guess I'll deal with it. And my children will deal with it."

She didn't want them to worry about her. She didn't want Ray to worry either; so, although she had agreed to tell him everything that Golbey told her and he had agreed never to seek out information and keep it from her, she was cozy with her fears around him too. Even with Ray, it was too early to start talking about "what if?"

64

She had too much going for her, she was convinced. She was a born fighter for one thing. And look what she had been through already, she said, as she began to list all her previous ailments, not just the stroke and the arthritis, but back through childhood, to a well-remembered burst appendix brought on, the story goes, by a badly timed enema administered by her determined mother. (Kak said of this event, "Ma sort of catered to her after that. I think she felt a little guilty.") This catastrophic catalogue was presented as evidence also of her belief that "God has tested me." She grew serious again as she made this claim, and the devoutness that was a part of her character as much—if not as conspicuously—as the dry-humored wife, the winking schoolgirl friend, the exasperated, intrusive mother, was made plain. "I think God has built up my resistance," she said, and though she left unspecified whether it was a physical or a spiritual resistance that she meant, what was clear was that at the moment she was thoroughly convinced of His succor.

Though less certain of her doctor's long-term ability to make things turn out right, she was equally convinced that he would do everything he could to save her. She decided at the start that she liked Golbey and trusted him, and as time went on, she got to like him better, becoming affectionate and effusive when talking about him to others, though in their frequent meetings she maintained a teasing, smart-aleck tone much of the time. "The doctor's the priest," she said to Raymond over the phone one day, meaning you buy what he says whether it sounds good or not. "It's important to have faith in your doctor," she said another day, "otherwise don't go to him." She meant such statements, but the fact that she liked Golbey personally came to count for more than her confidence in him professionally. She engaged him early on as her equal, partly because she preferred to like the people she spent any amount of time with and partly as a challenge. Superficially, theirs seemed an odd fit, as one of Terry's friends, meeting Golbey for the first time, pointed out. In Golbey, the friend concluded, "Terry had met her match." That was all she needed to hear.

Golbey is a solemn, slow-moving figure rarely seen inside the hospital without his white lab coat with his name tag showing. With his long, sorrowful face, and 1950s hair cut, he could pass for a cartoonist's version of the soberest of the joint chiefs of staff. Golbey is inadequately described as middle-aged; his face looks as if he has been around much longer, and when he smiles, or laughs, it is as if something deep and solid has broken apart. Toward Terry he observed a correct and tender attitude always, addressing her as Mrs. O'Brien, but giving the formal words a fondness with his tone. He was precise in his explanations of all that was happening to her and encouraged her to ask questions, which she did, up to a point, and to complain, which she did much less frequently. All of this she appreciated, but she spent a lot of time baiting him, trying to get him to laugh; she succeeded in unleashing a competitor. Golbey, it turned out, was almost as funny as she was.

When she was newly bald—or patchy, since her hair never completely fell out—she had very strict rules about people coming into her hospital room without warning. When Golbey surprised her one day when she wasn't wearing her wig, she scolded him and told him that if he had suffered a bad fright, he had only himself to blame. When he returned later in the day, she had her wig on again, and when he had finished what he had to say, she patted it and said, "This is better, isn't it?" Golbey stared at her blank-faced before responding in a dead-pan voice, "To tell you the truth, I hadn't noticed the difference."

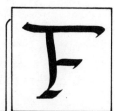 or years, the American Cancer Society has advertised a list of seven early warning signals for cancer. Aligned to form the acronym CAUTION from the first letter of each line, they read in otherwise forgettable order and phrasing:

Change in bowel or bladder habits
A sore that does not heal
Unusual bleeding or discharge
Thickening or lump in breast or elsewhere
Indigestion or difficulty in swallowing
Obvious change in wart or mole
Nagging cough or hoarseness

Popular notions about cancer would lead many people to add to this list sudden weight loss, extreme fatigue, or simply the absence of a former sense of well-being. There is reassurance as well as dread to be found in these checklist items, in that they run counter to the widespread and not unreasonable fear that cancer will sneak up on one without warning. To believe that one's body will signal the bad news unmistakably is surely a more comforting conviction, however naïve at root. In fact, sometimes it does; frequently it does not. And even when early symptoms do show up, their source and their significance can prove elusive. The process is not quite hit-or-miss, though it sometimes seems that way. Rather, as the diagnostic experiences of the eight subjects of this book illustrate, it is an imprecise and difficult process, dependent on many factors. Among them are the skill and thoroughness of the diagnostician, the persistence of the patient, the location and behavior of a tumor, the character of symptoms, and, not infrequently, simple luck.

Because it sometimes seems as if we have been pickled in information about cancer, one might be forgiven for thinking that it could be determined with certainty and rather quickly whether one has it. Yet obtaining an accurate cancer diagnosis anywhere outside one of the major cancer centers remains among the more difficult propositions in medicine.

As an example of just how far things can go despite the patient's best efforts, Johanne Johnson's case is deserving of a closer look. So, too, for very different reasons, is Howard Mindus's. His experience, ideal in many respects, not only reflects some of the real limits of diagnostic skill, but demonstrates how difficult it can be, under the best of circumstances, for a patient to find a doctor and a hospital to treat him.

Johanne Johnson is one of eight granddaughters named for her mother's mother, and the only one to survive into adulthood. She was born October 7, 1941, in the Bahamas, where her grandfather owned a small island of salt, which he sold bit by bit to the British all through World War II. When Johanne was seven, her family came to the United States, but there would be comings and goings between New York and the Islands forever, a parade of brothers and sisters, parents, grandparents, cousins and more cousins acting out a sense of family that is supposed to have disappeared with the village green. But family remains terribly important to Johanne, as is her sense of where she came from, which is in her voice and face still, a softness behind the city veneer. And the tenaciousness that life seems to have required of her is also intact, despite some bad moments in the last few years.

When things are not awful, Johanne is energetic—almost to the point of being hyperactive, intelligent, verbally extravagant, quick, playful, almost invariably direct. She has a gift for pursuing an argument aloud, singlehanded, and at high speed, that would be useful in the well of a courtroom; her soliloquies are sometimes hard to follow, but they are immensely persuasive. She talks gracefully, her huge eyes working harder than her hands as visual aids, her smile breaking unpredictably. Her face is oval and handsome, and closely filled with her features; when she is feeling well, her skin is lustrous, a brown the color of Gauguin's maidens, smooth and glowing. When she is feeling sick, it pales and grays slightly in immediate reflection. Her weight goes up and down accordingly; though she never gets fat,

68

she can grow very skinny in the wake of a bout of chemotherapy.

Since her divorce seven years ago, Johanne has lived alone with her son, Michael, who was twelve at the time of her diagnosis. She has remained on the best of terms with Michael's father, just as, until recently, she was on the best of terms with most of the world, enjoying life, working hard, and taking for granted, as most people instinctively do, her health, her ability to care for herself, to get around, to be independent. Not that she was unaware of stresses in her life. There are at least two sides of Johanne that have enjoyed prominence at different times of her life. One of these took her to a job on Wall Street, where she worked for several years under great pressure, overseeing the clearing of checks and other financial paper, until she knew she had to get out. Something of that same side frequently drives her to do more than she should, to push herself to exhaustion.

The other side of Johanne may have something to do with being "from the Islands," the phrase she occasionally invokes to explain her intuitive sense of what is right for her and what is not. That side of Johanne is alert to the messages given off by her body, believes that the maintenance of good health is largely one's own responsibility, is interested in nutrition, acupuncture, vitamins, herbs, and the power of prayer. The second side does not altogether approve of the first, regarding it as likely to get her into trouble. Whenever things threaten to get out of hand, as they sometimes do when her driven first side is in control, Johanne reminds herself that there is another way. "I believe we have a lot to do with making ourselves sick *and* well," she says. "It goes both ways."

It is hard for Johanne to say exactly when she became aware that all was not well. In January 1979, she made an appointment with a gynecologist because she was concerned about the severe menstrual pain that she was having. She had always had difficulty, but it seemed to have intensified lately, and she wanted to know why her flow should still be so heavy as she approached forty. The gynecologist she went to on the recommendation of a friend was "an adorable Italian," Johanne recalls, "with a deep, deep year-round tan," whose office was "just a sea of women. All you could hear was 'Next.'" After an exam that turned up nothing, she was given a prescription for Darvon and a second appointment for two weeks later, at which time the doctor told her that she had a tipped womb. He recommended surgery. That way, Johanne learned, she could have a baby. She told him that a failure to become pregnant was "not my complaint." Johanne kept a third appointment a month later, but the doctor, who she later learned had three separate offices in two different boroughs of New York City, was not there.

About the same time, Johanne began having difficulty moving her bowels. After trying bran, teas, herbs, hot baths and every other home remedy she could think of, she made an appointment to see an internist in the spring.

"I remember him telling me that constipation 'is the American pastime. You don't eat right, you don't take the time to sit on the toilet, talk to yourself—' Well, I thought, this makes sense. Then he prescribed stool softeners and another drug for coating the stomach. I went to the pharmacy and asked, 'How much are these stool softeners?' and they told me seven seventy-five or something, and I said, 'How much is this drug to coat my stomach?' and that was about nine dollars, and I said, 'Forget it,' and went back to the bran.

"But nothing was happening. So I tried enemas—very harsh, but I was desperate. And when I did move, the vitamins I had taken would still be whole." She went back to the internist, who ordered an upper and lower G.I. series. The X rays showed a shadow behind her navel, but, because he could find no obstruction, the doctor concluded that Johanne must have shifted position during the test. "Keep doing what you've been doing," he advised, and she did. When her bowels moved, infrequently, she would feel better for a while, but the feeling never lasted long.

"I was beginning to think that maybe something was wrong with me up here," she said, tapping her forehead as she told the story nearly two years later. "You know the expression, 'You have the solution within you.' Well, I thought, maybe I do need help. One day a friend in treatment suggested that I see her counselor. This particular day I was really down, I was crying, and I said, 'I don't know what's the matter with me. I just feel rotten. I've gone to doctors and they keep telling me there's nothing wrong. Maybe there's something wrong in my head.' We talked, and my friend said, 'Listen, you're healthy, you're normal. But I've noticed you're getting thin, you're irritable. Why don't you go get a checkup?' "

Johanne attempted to make an appointment at a clinic that tests for cancer and other illnesses and where she had had a checkup six or seven years earlier. When she was unable to fit any of the available times into her schedule, she made a third appointment with the internist. He did a repeat of the upper and lower G.I. series, but again found nothing but a shadow behind her navel.

By now it was the end of the summer, and in September, Johanne began taking classes in nursing at Bronx Community

College, commuting forty-five minutes to an hour each way by subway from her apartment on the upper west side of Manhattan. She had quit her job downtown a few years earlier and since then had worked for her brother and mother, who had opened a small grocery-delicatessen near Madison Square Garden. But she had become interested in a nursing career after working as a volunteer in the substance-abuse clinics at two hospitals, Roosevelt, in Manhattan, and Lincoln, in the Bronx. The program at Lincoln particularly impressed her, and she had become friends with the director, a young doctor named Michael Smith, who came from California. Smith was a psychiatrist but favored non-traditional, drug-free treatment methods of which Johanne approved. She found that she liked working with recovering addicts and alcoholics, and it was her plan to get her R.N. and then work full time either in Smith's clinic or in a similar one.

Lincoln is a big, busy municipal hospital in the South Bronx, the site of a lot of scary emergency traffic, and also a community hospital for the poor who live nearby. As part of her student training, Johanne spent the better part of forty hours a week there and got to know it well, though she arranged to spend as much time as she could in the substance-abuse clinic. One of Smith's techniques was acupuncture, and Johanne had tried it with some success in the past to relieve tension. When her constipation did not improve, "I went around for two or three weeks with pins in my ears," she recalls, but this time it brought no relief.

Sometime around the new year she returned to the internist a fourth time. After an examination once again turned up nothing, he recommended that she contact a psychiatrist. "He looked at me and I could tell he was thinking, This woman is really neurotic," Johanne says, torn between amusement at the memory and residual frustration. But Smith and her other friends were reassuring. Not only did they not think she was neurotic, they had begun to notice physical changes. "People started telling me, 'You're losing weight.' I knew I was thin, but it didn't faze me, because my weight fluctuates and I've never been a large person. But I don't think we really look at ourselves," Johanne says."You know, you're in the mirror, you're fixing your face, combing your hair, but you're not really *looking*."

One particular morning, she did look at herself hard and was shocked, "My breasts looked smaller and my face looked so small my eyes bulged in my head." In search of relief, she had been poring over Jethro Kloss's *Back to Eden* for months. Now she found herself returning over and over to the same section. It dealt with cancer of the colon. "But I said it's not the colon," Johanne

71

recalls. "I thought it was probably the intestines, because I'd been having this problem for a year and a half."

By the beginning of 1980, Johanne felt sick a lot of the time, caught between her certain conviction that she had cancer and her desire to believe the reassurances of the doctors, who told her she was fine. "But I knew it in here," she says, tapping her head. "I knew it was sapping my strength. I couldn't concentrate. I would sit down and have a cup of tea and feel as if I had eaten a four-course meal. At one point I realized after two weeks that I hadn't eaten at all. And I hadn't felt any hunger pains."

She noticed that her feet had begun to swell and that she was retaining fluid. "One day I was coming out of the apartment building and one of the security guards said, 'Congratulations.' I said, 'What for?' and he nodded at my stomach and raised his eyebrows. I said, 'Oh, come on. You know it's cold and I've got a lot of clothes on.' He smiled and said, 'Okay.' But as I was walking down the street, I got a glimpse of myself and I thought, Oh, my God. I came back, took off all my clothes and looked in the mirror. I said to myself, this is *something*. I thought back and I knew that I had had my menstruation. But the pain was there, and I was really worried. Everyone was asking, 'What's the matter?' 'Nothing, nothing,' I kept saying, but I was thinking that every time I lay down I couldn't sleep."

One night in early March, Johanne's cousin Evelyn called to talk. Evelyn, a couple of years older than Johanne, had had a hysterectomy and a colostomy the year before, and the two women had often discussed her treatment and her fears of dying. Johanne decided to confide in her. "I really don't feel well either," she said. "Something's going on." "Oh, my God, not you," Evelyn said. "You're the epitome of health." She would not hear of Johanne's being sick, and she kept insisting that everything would be all right. Johanne remembers that "I hung up and I went and sat down at the table, and I was struggling with philosophy—Kant or St. Anselm, or one of them, and I said, The hell with it. Tomorrow I find a doctor."

The next morning, March 11, she walked into the office of a general practitioner in the Bronx, not far from school, whom she had seen once about three years earlier, when she lived in the neighborhood. She had gone to him then with a variety of apparently unconnected complaints, and the day of the appointment, had been carrying a copy of *Back to Eden*. When the doctor spotted it, he made what she considered a crude joke. "Heal thyself," he had said, so annoying Johanne that she bolted for the waiting room. One of the nurses had persuaded her to return for her exam, but the experience had left a bad taste, and she went back to him really because she could think of no one else, because his office was near school, and because she was feeling desperate. She was convinced now by the swelling of her ankles and by her hard, distended belly that she was not crazy, that something was seriously wrong. The doctor examined her briefly and told her that, judging from the amount of swelling and from the weight loss she reported (30 pounds it turned out, from her normal weight of 120), he thought she probably had a perforated ulcer.

Johanne didn't think ulcers were the problem, but there was something in the doctor's tone that corresponded to her fears of over a year. He didn't act alarmed, she recalls, "but the sound of his voice alarmed me." Because he did not have the testing facilities to confirm his diagnosis, he wanted her to check into Lincoln immediately. By then, Johanne had seen enough of Lincoln to know that she didn't want to be a patient there. It was a place where people came to die, "of stab wounds, gun-shot wounds, and I had always thought *I* wouldn't want to die there." Roosevelt was not far from her apartment, and as she sat alone in this strange doctor's office, she kept telling herself, Go to Roosevelt, go to Roosevelt. "But I was worn out," she said. Lincoln was only a few blocks away, and she had the letter from the doctor in her hand.

She would remain at Lincoln for six weeks. In the first two and a half, she was examined daily: there were repeated, inconclusive internals, her blood and urine were tested, her abdomen X-rayed. She told her medical history over and over again, and every time she came to the part about constipation she would raise the idea of a problem with her colon or her intestines. The doctors listened to her and told her not to try to diagnose herself, suggesting that the little bit of training she had had as a student nurse had led her to leap to conclusions.

Even before Johanne was admitted to Lincoln, she was having trouble breathing whenever she lay down, because of the great accumulation of fluid, and she had spent several nights half-sitting in order to sleep. Once she was in the hospital, the nurses, several of whom she knew, kept her bed cranked into an upright position to relieve the pressure. "It wasn't painful, but I was gasping, and I could feel the fluid running up and down in my chest. One day I asked the nurse, 'Do me a favor, lower the bed a little.' She said, 'Josie, I can't,' but I said, 'Just for a few minutes. I'm tired of sitting up.' I remember she lowered the bed and I must have drifted off. I remember I felt something coming up into my nose and I remember jumping up and as I did, there was all this blood coming out, but it wasn't bright red, it was dark, and I said, 'Oh, my God, what's happening?' I couldn't get the buzzer so I started screaming. Everyone came running."

The blood that had been accumulating in her stomach cavity for weeks had backed up into her lungs. "They started to drain it off with a tube and a long needle right into the stomach. And they had this basin. I'm watching this; it was unreal. By then they had a tube in my nose, attached to a big jar. And as fast as they were pumping it out, the jar and the basin were filling up again."

Entering her third week, she had still not been told what was wrong with her. "I was worried. Three weeks and no one knows what's wrong. I was thinking, Shit, I should have gone to Roosevelt. I'll die here."

It seemed incredible to her that no one had been able to figure out what was wrong with her. Only when she threatened to leave—absurdly, given her condition—did she learn that several possibilities had been discussed with her family. Her mother, brothers, sister and several cousins, including "Tony the G.P." who had come up from Florida, had been visiting throughout and talking to the doctors. Now under pressure of her agitation and threats to leave, the doctors volunteered the word "tumor," its source unnamed, its actual location only generally understood. "Oh," Johanne says in a low voice, remembering those strange days, "okay, fine, a tumor, that doesn't sound so awesome. People have tumors every day. They can be removed."

As this information sank in, she began to study the faces of the people around her. "I looked at my cousin this particular day as we were talking, and something clicked in my head. I said, *Uh-uh*, no. Even though he's a doctor, we're family, and I can read him as sure as he can read me. His mouth was saying one thing and his eyes were saying something else. My mother and my niece came in, and I saw them and I thought, Oh my God. My mother had on her *shades*. The room was bright, but that's not my mother. Indoors? No."

Piecing together the story of Johanne's diagnosis from her account is like parsing a Cubist painting: all the facts are there, but they are presented in overlaid scenes, out of sequence, synchronized emotionally but not chronologically. It's as if the experience is recollected in freeze frames from a movie. Johanne's memory is remarkably accurate—in retracing parts of the story to confirm details, her original version is invariably correct—but because her presentation is disjointed, it is necessary to continually realign its elements to make sense of confusion. Yet this narrated, instinctive version—fragmented, punctuated by revelation and

74

after-the-fact recognition, alternately emotional and clinically calm—is most like the way it happened to her. There never was any clarity—not in the fifteen months leading up to her hospitalization, and not in the hospital either, until the very end.

What changed things, finally, to Johanne's mind, was the arrival of a woman gynecologist brought in as a consultant. Though Johanne had been examined internally many times while in the hospital, the doctors had found nothing. And although she stressed a lifetime of menstrual difficulty in every account of her medical history, even she believed the problem was intestinal. "The woman thing was last," in her mind and in the minds of her doctors. "When Dr. Durham* came in that morning and introduced herself," Johanne remembers, "I said, 'What are you here for?' She said, 'I know you're tired of this, but I'd like a little history.' I said, 'I told those morons some time ago about my menstrual problems.' She said, 'Oh, really? I'd like to hear about it.' And she asked me all the questions. How long have you had your period, how long have you had this difficulty? When you had sexual relations, did you have pain before or after? No one ever asked me that. They *never* asked me. That's why I say thank God for women in the medical profession."

Durham examined Johanne once again and ordered additional tests. Because everyone on the team of doctors now agreed that something lay hidden in the abdominal cavity, one more G.I. series was ordered. The significance of the "shadow" behind Johanne's navel—repeatedly attributed to a probable involuntary movement during the X-ray procedure—was to be determined once and for all. Johanne had insisted all along that she had not moved while the X rays were taken, and now seven doctors crowded into the X-ray area to see for themselves. Though she thought she would blow apart from the effort of holding a load of barium within her miserable, swollen insides, Johanne did not move. The shadow was there.

Later that day, Durham requested a rectal biopsy. With the patient on all fours and unanesthetized, a long needle with a flexible illuminated bulb at the end is inserted into the rectum. When fully extended into the bowel, the bulb opens and clips off a piece of tissue for biopsy. Johanne shakes her head and brings both hands to her face. It was a painful, ignominious, and in some ways preposterous experience, and telling about it, she can't seem to decide whether to laugh or cry. "Here they are,

---

*Pseudonym

75

going up inside me—these are men I've joked with and suddenly I can't look at them." She shakes her head again.

The next day, the procedure was repeated twice. Johanne was terrified. "I thought it had spread. I couldn't speak. I was just numb." The following day, she was lying in bed, when an intern came in with a clipboard and sat down and started talking very matter-of-factly about her condition. With no preliminaries, Johanne recalls, "He said, 'Well, you know, you have cancer, and the chances of you recovering from it aren't very good, and I'd suggest you take care of whatever business you have and just enjoy the time that you have left . . .'" Johanne was stunned. "All I could say—and I heard myself saying it and it wasn't my voice—was, 'Look at me.' And when he did—he stopped writing long enough to look at me—he was scarlet. His face was red, vivid, and I could see him saying, 'Oh, no,' and he got up and walked out of the room and I started screaming, and they all came in and said, 'What's the matter?' and I said, 'What's he talking about?' and then I saw all of them, and I knew.

"Well, they gave it to me in no uncertain terms. They put it to me this way: 'The chances of your surviving surgery aren't good. And if you don't have the surgery . . .' So, if I had it, I wouldn't make it, and if I *didn't* have it, I wouldn't make it. So there it was. It's up to you. What do you do? I cried. Not hysterical. Just a few tears. I said, I don't believe this. I don't *believe* it."

It was an ovarian tumor, of unknown dimensions, but unquestionably large. The decay in surrounding tissue appeared extensive. They could only guess at the damage done to other internal organs. Dr. Durham told Johanne frankly that she was afraid to open her up. Another of the doctors on the case, one Johanne had known for two years, came in to see her, "got down on his knees, cried and cried and said, 'I don't believe it. Not you.' And I was looking at him," Johanne remembers, "and thinking, What's going on? And I was like that all day. It got dark and I wouldn't permit anyone to turn on the light. Family came and a few friends came and some hospital co-workers. Everyone wound up crying, and I looked at them and I thought, Why are they crying? They're not dying, I am. But I couldn't believe it, I just couldn't."

As far as the doctors could tell, if Johanne did not have the surgery, she would live no more than three to six months. On the other hand, they could not promise anything if she did have it; until they opened her up, they were not prepared to say whether the tumor was resectible, nor how much damage it had already done. "I thought maybe I should go home and get my house in order," she remembers, but the idea of doing nothing but prepare for death was appalling. She decided to have the surgery, and took care of the only business that absolutely had to be settled. She spoke to Michael's father in California and told him that she wanted their son to live with him if she died.

The surgery was scheduled for the following Monday, March 31, her twentieth day at Lincoln. Johanne knew four members of the surgical team personally. Two of them were, like Johanne, Catholic and would later attribute their success to the workings of the "Master Surgeon." Having been, finally, as blunt as they had to be in outlining her situation, on the eve of the operation they were now reassuring, telling Johanne everything would be all right.

She was less sure. The night before surgery she dreamed that she had died. "I remember when they came in that morning about four o'clock to get me prepared, I was shaking, literally— my teeth were chattering. And I cried. I was so weak I couldn't really get a good cry, but it helped. Then they took me down, and all the doctors told me again that it was going to be all right. And I remember waiting to see Dr. Guttierez*—he's my heart—and I asked him if I could see the thing that was killing me. I was pretty groggy, but I asked him and he said to me, "Do you know what you just said?" and I said, 'Yeah. I want to see this thing that's killing me.' And he said, 'You will.'"

Johanne was in surgery for seven and a half hours. When they opened her up, Guttierez later told her, the tumor was "waiting there" for him, the "healthiest" tumor he had ever seen, vitamin-fed and nurtured through fifteen months of mystery. It was cradled in the intestines, which helped to explain how it had eluded detection so long. The ovaries, uterus, and fallopian tubes had been completely subsumed by the tumor and were removed along with it. The rectum and intestines showed extensive malignancy as well, but the position of the tumor had effectively shielded the remaining nearby organs—kidneys, liver, stomach. The intestines required most of the surgeons' attention. They were spread out like lengths of encrusted clothesline, hosed down and gone over inch by inch. Areas of malignancy were cut away, and the remaining segments of healthy tissue were stitched back together. In anticipation of follow-up chemotherapy and radiation, if needed, and because they did not want to perform a colostomy on this young woman if it could be avoided, the rectum was spared, and Johanne was assured that if the first few

---

*Pseudonym

treatments failed to reduce the mass in the rectum, they could always go back for it.

Before Johanne was wheeled out of the surgery into a recovery room, she emerged from the anesthetic, and Dr. Guttierez kept his promise. He lifted the tumor and showed it to her. Johanne was transfixed. "This thing was tremendous," she recalls. "It weighed sixteen pounds and was shaped like a piece of beef—not oval, but sort of squared away at the ends, I suppose because they had to cut it away to get it out of me." Groping for a better description, she suddenly says, "It was like an eye round, an eye round of beef." She looks amazed still as she tells the story. "So that's what it was, I thought. My God, that's what was killing me."

Howard Mindus first touched his hand to the lump on his neck while talking with guests in his living room, the evening of September 10, 1980. It was about the size of a shelled peanut, hard to the touch, located on the left, an inch or two below his jaw. In "as short a time as it took to reach for the other side of my neck and determine that this was not a normal part of my anatomy," Howard, a lawyer who negotiates multimillion-dollar contracts between industrial clients and the big banks that lend them money, concluded that he probably had cancer, or more specifically, a lymphoma of some kind.

This was not the imaginative leap of a hypochondriac, but a fairly reasonable deduction, considering his family history. His father had been diagnosed with lymphoma seven years earlier, and his paternal grandfather had died of leukemia at the age of forty-three, when Howard's father was ten. It would be an overstatement to say that Howard had been waiting for his cancer for years, but he was certainly not surprised when it appeared. A few seconds after he found it, he considered his age, thirty-six, and further refined the diagnosis as possible Hodgkin's disease, a relatively rare type of lymphoma that usually occurs in young adults. As it happened, the almost instantaneous self-diagnosis was correct, but its confirmation would take close to a month, while a determination of how far the disease had advanced, a process called "staging" that is an essential prerequisite for proper treatment, would take almost two months. And in the end, because of a precondition of a bad back that would, in the absence of Hodgkin's, be regarded as of no consequence medically, there remained a small doubt—in the minds of his experienced diagnosticians, and therefore in Howard's mind, and in that of his wife, Myriam—that his disease had been accurately "staged." If it had, then Howard was among the most fortunate of cancer patients, Hodgkin's being one of the most curable of cancers: when caught early, properly diagnosed and treated, there is better than a 75 percent chance of a full cure. But if Howard had not been correctly staged then he had lost the "best-case" chance; the disease would almost certainly recur in time, and the treatment for it would be harsher and less effective, the prognosis less favorable.

That such confusion should arise in a case of Hodgkin's is ironic, since it is otherwise so predictable a cancer, but it is only one of several, conspicuous ironies of both a personal and an existential nature that marked Howard Mindus's experience, and that are characteristic of cancer generally—suddenly meaningful juxtapositions of dates, facts with new meaning, words with new impact. Cancer is a disease that stimulates barbed reflections in great number. And if nothing else, the uncertainty characterizing Howard's diagnosis could stand as a paradigm for the ambiguousness of having cancer as a whole: Do I or don't I have it? (Or this particular form of it?) Will I or will I not be cured? Do they (the doctors) know what they are doing? If they don't, what can I possibly do about it?

Howard Mindus may have been temperamentally better suited than most to deal with the ambiguities of such a circumstance, but the month that he spent waiting out a firm diagnosis took its toll. It's a bit hard for him to concede how peculiarly threatened he felt during that time, which he describes as his only real period of alarm. In retrospect, he says of his anxiety, "My principal psychological reactions [that is, fear of death] all took place between discovery and diagnosis." In more emotional moments, he allows as how he would occasionally find himself gazing at his fifteen-month-old son, Daniel, with a mixture of sadness and disbelief, trying to imagine the possibility that he might not live to see him grow up. Myriam's version of the same period is typically thicker with emotion, and when she hears Howard dryly recounting his memories, she is inclined to blink patiently and smile and say very gently, "Howard."

The day after Howard discovered his lump happened to be Rosh Hashanah, a Jewish holiday, and so he did not reach his internist, Morton Davidson, until the next day, Friday, September 12. He made an appointment for Monday, the fifteenth, at which time he recalls telling Davidson "that I was greatly concerned that I might have cancer, because of my family history." Although interested in the cancer history that Howard outlined, Davidson's initial assessment was more conservative. He told

Howard that he thought the swollen lymph node—for that's what the lump was—probably represented a response to some kind of infection. If antibiotics did not cause it to disappear in a week or so, however, Howard should return, and he would start some tests.

"Maybe I saw him September 17," Howard says, recalling the sequence of events leading to a diagnosis. "When it hadn't gone away by, say, the twenty-fourth, I went back, and he did an X ray, which showed a shadow near the heart. The next thing he ordered was a gallium scan, which is a general diagnostic test, very nonspecific. You're injected with a radioactive isotope, which settles in areas of high metabolic activity, such as cancer, scar tissue, or simple infection. After three days, you go in and are read. They injected me on a Thursday or a Friday, and then I went in the next Monday, and they took pictures with a nuclear camera."

Sitting in the near-empty waiting room of the fourth-floor clinic at Memorial six months later, Howard is calculating without reference to a calendar and after a long morning's work, and so he is slightly imprecise about these landmark dates. Everything else about his account, however, is concise and thorough and exact, and yet somehow he does seem a little offhand about the larger subject. It is hard to say how much this reflects his confessed habit of minimizing or the fact that, despite the difficulty with his diagnosis, he has consistently believed from the start—with only moments of wavering doubt—that what he had was "not life-threatening," given what he knew of current treatment.

Perhaps certainty about the outcome made minimizing possible, but there is no question that Howard has made it his consistent policy to take the most optimistic reading of events. He did it from the first moment, when on the shortest notice, he came up with a diagnosis that was not only plausible but, given the range of possibility, the most favorable, barring a bad case of flu. That he knew of Hodgkin's may have been a bit of luck—a friend and co-worker of Myriam's had been diagnosed as having Hodgkin's a few years earlier, and it had been raised as a possible cause of an ultimately undiagnosed illness of Myriam's before that—but it took more than a bit of resourcefulness and self-protection to call it to mind on feeling a lump one evening in the living room.

Hodgkin's is a cancer of the lymph system, a network of glands that is part of the circulatory system and that extends upward from the groin through the central trunk of the body, with extensions into the neck and armpits. The lymph glands produce a type of white blood cell, called lymphocytes, that the body needs to fight infection. In Hodgkin's, irregular and fast-growing lymphocytes begin to be produced, resulting in tumors that crowd out healthy working cells.

When the disease is confined to one area of the lymph system, it is called Stage I. If it appears in two or more locations but is contained either above or below the diaphragm, it is called Stage II. In Stage III, tumors appear both above and below the diaphragm. In Stage IV, the disease has spread beyond the lymph system, to the bones, kidneys, liver, lungs, or other tissues.

These stages, called clinical stages, are further characterized as A or B according to the presence of such symptoms as weight loss, fever and night sweats. A second, more detailed staging process, called pathological staging, further refines and sometimes alters the diagnosis. In addition, Hodgkin's is classified by cell type. Each of these diagnostic nuances has an important and specific application in treatment, and the more refined the diagnosis, the more certain one can be of streamlining the treatment to the particular patient's circumstance. The time to get it all straight is early on, before treatment is begun: one does not want to overshoot, resulting in more treatment than necessary, and most emphatically one does not want to undershoot and risk missing anything.

The results of the gallium scan in late September showed the presence of something unusual in three places: the mediastinum, a cavity between the lungs that contains the heart, several smaller organs, and a dense cluster of lymph glands; the neck; and the lower back, referred to technically as "the lower right iliac." When Howard read the report, he noted only the mediastinum, corresponding to the area shown on the X ray, and the neck, corresponding to the visible lump. When Myriam read the report, she immediately remarked on the third location. "That's the pain in your back, Howard," she said.

Davidson arranged for Howard to be admitted to Beth Israel hospital in Manhattan for a biopsy, and "four or five days later," Howard's account continues, "the results indicated Hodgkin's."

What they knew now was no more than what Howard had guessed that evening, but knowing it was a big relief. Still to be determined was how far the disease had progressed. And because Howard's case had been managed up to this point by his internist, he had yet to find an oncologist to treat him. Selecting a doctor, deciding where he would be treated, and obtaining a more refined diagnosis would take almost another month.

At the time his illness began, Howard Mindus was eleven years out of Yale Law School and a junior partner in a big law firm. His wife, Myriam, who still uses her maiden name, Ellis, is, like Howard, extremely bright and beautifully educated, and until shortly before Daniel's birth Myriam worked for the City of New York's Department of Housing Preservation and Development. Howard had worked briefly for the city, too, before joining his present law firm in November 1973, a year after he and Myriam were married.

In important ways, the Minduses' life was full and happy, and outwardly it appeared orderly and safe as well. But in the five years leading up to Howard's diagnosis, they had been through two mysterious and unsettling health scares—one involving Myriam, another involving Daniel—that had left them unusually aware of the tenuousness of health in such young and healthy people as themselves, and conscious, in a way in which most people are not, of the real limits of medicine and the medical profession.

Myriam's trouble started in December 1975, when she was twenty-nine, and did not end until April 1977. It was essentially an intestinal disorder, but the closest it ever came to being diagnosed was to be termed an "intestinal inflammation without identifiable cause." In the meantime, it brought on painful abdominal attacks every three weeks, causing Myriam, who was small and light to begin with (her normal weight is 90) to drop to a low of 77 pounds. She was repeatedly tested, sent to an endoscopist for a biopsy, and hospitalized once at Beth Israel, to rule out, among other things, Hodgkin's. (Myriam remembers the exact moment when she learned that she did not have the disease. Her reaction, and Howard's on hearing the news, was, predictably, "Thank God it's not Hodgkin's." Four years later, waiting for word on Howard's biopsy, performed in the same hospital, their reaction on learning that of all cancers, Howard had this one, was again predictable: "Thank God it *is* Hodgkin's.") Throughout this long process, however, both Myriam and Howard felt that they were being given careful attention by the doctors they consulted: the problem was not lack of thoroughness and it was not incompetence—whatever Myriam had, it could not be reliably identified or classified, and in the end, it was treated, successfully, with aspirin.

It was tougher when Daniel became sick, two and a half years after Myriam's recovery, when he was about six months old. He suffered from what was eventually diagnosed as "chronic irritable bowel syndrome," characterized by nearly constant diarrhea and a slowing of his normal growth and development. In Daniel's case, the Minduses were less sanguine about the failure to obtain an early and definite diagnosis—and cure—than they had been in Myriam's case, because they saw their formerly thriving child faltering badly. Looking back, they feel that Daniel's care was not the best and that they should have been more aggressive in seeking out new treatment more quickly. For almost six months, they followed a minimum diet of rice and chicken prescribed by their pediatrician and intended to relieve the diarrhea. Instead, Daniel became weaker and weaker, suffering also a bad virus during this time, until the late spring, just before his first birthday, when he was hospitalized for rapid weight loss. Baffled, their pediatrician recommended that the Minduses take Daniel to a specialist on Long Island, who diagnosed Daniel at the first and only consultation and prescribed a complete diet—the opposite of what had been tried up till then. Daniel was soon thriving again.

Surprisingly, these back-to-back experiences did not leave the Minduses disillusioned with the medical profession. Despite the fact that in both instances they went for long periods without obtaining clear answers, they generally believed that they were dealt with in good faith by the professionals with whom they came into contact. What they learned is that sometimes there are no answers, or the wrong people are asked the questions, or the questions are asked at the wrong time. Knowing the limits of their own professions leavened their judgment as well; they did not hold titles, even medical titles, in special awe; they expected good care and careful care, but they did not expect infallibility. And so they came to Howard's illness, undeserving of another bang on the head, but prepared.

Which is generally the case with Howard. He describes himself as being, among other things, "not a risk taker," and there is absolutely nothing rash about him, in manner, or appearance. His dryness, even in humor, signals a habit of caution. His language is precise, reflecting a determination that nothing important should go unremarked, nor anything not meant be suggested. He says he has a "bathtub memory," meaning it can hold great quantities of fact for the required time, then empty at the pull of a plug. He likes his work, because it is demanding and because it suits his brain and his personality, but he suspects it a little for the same reasons. Although his firm is "not the kind of place where one is required to give one's whole being, the demands are heavy, the professional standards are exacting."

The work itself, detailed and complex, it perhaps too easily sunk into, offering too attractive a hiding place from other, less tidy areas of life to be altogether trusted. Myriam was the one who pushed for a child; in retrospect, Howard sees it as something of a redemptive act, pulling him away from his work and calling out some of his better qualities. One is often conscious that there are things about his personality that Howard does not admire and there is a corresponding touch of self-improvement in his eminently decent character.

Physically, he is in good shape—trim, and if not athletic in the active sense, "fit" in the broader sense, as if ready for a long hike or an all-night negotiation. His long triangular face is framed by thin but still curly hair that has begun to retreat from his face on all sides. Wire-rimmed glasses anchored to prominent ears give him a stern appearance until his smile, surprisingly open and broad, transforms him quickly from middle-aged to boyish. He looks very much the wholesome intellectual, more believably cast as a professor of Russian literature or an interpreter of the sonatas of J. S. Bach (of which he is especially fond) than as a lawyer who draws up contracts between tanker companies and financiers.

When it came time to choose a doctor to treat him, Howard quite naturally drew on his long habits of caution and consideration. At the time of his biopsy, his internist had recommended two specialists, one affiliated with Beth Israel, the other with Memorial Sloan-Kettering. Had he felt unwell, or had Hodgkin's been a faster-moving or more potentially threatening cancer, he might have accepted either recommendation quickly in his eagerness to begin treatment. But "I felt I was going to be in with this guy for some time. I had already lost a few days. A few more wouldn't hurt." He decided to look around.

Over the next few days, he and Myriam talked to everyone they knew who had ever had or knew anything about cancer. "We got a lot of advice to go to Memorial," Myriam recalls, and specifically because of the extensive radiation treatments he would most likely be having. "Everyone who knew anything was very strong on my having the radiation done here, even if I chose a doctor somewhere else," Howard remembers. Furthermore, his father had been a Memorial patient for several years, after beginning treatment elsewhere.

For some patients, a place like Memorial is simply too appalling to contemplate; as with the Victorian almshouse at the end of the lane, to go there is to be counted among the damned. But Howard felt none of this, and not simply because his father had been a patient there. He saw it for what it was, a highly regarded specialty house, and he happened to have one of the specialties it treated. In fact, he could have been treated almost anywhere in New York, as the Hodgkin's protocols are now standard and widely disseminated. From discussions with his internist,

Howard knew that most of his treatment would take place on an outpatient basis, on something approximating a monthly schedule for chemotherapy, daily for the period of radiation. If he was to be treated at Memorial, despite being a private patient, he would always be in a crowded clinic setting, as he knew from accompanying his father to appointments on occasion. Were he to go to a private doctor, his treatments would take place in small, presumably more peaceful offices, with less waiting, greater privacy, fewer reminders of other people's illness. Though this was not a major issue with Howard, it seemed worth considering at least, and so he made an appointment with the specialist recommended by his internist and affiliated with Beth Israel. Howard found the man responsive to his questions, likeable, intelligent, more than acceptable as someone to sign up with for the long haul. "If it had been strictly a personality thing, I would probably have gone with this guy," Howard says, but he was reluctant to give up the edge he believed he would have at Memorial.

Focused on Memorial again, and despite having two names in hand—the one given him by Davidson and that of his father's doctor—Howard ran into a problem. One doesn't just pick a hospital, one picks a doctor, and finding out the right category of specialists turned out to be tricky. He had mentioned the name his internist had given him to several people and had gotten reports that the fellow was both accessible and brilliant but also a bit independent, not known as a "team player" at Memorial, though highly respected. Howard was interested in meeting him, but the man was out of the country and was not expected back soon. His father's doctor he had met, and he knew him to be well-regarded and thorough, but the "personal vibrations" on those occasions when Howard had accompanied his father and asked about his treatment "were not good"; under the circumstances he was "not keen" on signing up with the man. And although Howard knew that he wanted a hematologist, even that didn't narrow the field sufficiently since as a rule hematologists at Memorial further specialize in either lymphomas or leukemias. A friend of Myriam's family who worked in the lab at Memorial, for example, produced several names of doctors, but they were inappropriate for Howard's disease. From other friends came totally blind leads—names of oncologists who were not hematologists and who treated other diseases exclusively.

This inefficient probing might have continued even longer if Howard had not finally been put directly in touch with the doctor at Memorial who had treated Myriam's co-worker for Hodgkin's. The man had since switched to another specialty but was willing to speak to Howard frankly about names and specialties, and he proved "unusually forthright and candid. He was complimentary about the professional qualifications of all the people we discussed," Howard recalls, "but what he told me about individual style and openness helped me get an idea of who I was choosing among. But the most important thing was that finally I had real names of real doctors who specialized in Hodgkin's."

Roughly a month and a half after he first felt the lump in his neck, Howard, and Myriam as well, sat down to talk with Benjamin Koziner. Koziner is a man of startling handsomeness and a soft, difficult-to-place accent that does, however, put one sharply in mind of ski slopes. The Minduses had him privately pegged as the "insouciant Israeli," a probable product, in their fantasies, of the same exodus that brought their German and Jewish parents to the United States in the 1930s. (In fact, Koziner is of Austrian descent, born in Argentina, and roughly their contemporary.) The Minduses found him frank, willing to answer their questions, unintimidating, and thorough. After the meeting, they went home, talked it over and decided to go with Koziner and Memorial, conscious that despite their diligence and their fortunate contacts, in some respects they were as much in the dark about their choice as two people who stumbled in off the street. As Howard put it, "My clients can read documents I prepare for them. But there was no way I could properly interpret Koziner's abilities." In the end he went with reputation, recommendation, and hopeful instinct.

Howard spent twelve days as an inpatient at Memorial while his disease was staged and typed. He had a lymphangiogram, a CAT scan, a bone scan, and several bone-marrow biopsies. All his major organs were found to be free of disease, and only concern over Howard's recent history of back pain prevented Koziner from viewing this as a fairly clear case of Stage II Hodgkin's.

The trouble had begun in November 1979, when Howard first experienced sharp, episodic pain in his right lower back. He consulted an orthopedist and, although no diagnosis was ever made, a corset was prescribed for relief. By the time the corset was ready, however, the pain had let up and Howard never wore it. In January, the pain returned "with a vengeance," accompanied by bad night sweats. In April and early May, he underwent physical therapy, which was no help, but the pain again subsided on its own, and Howard spent most of the summer of 1980 without discomfort. In August, when he and Myriam and Daniel were at the beach, the pain came back, aggravated by hours of carting Daniel in and out of the water. Just before he discovered the lump in his neck, Howard had gone to a chiropractor for his back and had gotten some relief. But the condition, whatever it was, was still very much on his mind and he mentioned it on his first visit to Davidson and in every consultation thereafter.

As part of the staging process, several bone-marrow aspirations and biopsies were done, the marrow being drawn from both the lower left and the lower right of Howard's back, with repeat marrows on the right side, where he had had the pain. What Koziner was looking for are what are called Reed-Sternberg cells, indicators of a fibrotic condition that is one of the hallmarks of Stage IV Hodgkin's. Though there was some evidence of fibrosis in the marrow, and although the gallium scan done a month earlier had showed unusual activity in the area, no Reed-Sternberg cells turned up; nor, on testing, did Howard's blood show signs of a type related to Reed-Sternberg.

The circumstantial evidence—pain present in the back for almost a year prior to diagnosis, indications of fibrosis in the marrow—were certainly suspicious and worrisome. But when repeated testing turned up no hard evidence, Koziner concluded that a diagnosis of Hodgkin's Stage II was appropriate. His account to the Minduses was detailed and frank as to the limits of diagnosis. Although Howard did not remember him putting it so flatly, Myriam recalls Koziner's saying that if Howard's case were presented to a panel of Hodgkin's specialists, easily half could read it the other way.

In effect, they had to choose to go with Koziner's judgment (backed by his staff colleagues) or start over, which they were free to do. But the fact that it was a matter of professional judgment and that there would likely be no more clinically definitive evidence uncovered were they to go somewhere else was something the Minduses recognized. They would always be in essentially the same position of having to accept someone else's best judgment; certainty was never going to be offered them—in this matter, at any rate.

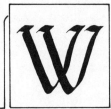ithin a few hours of Terry O'Brien's February 9 admission to Memorial, an intravenous needle had been inserted on the inside of her right forearm. Three days later, her I.V. infiltrated while she was getting blood and had to be removed, but Terry considered this a lucky break, since it allowed her to abandon her bed for an hour or so while waiting for one of the specialists to show up to replace the needle. She was supposed to stay in bed while she was getting blood, and the restriction was getting on her nerves, so she was happy to be able to settle without her I.V. pole in an armchair next to the window. Sitting in her bathrobe with her face raised gratefully to the winter sun, she glanced across her empty bed and sighed. "Oh-h-h—I know I'm going to be spending a lot of time in that. I don't want to get back in any sooner than I have to."

Her son, Raymond, a handsome young man who resembles his father in bulk and feature, has come to visit this afternoon. He sits on the edge of her bed, his eyes lowered against the glare of the sun behind her head. After a while, the I.V. specialist appears. She seems harried, less relaxed than the floor nurses, who rarely rush and are invariably friendly. She asks Mrs. O'Brien to spell her name. "O-B-R-I-E-N, T-H-E-R-E-S-A," she chants, practiced by now. The name check is a safety measure, to prevent one patient from getting another's chemotherapy or blood order.

Satisfied that she has got the right O'Brien, the nurse kneels and begins tapping the inside of Mrs. O'Brien's left arm with her two forefingers. Mrs. O'Brien, who has been joking and talking up to now, winces and tries to say something to the nurse, but the woman, who is dowsing for a vein, is concentrating so hard she doesn't hear her. Mrs. O'Brien rolls her eyes and tries again, saying, "I don't think you want to use this arm. It's the one that swelled up already." The nurse, still tapping hard against the tender surface, cocks her head as if listening for some faint emanation that only she can hear. She nods briskly in confirmation and swabs the spot with alcohol. Mrs. O'Brien lifts her eyes to the ceiling and presses her lips together. The nurse takes a fresh needle from her kit and, pressing down, inserts it expertly into the vein. At the moment of contact (she too is something of an expert now), Mrs. O'Brien covers her eyes with her right hand. Still, it hurts. "Oh-h-h," she says, half moaning, half grunting. "I never look."

Attached to the needle is a small length of I.V. tubing stopped at the end with a plug. The I.V. nurse presses a small bandage over the spot where the needle enters the arm, packs up her kit and departs. One of the floor nurses will come in later to hook Mrs. O'Brien back up to the remaining packets of blood that hang from her I.V. stand. It's a routine by now, familiar and likely to be repeated many more times. Mrs. O'Brien takes a certain interest in the technical details, sometimes quizzing the nurses about procedures, sometimes responding with indifference. Generally she gets what she needs to know straight and, depending on her mood, chats about it with interest. Today she is the instructor, describing the type of needle she had just been given—a "butterfly"—and demonstrating, by raising her freshly pierced arm, how the main I.V. line will be attached to the bit of tubing taped to her arm.

Her grasp of chemotherapy is basic and correct, and it reassures her. She reports with satisfaction the explanation one nurse gave her, that there are thirty-five different drugs used in chemotherapy (the actual number is closer to fifty, though it is always changing, as new drugs are added and old ones are dropped) and that they are combined, like the letters of the alphabet, to form treatments for specific types of cancer. The simplicity of the concept appeals to Terry—it takes a lot of the mystery out of the big, opaque word. And she finds it exciting, the way getting to the moon is exciting. "Isn't it something, what they can do," she says of the many procedures attempted in her behalf. "I hope it works."

It is all said casually, but, although she treats everything connected with her disease—the repeated hospitalizations, the tests, the tubes, the packets of blood and bottles of poison, the sharp needles and the confinement—as so many nuisances, like having to clean rooms to have them painted, she pronounces the word "cancer" easily. She has thought up no euphemisms. Once in a while, she says, "this thing," but usually it is "my cancer." It's as if by saying it out loud she reduces its importance, its threat. She mixes it up with less scary words all the time, until it does almost seem as if it is just one more item on a long list, not the item that will overwhelm all else.

Talking to a friend from Colts Neck on the phone one afternoon she warned, "I haven't changed. I'm still mean." She gossiped about local news, the emphasis being on the country club. "I guess I'm going to miss the St. Valentine's Day dance tomorrow night," she said, in the voice of someone who's been to plenty of them already. "Yes," she says, "it looks like I'll be right here in this room. I don't know whether I'll let Ray go without me."

She tells the friend with delight, her voice rising and falling in hoarse giggles, of how last night her daughter Susie, "my doctor-daughter, started fiddling with my tubes,"—meaning the I.V. tubes regulating the flow of blood. "I told her," Mrs. O'Brien said with fake disapproval, "'Susie, you can't touch any of these devices. It's not your hospital.' But she said, 'Ma. I know what I'm doing.'"

Eventually, her caller worked the conversation around to when Terry would be getting out of the hospital. Terry said she didn't know, since all the test results were not yet in. "You never know from one day to the next with this thing," she said casually, "but by tomorrow, I should have a general idea of what my future is."

By the end of the day, at least her immediate future had been decided. She would go home on Sunday, the fifteenth. Golbey's discharge summary concluded that her symptoms were more likely of viral origin than the result of chemotherapy, but because of her generally weakened (though improved since admission) condition, she was not to come back to the outpatient department until February 24, to give her body another week's rest from chemo. Her long-term future was for the moment left unexplored.

The Saturday following Terry's discharge, February 21, the O'Briens went to a wedding. At one point during the Mass, when the seated congregation arose, Terry discovered she could not. "I had no strength in my legs at all," she said later. "I had to push myself up off the pew with my hands or get Ray to pull me up. It was terrifying. All I could think of was being in a wheelchair next." The condition persisted all weekend long, and she had the kids pulling her out of chairs, Ray helping her up the stairs. Once she was on her feet she was all right, but she could not propel herself to her feet without great effort or assistance.

She arrived early for her appointment with Golbey on Tuesday. The strain of joking about her condition—"Isn't it ridiculous?" she said several times, "I mean I couldn't get *up*"—was showing and she was visibly shocked by this turn of events. After he completed his regular examination, Golbey told Mrs. O'Brien that he wanted to consult with a neurologist. She nodded and then asked, "What about chemo? Am I going to get any today?" Golbey said he preferred to wait until this new problem had been checked out. He disappeared, to return in a very short time with Dr. Kathleen Foley, a young woman who appeared to be about twenty minutes out of high school but is in fact an experienced neurologist who has been on Memorial's staff for eight years and now heads its pain service.

Dr. Foley is tender with Mrs. O'Brien from the first word. Either she reads her instantly or has been warned by Golbey that Mrs. O'Brien is suffering a rare panic and trying not to show it. She faces Mrs. O'Brien, who is seated in a straight-back chair in the examining room, and bends deferentially forward as she explains that she and Golbey would like to put her back into the hospital for tests. Mrs. O'Brien nods and looks up at the younger woman. "How long do you think I'll be in?" she asks. "Six or seven days," Foley answers. "Okay," Mrs. O'Brien says. "One thing, though. We're going to Florida from the sixth to the fourteenth. That's definite. I can't come in during that period." Foley nods and starts to leave the room to arrange an admission when Mrs. O'Brien says something that suggests she thinks the tests will be done after she comes back from Florida. Hearing this, Foley steps back into the room and as gently as possible makes it clear that she was talking about admitting her right away—today, if possible.

"Today?" Terry is horrified. "I can't come in today. You mean right *now*?" Her face contorts in disbelief. "I have to go home. I haven't got any clothes with me. There's no one there to pick up the girls after school. My husband's out of town till tomorrow." The protective barrage of objections is automatic, as nonsensical and instinctive as those of a kidnapping victim. Foley smiles tentatively at Mrs. O'Brien, who looks up at her and asks, "Are you serious, really? Is it that important?" Foley bobs her head and says soothingly, "We'd like to help you feel better, and it may be something we can take care of. I promise we'll get you in and out as fast as we can. Then you can go off to Florida and have a good time."

Mrs. O'Brien bargains. "How about tomorrow? If I could just go home and come back tomorrow—get everything organized at home, pack a bag, see that everything's all right—I'd feel a lot better." Foley agrees to this and goes off to see about getting a bed for tomorrow.

Though she is relieved to have won her point, Mrs. O'Brien is shaken by the urgency of this admission. "Neurology is the brain, isn't it?" she asks, knowing exactly. She exhales, starting to laugh. "That's all I need," she says. "What's next?"

By the time Dr. Foley returns, she has humored herself into relative calm again, and she grows friendly. She tells Dr. Foley that her daughter, Susie, is a doctor too, and is surprised when the neurologist says, "Yes, I know." It turns out that Dr. Foley's father worked with Ray at Emigrant and the two families have heard reports on each other for years. Mrs. O'Brien is thrilled. "I've heard your father talk about you," she says. "He's *so* proud of you." All her sociability is restored for the moment. Dr. Foley is a gift, perhaps the one doctor on the premises who could make her forget the implications of neurology, and Mrs. O'Brien leaves the clinic with a good piece of friendly gossip as ballast for her premonition of disaster.

On Wednesday, the twenty-fifth, she returned to the hospital at about noon, was processed and sent upstairs, but the room wasn't ready, so she sat in the seventh-floor lounge with her hard canvas suitcase until four o'clock. By the time she got into her room and settled, it was too late for any tests to be started. "They've wasted my whole day," she grumbled. And being on the seventh floor, the neurology floor, made her nervous. She eyed the door to the hall as if expecting a platoon of patients to parade past with big, baseball-stitching seams in their shaved heads. The urgency of this admission and the problem with her legs had unnerved her. Still, she managed to joke, a bit sourly, with Golbey when he came by, and she had a suitable remark for each of the floor staff as they appeared.

The next day, Thursday, she had a myelogram and a CAT scan. In the first, a dye is injected into the spine, and multiple X rays are taken to see whether anything is pressing on the nerves. In a CAT scan, the entire body is slowly surveyed, head to toe, for tumors. On Friday, one specialist probed with long needles for feeling in her limbs, hands and feet, and another made her spell "world" first forward, then backward. She was asked to figure the number of nickels in $1.35, but was disappointed when no one asked her her address, a question that Golbey, in trying to give her an idea of what the tests would be like, had suggested as probable. She remembered this in reciting the tale of the tests later on, when she was feeling cheerful once again. "Nothing is pressing on your nerves," she quoted the neurologist, who gave her the report late Friday.

Her brother, Brian Sweeney, was visiting from Connecticut. He had brought a bottle of white wine, one mark of the generational difference ten years made, and she chided him for his choice. "Why didn't you bring scotch?" she asked. Ray arrived and she grew more boisterous, her tumor-free brain whizzing with questions and relief. By the time Golbey arrived to tell her that she could go home the next day, she was flooding the room with talk, urging Brian on to tales of the Sweeney family, grilling Ray on his work and plans for the weekend. After a few minutes of this, Ray looked to Golbey in appeal. "Can't you give her something that'll keep her quiet?" he asked.

On Tuesday, March 3, Mrs. O'Brien received three milligrams of Vindesine as an outpatient but no Methyl-GAG, which Golbey had decided to discontinue as "possibly toxic" to her system. In its place, he prescribed a drug called Cytoxan, for her to take in pill form while she was in Florida. One of the most widely used cancer drugs, Cytoxan has not been terribly effective against lung cancer, but it did sometimes slow the rate of tumor growth. And even though the tests of the previous week showed no new tumors specifically interfering with her motor nerves, the steady growth of the multiple tumors already identified throughout her bones had not been slowed by the Methyl-GAG or the Vindesine. It couldn't hurt to add a small dose of Cytoxan, Golbey decided, and it might help.

On the sixth of March, Terry, Ray, Carol and Nancy flew to Florida to spend ten days in the condominium that they share with another family outside Jacksonville. Terry began taking the Cytoxan and had an immediate, violent reaction. "In all my years of living, I've never been so sick," she reported to Golbey when she got back. She threw up every fifteen minutes for four hours. "And the *pain*," she said, squinting hard. She had stopped taking it, she said. "I was on vacation. I felt bad enough already." When she told this to Golbey, he said he didn't think the Cytoxan could have had such results at the level she was getting, and he persuaded her to try it again, in half dose.

This was the seventeenth of March, St. Patrick's Day. Mrs. O'Brien had arrived at the clinic early, as usual, wearing a huge button on her white sweater that said, "Kiss me, I'm Irish," and she cheerfully told the nurse in the chemo room a story about her telling a friend that she wants the coffin shut at her wake. "I said to her, don't you peek, but if you do, and I answer, for God's sake don't shut it again." The nurse asks, casually, since there are no other patients around this morning, what I'm doing there with her, and Mrs. O'Brien says, "She's writing a book about cancer patients. She's going to put me in her book." She waits a beat. "I want to be famous before I die."

Complimented on her good color—she really looks as if she's been somewhere warm—she says that she feels tired. Pointing to her pinkish-tan skin, she says, "You know you can get this in a gel now."

The trip to Florida has had a mixed effect. She had looked forward to getting away, to forgetting about the hospital and medicines and feeling lousy. Florida was far enough away and so much a place to have a good time in that she believed in it as a child believes in the power of a trip to the zoo. But it turned out that she felt sick there, too. She could hardly enjoy a drink at night, and dinner was impossible. She was tired most of the time and found it hard to get down to the beach. And she felt guilty for being such poor company for Ray and the girls. Coming back was almost a relief. The visits to the hospital permit her to let down, to pursue a routine that makes more sense in terms of how she feels. She has begun to notice this and isn't sure what to think of it.

As he does every few weeks, Golbey has ordered X rays today, to monitor the progress of the cancer in her bones. Mrs. O'Brien takes the slip his secretary, Mary Ann Barletta, has filled out, and she leads the way to the second floor, to a waiting area outside the X-ray rooms. There is a women's section, and a men's farther along the passage. A door leads off each to a changing room, much like a health-club locker room. It is carpeted and pleasant, with a private bathroom and, along the wall as you enter, shelves stacked with medium-blue wrappers. Mrs. O'Brien changes into one of these, which dwarfs her, hoists her bag onto her shoulder and returns to sit outside. Some days, half the chairs are filled with patients waiting to be X-rayed. Today, the lounge is nearly empty, and we wait, talking about her children, for twenty minutes or more. Once she is called, she is gone for just a few minutes. She is having pelvic and lumbar X rays today, both routine, as she points out. This is where she came every three months or so for chest X rays before the metastases were discovered, every time she had an appointment with Dr. Beattie. There are fewer and fewer places she has not yet seen in the hospital, it seems. As we get back into the elevator when it is time to leave, she says, with good humor, "I tell all my girlfriends, 'You know, you feel sorry for me because I have cancer and have to go to the hospital. But to me it's normal, it's what I do.'"

She has become a weekly commuter, an occasional overnight guest. She insists on coming alone to the clinic, though many of her friends have offered to accompany her. "It would be different if I had to drive in or take the train," she says, but she comes in for her weekly appointments with Ray early in the morning, driven by Ray's driver, Gene Hopper, who waits for her and drives her home again. This is luxury enough for Terry O'Brien, and she is not about to complain of her journey.

The following week, I find Mrs. O'Brien not in the clinic but in Golbey's office, on the same floor, beyond a pair of swinging doors behind the chemo room. Her face is dry, skin stretched tight across her bones, with tiny lines showing everywhere, not just at the sides of her mouth, where they are worst, or at her eyes, but on her cheeks, forehead, chin. Her laugh is forced and gravelly. She retreats into Golbey's office again, without explaining.

A few minutes later, she emerges from Golbey's office a second time. She seems to sag from the shoulders and holds herself erect with great effort. She shakes her head and tries to speak lightly, but it doesn't come out that way. "I don't *believe* my body could be doing this to me," she says. "I can't believe my body could have what he says it has inside." She hesitates. "Can a person have two cancers?" she asked. "Wouldn't you know I'd be the one."

It turns out that the most recent X rays, taken the week before, showed a hardening of the bone from the tumors, not the brittle textures usually consistent with lung-cancer metastases. It is pretty clear that the Vindesine is not working, and Golbey has now given fresh consideration to the possibility that a second primary—most likely breast cancer—may have been missed. As he explains, one in twenty lung cancers behave the way Mrs. O'Brien's cancer is behaving, while one in two breast cancers behave this way. It's worth looking at again. "So," Mrs. O'Brien says, squeezing one small breast and making a face, "I'm gonna have a mammogram."

"He had me in shock," she says at first of Golbey's theory. "I asked him if it was possible to have two separate cancers, and he said, 'Yes.'" She lifts her shoulders in astonishment. "So then I asked whether it was easier to treat breast than lung, and he said, 'Usually.'"

Telling this, she is still shaky. Her lips are parched and the slip of paper that she carries—the mammogram order—flutters erratically in her hand. It turns out that she was up much of the night because of a sudden increase in pain, mainly in her ribs and lower back. She's been taking Darvocet, a moderate-strength painkiller, since January, but now, she says, it's doing nothing for her. "I used to take one every four hours, now I'm taking two every four hours, and it doesn't help."

We go downstairs, to the second floor, to a Dr. Watson's office, for the mammogram. As we enter the reception area for Watson and several other doctors, Mrs. O'Brien stops and points at a dapper-looking fellow dressed in a creamy-tan suit, light shirt, and pale-golden-orange tie. "Look at those shoes," she shouts, pointing to his feet. In sharp contrast to his elegant suit, Watson is wearing a pair of beige suede casual shoes, and he looks down now at his feet, laughs and says, "I remember you!" He and Mrs. O'Brien approach each other, laughing, occasionally shrieking as each tries to be the first to explain to anyone within earshot why they are being so silly with each other. It seems that Robin Watson did her original lung biopsy two years before, the needle biopsy that confirmed her cancer before surgery. They had met a second time about a year later at a big fund-raising affair that she and Ray had attended. At that meeting, Watson says, Terry chased him across the room with a friendly greeting of "You're the one who did my biopsy." Later, she had pursued the subject of his dress shoes, which she thought unusual, and neither had forgotten.

So now Terry has discovered another old friend, and she is pleased. Golbey has discussed his suspicions with Watson, who now chats with Terry quite sociably about the possibility of a breast cancer. He tells her that they were unhappy with the results of the other mammogram, taken in January, and Terry says, "I'm not surprised. Does it have anything to do with size?" Watson ignores her self-disparagement and says, "It has to do with several things actually." There is a bit of excitement in the air— won't it be terrific if she has breast cancer after all?

When the mammogram is done, she returns for her bag and book, miming the twisting of a breast that is required for the procedure. "I did my best," she says as we leave. There will be no chemo today, she says, Golbey having put it off pending some decision on her primary cancer.

By the time she gets home, she has persuaded herself of her possible good fortune. The idea of breast cancer catches hold. She explains it all to Ray, stressing the positive aspects, how it could account for the failure of the lung treatment to slow the metastases, how breast is more successfully treated with chemotherapy. She calls Susie to tell her the news, and Susie would later recall that her mother "seemed very happy about it, which was wise, if it was true."

The following Sunday was Terry's fiftieth birthday. She and

Ray had planned a quiet Saturday-night dinner with three other couples to celebrate it and their twenty-ninth wedding anniversary. When they arrived at the club, she was greeted with a surprise party thrown by a group of friends, several of whom took pictures that showed Terry looking tiny and pursed around the mouth, but gay and very much in the center of things. There are shots of her wiping tears away while holding her glasses, of her bent double with laughter, of her holding a drink and talking. It was a great party, she said afterward, though she got through it in a way unusual for her, with very little to drink. She had lost the taste, she said. "I told Ray, 'It's bad enough that I can't eat, but not to be able to drink!'"

Her weight, in fact, had been dropping steadily. Her weigh-in on January 14 had been 122. Now she was down to 109, and very much looked it. Except in the middle of a birthday party, she almost never felt good anymore. She says the pain of the week before disappeared a few hours after she left the hospital but had since been replaced by a worse one in her neck, which has been stiff for five days, she says. She's sure it's not the result of a draft.

She explains the change to Golbey when she is called for her exam, and he tells her that he has decided she should get radiation for her pain. Mrs. O'Brien asks whether the radiation will have any effect other than relief, and Golbey says that it should correct some of the damage to the bone that the cancer has done.

She wonders why her appetite should have so thoroughly disappeared. "Is it because of chemotherapy?" she asks, though she has had so little actually. "There are times," Golbey tells her, "when chemotherapy is like a crutch—everything bad that happens can be blamed on it. And yes, it can depress appetite," he adds. "But pain can as well. It can make you lose appetite. It can make you throw up. That's one reason I'd like to try to relieve it some." He tells her that the pain medication that she has been taking is the mildest he is permitted to prescribe. Terry says, "And I'm so good, too—I wait the four hours." Golbey chides her. "I've told you you didn't have to wait." He explains that the four-hour rule has to do with the average length of time it takes for a medication to be excreted, "but if it looks like it's wearing off in three hours, you can take more. With some medications it matters more that you observe the time limit. With this it doesn't."

Mrs. O'Brien nods, trying to accept this, then asks him, with mild irony, "Have we decided where the cancer is coming from yet?" Golbey says, "There is absolutely no suggestion, from the mammogram, that it is from the breast. But its behavior is still perfectly compatible with its coming from the breast. Things are not that stereotyped that it has to be one or the other by what we can see. It would put me on firmer ground if we knew for certain. But we are going to move toward breast." Though Terry is slightly mystified by the possibility still, she has no inclination to doubt Golbey's judgment. She hopes he's right.

Golbey has told her that she will probably go for radiation every day for a week or so, and when he leaves the room to arrange an appointment for her with one of the radiologists, she leans forward in her chair and whispers, "Every day? He's got to be kidding." I tell her I think it's the usual thing and encourage her to ask Golbey more questions. When he returns, she says she would like to ask him more about what she calls radiology, and Golbey says, "Good. The questions often don't occur until after you've left the room." She asks whether it's painful. "Not if it's done properly," he answers. "Does it burn?" she asks. "Possibly, but very faintly, like a light sunburn," he says, and then elaborates. "In the hands of an experienced radiologist it's very useful. In the hands of someone inexperienced, yes, it can be a very dangerous tool."

"It should relieve the pain, though," Mrs. O'Brien says. "There's a good chance of that," Golbey tells her. "Good," she says, "because it seems to be getting worse."

Waiting for Gene Hopper, Ray's driver, to return to pick her up, she lowers herself carefully into a chair in the first-floor waiting room. Her stiff neck catches her like a nun's coif when she tries to turn her head to look out the window. She winces. "I hated to have to tell Golbey I've got a pain in the neck," she says, stroking it. "I hope this radiation business helps." She feels "lousy," she concedes, her guard truly down. "The worst thing is I'm tired all the time. I could sleep twenty-four hours a day. I don't know what that means," she says vaguely, then leans forward suddenly, as if about to impart a secret. "Ray says to me, 'You're not going to quit on me, are you, Te?' No," she says, and sits back in her chair. "I want to fight. I want to live."

She is silent and seems perplexed. It's as if she can't believe her own words—that they are necessary, that her life is seriously in question.

"My friends tell me that only the good die young," she says, trying for a tongue-in-cheek tone. "And they say, 'Terry, you're too mean.'" She says that she and Ray have decided to redecorate the house—just the downstairs rooms, she says, where nothing's been changed for thirteen years. "Actually," she says, "I told Ray, the reason is that when it's all done and I'm gone and another broad moves in she can't change it all around. He won't have any money left." She laughs at this and seems genuinely tickled by her joke—perhaps there is a bit of wishful thinking in it, too—but it is hard to miss the symbolism, or superstition, contained in such a grand plan for the future. It reflects the blind faith of which she is rarely guilty, but which is growing more and more tempting all the time. And though she usually leaves her fears unspoken, she can't seem to let go of the subject of death today.

"I've thought about it," she says quietly. "About what it means. What scares me is, what is it like when you go? I wish I knew. Like everybody else, I'm scared of the unknown."

She says this calmly, perhaps a bit nervously, but it is such an ordinary day, muggy and thick like summer, rather than the first days of spring, that it is hard to believe the subject of death has any immediate application.

"What about heaven?" I ask. "I believe in heaven," she says, not doubtfully, but as if she might be challenged or teased. "But will everyone be there?" she asks, meaning "Is it what I've been counting on?" I ask her what her image of heaven is, and she answers, smiling but cautious, "Well, that it's peaceful. And that you see Christ." Responding to her tentativeness, I ask, "Do you really believe in it?" "Well, I should hope so!" she snaps.

She changes the subject abruptly to the party, but finds the same theme again. "My friends joke about turning fifty—they say, 'Don't tell, nobody needs to know.' 'What do you mean?' I tell them. Believe me, I'm counting. And I'm going to count fifty-one and fifty-two, and just hope I keep on counting."

Gene appears on the ramp leading from the front door and she starts out. The week before she had said she was going to order a second wig, the one with the streak, and I ask her whether she did. She nods and says, "Didn't I tell you? I went into the store, and the woman there looks at me—she's talking about the one I've got on, you understand—she looks at me, and she says, 'Mrs. O'Brien, I think you've got your wig on backward.'" She shrugs and laughs, gives the wig a pat of the hand and is gone.

The radiation department at Memorial operates five days a week from 7:30 A.M. to 6:00 P.M., and from 7:30 to 11:30 Saturday mornings, and may well be the most repellent quarter in the hospital. The small waiting room is cramped and uncomfortable, and the sights on an ordinary day make one gasp. A rough segregation by disease prevails in the chemotherapy clinics on the fourth floor and their annexes elsewhere; no young children mix with the adults (pediatrics is an entirely separate division in the hospital, with one inpatient floor and one outpatient floor reserved for children through the age of fifteen), and patients tend to be scheduled by the type of cancer they have. In radiation, everyone is jumbled together, individual time slots arranged without regard to specific diseases. A lot of face-cancer patients get treatment here, children with tumors both visible and invisible, adults with frightening sunken cavities, hollowed-out necks, cut-away jaws. They all sit side by side with the less conspicuously scarred patients, because the machines are there. Patients with canes and walkers move awkwardly past an obstructing pillar on the way to treatment rooms, the magazine tables spill over with beat-up copies of *Newsweek* and *Family Circle*. Shelves of children's toys chill rather than cheer. It is a windowless, cell-like room, and though it is actually on the second floor, it has the underground feel of a cellar.

Mrs. O'Brien was scheduled for five treatments, Wednesday, Thursday, and Friday of that first week, plus the following Monday and Tuesday. She arranged to have them at five-fifteen in the afternoon, figuring that Gene could bring her into the city in the middle of the afternoon, when traffic was light, and pick up Ray while she was getting her treatment. When there was no backlog, she could be in and out in a half hour or less.

The treatments were aimed at her upper spine, where a tiny cluster of tumors at the neck was giving her trouble, and at her right hip, where the metastases had first caused her pain. The exact areas to be radiated were outlined in purple ink, and she was instructed not to get the markings wet while bathing. Golbey had warned her ahead of time that she might have some nausea from the treatment, and after the first one, she did. Nancy and Carol cooked dinner, she reported, but the treatment didn't bother her the following day, and she cooked. Still, coming in daily was "a pain," she said, and in the middle of it all, she had managed to produce a mild fever. She asked Golbey whether that was a normal side effect of radiation, and he told her no. "Then he said to me—get this—'When we doctors talk about side effects, we're talking about *normal* people.'"

Intended as a palliative for pain, the treatment did give Mrs. O'Brien some relief at the neck and hip, but by the middle of treatment, her feet, which had bothered her in a low-grade way all winter, suddenly hurt a lot. On Monday afternoon, I came upon her heading into the clinic in white sneakers at around 5:45, a half hour late for treatment. She was carrying a brown leather briefcase and was scurrying, looking distinctly like someone hoping to avoid arrest. She told me to be quiet as we walked past the guard and headed for the elevator. "Going for radiation," she called to him and stifled a smile.

In the elevator, she pressed the twelfth floor, said she had already been for her treatment and was heading to see Ray. She waited for a reaction, and then said, "It's not cancer. Would you believe he's got a bleeding ulcer?" All this was delivered in an excited, conspiratorial whisper. We got out on twelve, an office floor empty at this hour, and crossed over into the hospital proper, a circumvention of the rules—we had no passes, which are doled out two to a patient on the ground floor of the hospital—that she seemed to enjoy.

Ray O'Brien was sitting up in bed reading and looking, despite the tethers that connected him to an I.V. bottle, rather fine. For such a big man, he looked unconfined by his circumstances, and only a bit sheepish. He had landed in a bed at Memorial because six months earlier he had started going to the internist that Terry had acquired when she was in for her surgery. When Ray reported to him over the weekend that he had had blood in his stools, the internist had insisted he come in immediately. So now Terry hovered at the foot of *Ray's* bed, clucking at their reversed positions. Ray in turn called attention to her sneakers, which, he observed, did not match her outfit.

Terry seemed both upset and relieved by Ray's hospitalization that week. She felt that he didn't take care of himself, that he worked too hard, accepted too many responsibilities. And while she believed that she could protect him from the more aggravating aspects of raising children and, amazingly, from some part of what was happening to her, she had no control over his work life. And this was not a good year for the savings-bank business in New York. Emigrant was one of the five largest savings banks, with assets of $3.1 billion in 1981, but, like its competitors, it was withering under the pressure of high interest rates and a backlog of long-term, low-interest mortgages. When one of the specialists who had been called in to treat Ray O'Brien's ulcer asked Tom Fahey, his internist, whether Ray was under any special pressure, Fahey replied, "Other than that his wife is dying of cancer and his bank is going under, no."

In a sense, his business life had taken on much the same character as his personal life; he had always been able to make things happen, but now he was blocked. He could do virtually nothing to save his bank; he could only try to protect his employees and depositors. He could not save his wife; he could only comfort her and pay the bills. But at least the bank was his problem; Terry very much regarded her cancer as her problem, and despite their closeness, there was a limit to how much of it she would share with him.

Terry was no diplomat with her friends—"My father loved the way she used to zing 'em at Navesink," Sean put it; but with Ray she was a mix of blunt and careful. She wouldn't dream of keeping anything of substance from him, but she believed absolutely in the prerogative of a wife to pick her moment. Her response to Ray's ulcer was to corral him and get him well by force if necessary, and to take the opportunity to make light of her own deterioration. Except for the sneakers, and the occasional tipping to one side of the hair on her head, it was easy to forget during Ray's week in the hospital that Terry was usually the one in bed. And she enjoyed the illusion, if only for a week.

One afternoon, while Ray was being examined, Mrs. O'Brien and I went down the hall to visit Jimmy Polack, who was in for a fever for the second time, and in an uncheerful frame of mind. In his fourth month of treatment for leukemia, his thoughts this week have to do largely with such uncomfortable subjects as quitting treatment, the pointlessness of life, his in particular, and death. When I introduce Mrs. O'Brien as someone who also has cancer, he stares at her in disbelief. She is breezy as a debutante, talking to him in an excited, friendly voice.

"So, you've got leukemia," she says. "I've got something worse. Yes, I had surgery two years ago—they took out part of my right lung, and everyone thought I was fine. Now I'm back because it's spread a-l-l through my bo-ones." She stretches the last few words out as if telling a child a fairy tale. There is no menace in her account, only awe. When she finishes, she remarks on Jimmy's bald head. "I lost mine, too," she says, giving her wig a jerk. "But you guys have it easy; we *have* to wear these things or we can't go out on the street."

Of all the things that leukemia has meant to Jimmy, his baldness is perhaps the most difficult to tolerate, but he smiles at Mrs. O'Brien's comment. "I see you have your ears pierced," he says. "I think I'll try that before I get one of those." They kid about whether pierced ears will cure cancer. I say I've heard the Irish used to believe that pierced ears improved eyesight, like eating carrots. Mrs. O'Brien says it didn't help her, and Jimmy says he can see just fine. It's a silly conversation, but it boosts Jimmy for the moment.

Back in the hall, Mrs. O'Brien sags. "Oh, the poor, kid," she says in a hollow voice. "What a thing to have to go through at his age."

Ray is released from Memorial at the end of the week, and the following Wednesday, April 15, the O'Briens take off for Florida, where they will spend Easter. Nancy and Carol, Mrs. O'Brien has said, are going mainly in the hopes of getting tans for the dances at the end of the school year. "There's not much for them to do down there," she says, somewhat guiltily, as if she feels she shouldn't be dragging them away from their friends. And a few weeks earlier, Ray had called Terry's older brother, Jimmy Sweeney, in Chicago, and invited him and his wife to join them in Florida for part of the time. It had occurred to Ray that if Jimmy wanted to see his sister before she died, he had better make a point of it. He did, and he and his wife joined the O'Briens in the middle of their stay.

But it was not a jolly holiday. Terry felt sick almost from the moment they arrived, although she did all right, she claimed, until Sunday the nineteenth, which was Easter. She made it down to the beach a couple of times, but she had no appetite, and whenever everyone else wanted to go out to dinner, she didn't. She couldn't drink, which annoyed her, and the worse she felt, the more scared she got.

She was up all night vomiting on Tuesday, the twenty-first; and on Wednesday, "I wanted to come home."

She called Golbey and told him of her nausea and vomiting. Since it was unlikely that her condition was a response to the Vindesine she had had a week before, there was a possibility of a blockage of some kind. Golbey told her he would arrange for her to be admitted as soon as she could get back from Florida. Ray was to leave for New Orleans on a 5:30 A.M. flight the next morning, to attend a board meeting, and he arranged for Terry and the girls to be on a 6:30 flight to New York.

They arrived in Bedholding at ten after one, Thursday afternoon, the girls wheeling their mother through the door. Mary Ann Barletta, Golbey's secretary, came down to help with the admission, and she was shocked by the change in Mrs. O'Brien. "I'd never seen her cry," she said. "But she did today."

"She presents with intractable nausea and vomiting," Golbey's notes read, "with a five-pound weight loss in the past week and abdominal pain and tenderness. She is mildly dehydrated and has headache and neck pain. Patient is now admitted for further evaluation and treatment."

Both her red-blood and platelet counts were low, possibly as a consequence of the radiation treatments, possibly the result of the cancer's progress, which, Golbey's notes indicate, had continued despite chemotherapy.

In Florida, all Terry could think about was closing the 700-mile distance between her and her doctor. She came in thinking that she was about to die, but also hoping that something extraordinary would be attempted once she was back at Memorial, as if some powerful resource had been held in reserve for when things got very bad. In fact, her treatment this time was modest: she was given blood transfusions, intravenous "hydration," and enemas, which ameliorated the most unpleasant of her symptoms—headache, constipation, vomiting, dehydration, exhaustion. No blockage was found, no life-extinguishing tumor had sprouted since she had last seen Golbey. Her condition was worsening, but by inches still, or feet, not by the miles she had imagined. Nothing markedly new had occurred; her system was simply breaking down at a steady rate.

Dr. Golbey did not put it to her quite that way. He focused on the parts rather than the whole in their discussions. And she did not ask for a larger picture. She asked instead about chemotherapy. It had become for her, and for Ray, an *idée fixe*. As long as Golbey was prescribing it, there was hope. They were equally aware of how sporadic her chemo had become, and though they did not like to dwell on it, once Terry's first flush of enthusiasm had worn off, neither she nor Ray believed in the breast-cancer theory. She had lung cancer, and the chemotherapy used against it had not worked.

Like his wife, Ray O'Brien had finally begun to let himself think she might not make it, although, barring his appeal to Jimmy Sweeney, he did not articulate his fear readily. He returned from New Orleans late Thursday night and was at the hospital Friday, by which time Terry was greatly improved, and optimistic once more. She began recalling the trip to and escape from Florida in hilarious flashes, describing her misery from being unable to eat and her frustration at being on vacation and having such an awful time. She reenacted a scene in which friends were urging her to go out for cocktails despite her protests, and then suddenly remembered a dream she'd had the night before.

"Oh, it was such a wonderful dream," she said. "I suddenly got very hungry and I was dying for a corned-beef sandwich on rye, with a pickle. I could hardly stand it," she said, describing the dimensions of her vision in the air with her hands. "I started picturing the paper it came in, you know, that pale-brown deli paper. I could hear it rustling as the man wrapped it for me—" Her voice trailed off, and Ray leaned forward and said, "Te, take the Amphogel." She ignored him, and sighed. "It's been six months since I've been really hungry," she said. "Will I ever have an appetite again?"

She turned to the subject of her children after a while, reporting on Chris, who had been home alone, and sick, while they were in Florida, and on Sean, who had called from school to see how she was doing. She kept saying how wonderful Carol and Nancy had been in bringing her back from Florida, and she seemed to want to believe that the experience hadn't frightened them too much. "My two girls," she said, looking to Ray for confirmation, "I don't think they know what this means."

"No," Ray said. "They think about it, but they get used to it. You're their mother. This is what's happening and they adjust."

Out of his wife's hearing, Ray O'Brien's attitude is not much different, but he lets himself voice his worries more openly, his booster's role temporarily suspended. "What goes through my mind, and hers," he says as he waits out his wife's daily examination one afternoon in the lounge down the hall, "is, why is Golbey going so slow with the chemo? Does he think it won't do any good?" O'Brien is a man used to making things work out, but in this matter he is powerless, and he knows it. The possibilities for Terry are narrowing, the chance of a big change nonexistent. And with treatment less and less likely, he begins to dwell on the more immediate details of her condition. "What I'm really worried about," he says, "is that she's literally starving herself to death. Sue says the same thing. She never was a big eater, but now she's been taking painkillers for four months with nothing in her stomach. That's why I keep trying to get her to take the Amphogel."

O'Brien talks admiringly of his wife's strength. She resists taking her painkillers, he says, despite terrific discomfort, because "she doesn't like the idea of losing control." All her jokes about drinking add up to a very moderate habit; she is not one to blot out consciousness. So she is heading into this with a clear head, O'Brien says, and he knows, if perhaps she doesn't, how bad it could be. He remembers that when his mother died twenty years ago, rather suddenly, his father simply faded. "Within six months, he had cancer. At first we thought it was depression. He never mentioned the word *cancer*. But it was in the liver."

The idea of the disease being unspeakable offends O'Brien. It is ominous, dreadful, but not shameful. He thinks people's ideas have changed since his father died, but not completely. A good friend of theirs had died of cancer a couple of years earlier—in fact, the same weekend Terry had her lung surgery. He hadn't talked about it, not even to his wife after the first couple of weeks, and his children didn't understand what was going on until it was over. His was a kind of stoicism—or, more correctly, denial—that went too far for the O'Briens. Though they have to some degree distinguished among their children by age and situation—discussing Terry's cancer somewhat differently with each—the O'Briens are trying hard not to make the mistake they believe their friend made. It is a fine line for them, between conceding just how bad things look—when conceding might mean giving up—and fostering false hopes.

Sean O'Brien would later say that while he felt the subject was not exactly taboo, he got the impression that his parents weren't eager to talk about it. He imagined that his mother was talking to his father about it "all the time, and that she was probably sick of talking about it, since she didn't bring it up. So I didn't either, though I wanted to always." Susie O'Brien remembers it differently and suggests that Sean may have felt left out because he was away at school all spring and returned to see a change more pronounced than would be obvious to the others. "And my parents didn't want to call him up at school and report every crisis, every change of status, it's true." Carol and Nancy, on the other hand, could not help but feel, living in the same house, that, spoken or unspoken, their mother's cancer was the only thing on their parents' minds. Certainly, Terry O'Brien's cancer was never hidden, but it was not dissected at the dinner table nightly, and in the early spring its speeding-up was minimized whenever possible. But it wasn't only for the children. Neither of the senior O'Briens was ready to quit. So Terry perked up after a couple of enemas and a fix of somebody else's blood, and Ray kept on trying to get her to eat.

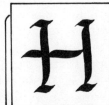ealthy, Lou Finkelstein is a lean 5 feet 10½ inches, with a thin, unlined face that is tan much of the year from trips to Florida. His eyes are dark and round and heavily lidded, and his mustache grows neatly and close to the line of his downturning, expressive mouth. His nose is thin, and he occasionally strokes it as he talks, pinching the top of the bridge absently and running his thumb and index finger along its length as his eyes widen slightly. He smiles easily, showing teeth too perfect for a Brooklyn boy, which is how he occasionally refers to himself despite twenty-five years in suburban New Jersey.

He likes his body and dresses well, most of the time in cream-colored conservative sports clothes, with beautiful, monochrome socks to match and soft, polished shoes. His brown scalp is bare to the sun year round, but when he is not chemo-bald he is only half-bald, with a thick fringe of gray hair that begins halfway down his skull.

Every year, Lou and his wife, Anita, who is round-faced and soft, trim and small, and perpetually and cheerfully on a diet, attend a fund-raising dinner for cerebral palsy, and every year they have their picture taken in a sweet, prom-style pose, three-quarter length in front of a ballroom swag. The picture from November 1980 is much like earlier ones: Anita is wearing a simple black evening dress, her hair full and blond, her smile also full. Lou is wearing a midnight-blue tux with gleaming lapels. But his face is close to unrecognizable. Male cancer patients often joke about their Kojak looks, but in the picture Lou looks exactly like Daddy Warbucks. His face is as round as a medicine ball, his eyes are dots without the anchor of eyebrows, the mustache is gone, and the top and sides of his head are uniformly covered with skin, not hair. His color is slightly orange, and though that could be the photographer's fault, Anita looks perfectly normal. The one feature on Lou's face that is unchanged is his smile—it is broad and white in the center of that puffiness, and he looks like a man who is thinking positive thoughts.

Anita's chin is up as well, a show of nerve as well as optimism. Whenever friends would begin to croon morosely about Lou's condition in that period, she would say firmly, "He's alive. I'm not in mourning."

Nor was there any need to, rough as things were for a while. Lou Finkelstein's is the sort of story the American Cancer Society would like to publicize, the sort of triumph of modern medicine that we would all like to believe in, and that in part leads to shock when things go otherwise with one's own medical life. When he says of his ten-month experience with cancer that "it's as if it never happened," he means it literally, and it is easy to see why. He is a man risen from the grave, hale, fit, happy, perhaps happier than ever before. He loves his wife, he loves his doctors, he loves his son and daughter, and he celebrates his friends as the best a man could know.

Cancer didn't make all these things happen for Lou Finkelstein; and though he is a sentimental man, he does not go so far as to suggest that it did—only that in its aftermath, the things that have always been precious to him are more so, the pleasures that he most enjoys have ripened slightly, and "the reds are redder."

When he first noticed that "one glass of wine at dinner started to conk me," he figured, "okay, I'm getting old." At fifty-two he was too young and in too good shape generally to be nodding off in the middle of a dinner with friends, but as his wife, Anita, who is in some respects the more reliable historian of the two in the matter of Lou's illness, says, "You don't notice things about yourself, and you don't read their meaning, until something happens." And besides, Lou says, "I didn't believe in illness." It was easier to believe in the premature arrival of his dotage.

The next signal was as easily misread. "I was moving a heavy piece of furniture, and as I finished, I felt a sharp pain in my groin. I thought, You dummy, you must have pulled a muscle. I went to my internist, who looked me over and said that he thought I probably had a full bladder at the time and that the movement forced urine back into my kidneys. He gave me some painkillers. We went off to Florida, and the pain persisted. I was running out of painkillers, so my cousin in Florida arranged for me to see a urologist there. The guy examined me, said he thought I should have an X ray, but that if I was going home, I'd be better off seeing my own doctor. So I took the painkiller, and when I got home, I went back to the internist."

He left Florida thinking he had one complaint for his internist, and arrived home with a second, which he took to be unconnected—a small lump in the hollow of his left collarbone. "I didn't connect it with the groin pain," he says, and, despite the fact that both of his parents died of cancer, he never made that connection either. "The reason is that I'd already been through that—I've had a bump on my back for years that alarmed me when I first discovered it, and the doctor had checked it out. So I thought, a bump, a lump. I was very nonchalant about it. I just said, 'Oh, by the way, I have this lump you might want to look at, too.' When he said to me, 'How long have you had it?' I said, 'I don't know.' But I knew that I'd been in for a checkup two or three months before, and that he'd done this thing of feeling my shoulders and my neck—if it had been there then he would certainly have found it."

His internist told him that the lump was in fact an enlarged lymph node, and he was concerned. "He sent me for an upper and lower G.I., and then for a biopsy, which I had as an outpatient." Lou's doctor advised him that the chances were that it was one of three things: a malignancy that was untreatable, a malignancy that was treatable, or nothing. And so the worst period started. It was a few days' wait between the biopsy and the consultation, at which his doctor "made it quite clear that this was a very, very serious type of cancer." Though Anita remembers almost everything else, she has a hard time remembering that awful scene in the doctor's office, but between them they remember the word "seminoma," and their instinctive decision that they would seek expert care. "I said I wanted to see Beattie," Lou recalls, speaking of Edward Beattie, the chief medical officer at Memorial, whose name Lou had heard from a friend. He was able to arrange an appointment with Beattie for ten days later. In the interim, the lump got bigger and Lou waited. He felt lousy, really sick for the first time, though he would forget that eventually and have to be corrected by Anita when he said he spent the time going to his business as usual. "Don't you remember you didn't feel well?" Anita interrupts. "You were home that week. Betty and Joe came to visit, and Marty. I can't believe you don't remember." Lou lowers his heavy eyelids till they are nearly shut and shrugs—"I really couldn't tell you. But I do remember that the biopsy gave me more grief than the major surgery."

It gave Anita grief as well. The Saturday before they were to see Beattie, she called Lou's doctor to say, "I don't like the way he's feeling," and was stunned to hear the doctor say, with the kind of sympathy that in itself seems terminal, "What he has is very serious. But it'll be over very quickly. He won't suffer much."

This ghastly prediction Anita decided to spare Lou until they had seen Beattie. In part she didn't believe it, but looking at him—suddenly pale and sick, and utterly changed in a period of weeks—she could not disbelieve it totally. She confided only in their son, Andrew, who was twenty-four at the time, and got through a big family dinner the following night with her mind fixed on their upcoming appointment in New York.

They saw Beattie early in the week, and after he looked at the pathology report on Lou's biopsy and examined the X rays, Lou recalls him saying, "You're lucky. You've got a 30 to 50 percent chance of making it."

"We danced out of Beattie's office," Lou says. A thirty-to-fifty chance of survival was suddenly wonderful news. "Let me put it this way," he adds, "I didn't think it was a 'Dear John.'"

Beattie scheduled Lou for a second biopsy and a total diagnostic workup early in June 1980. From the biopsy, it was clear that the lump in Lou's neck was not the primary tumor, and a search for the primary was begun. The biopsy had indicated seminoma, a form of cancer also called a germ-cell tumor, that accounts for about 40 percent of all testicular malignancies, but there was no sign of tumor in either testicle. A series of tests was done to try to find the tumor, among them one called an IVP, for Intravenous Pyelogram, in which dye is injected into the patient and fluoroscopic X rays are taken of the kidneys, ureters, and bladder in a search for obstruction. The IVP showed a tumor tucked up and away behind one of Lou's kidneys, in what is called the retroperitoneal cavity. Like an ovarian tumor, it was well hidden, and like an ovarian tumor, it had grown huge in the dark, actually rotating a kidney before it was detected. In its found state, the tumor was considered too big to remove surgically, but its type was a prime target for chemotherapy. Of all serious cancers, germ-cell tumors are at present the most curable.* When they are caught early and treated surgically, the cure rate is 90 percent; even in later stages, the chemotherapeutic regimen is so effective that a rate close to that prevails. Lou's case was somewhat un-

---

*Two categories of very high-incidence cancer, skin (excepting malignant melanoma) and cervical cancers *in situ* (detected early) have higher cure rates, but are not counted in cancer statistics as major cancers.

usual in that his tumor originated outside the testes, but there was good reason to think that it would respond well to chemotherapy.

Lou received his first dose of chemotherapy while he was still an inpatient. His doctor was Terry O'Brien's doctor, Robert Golbey, head of Memorial's Solid Tumor Service, and one of the principal originators of the treatment that Lou would be getting. Golbey had spent much of his career on germ-cell tumors, and his work in that area had been most rewarding; when he began his work in chemotherapy, 10 percent of all germ-cell patients survived; now 90 percent did. No other category of tumor had yielded so much ground to chemotherapy and some, like the majority of lung cancers, remained effectively immune to chemotherapeutic innovation. So, the victories possible with germ-cell tumors—even though they account for fewer than 1 percent of all cancers—were especially valued, both for the real lives they salvaged and as proof that some ground was being won.

Lou cannot remember the names of the drugs that made up his protocol, only certain terribly vivid memories over the course of treatment. But when he asks Anita which drug it was that made him so cold, she answers instantly, "Bleomycin." The other drugs she names as easily: cis-platinum dichloride; Actinomycin-D, Vinblastine and Cytoxan.

Each of the five alone can result in mild to severe nausea and vomiting, with cis-platinum producing the most notoriously violent reactions. In combination, they can be brutal, and Lou Finkelstein's experience was no exception. Yet, when the truism so knowledgeably invoked by noncancer patients—that "the treatment is worse than the disease"—is suggested to him he simply flicks his head from one side to the other disparagingly, and says, "I don't believe that's true. There's discomfort. There's a feeling of What are they doing to me? But I found—and I suppose it's my own way of pretending, my own defense—but I found myself telling jokes, trying to be humorous throughout. I guess it was for my sake, for my own sense of balance."

Some patients like to be sick in private. Lou longed for Anita to arrive at the hospital, and she did arrive, every day at noon. Sometimes Lou's aim was not so good, and one night Anita had to wear his bathrobe home, having lost her clothing to one of his attacks.

Food became the enemy. "I was hospitalized four times," Lou says, "and every time, the food became less palatable. The sight of that yellow tray—they could put filet mignon on it and I wouldn't look at it." Favorite foods he made the mistake of eating before chemo were transformed. "I used to be a hot-dog freak, I couldn't pass an umbrella without having one," he said more than a year after he was first innocent enough to eat one before a treatment. "For months I couldn't smell one without feeling sick. Only recently have I been able to eat one again. Eventually I tried to get a private room, even though I liked having someone to talk to, just so I wouldn't have to see my neighbor eat. When I first came out of the hospital, I couldn't go to a restaurant and watch *you* eat."

Every time she got him home, Anita would try Lou on new foods one at a time, as one would do with a baby, to see what he could stomach. He could take spaghetti—but only without meat—cereal, chicken soup, Italian ices, and little more. Anita became a diligent nag, rightly convinced that he required nourishment and solicitude. And through six months of chemotherapy, he never dropped below 170 pounds from a normal weight of 180.

Anita saw that he had his way whenever he could, and care and rest, but in every other respect, they conceded as little as possible to his illness, pushing it aside whenever they could between treatments, holding tight to family, friends and work. Lou had started his own retail furniture store in New Jersey twenty years earlier, after working as a wholesale furniture representative most of his life, and in the last decade it has prospered sufficiently to make it possible for them to live life much as they like. Their son, Andrew, and daughter, Claudia, are on their own— Claudia is married and gave birth to a daughter just after Lou's treatment came to an end—and Lou and Anita are free to pick up and go when they want, which is Lou's definition of success. He has arranged things so that his business can run in his absence, and maybe that is why he seems to enjoy it so much while he is there. He brought his work with him to the hospital, and he planned the store's ad campaign between attacks of nausea. "I had my ad guy and the I.V., and we just moved into a conference room down the hall." Lou used the bedside telephone like a movie mogul and sometimes had to take it off the hook to get some rest. And he used his friends, nakedly and affectionately, to keep in close touch with the world. When one friend said, "I'll do anything for you, Lou, just tell me what to do," Lou said, "Call me. Just call me every day to talk. You don't have to come, just let me hear your voice." All through treatment, he and Anita were busy making plans to celebrate when it was over. They wound up scheduling three separate vacations with three separate couples for the year after. But Lou's favorite story from his illness is about his friend Sydney.

Sydney and Lou go back over thirty-five years, to Brooklyn. Lou was best man at Sydney's wedding, but over the years, Lou felt that the relationship "had deteriorated into a fairly one-sided thing." He felt he was the only one who made an effort, that all the calls were going one way, and he got to be pretty upset with Sydney, stewing over it and complaining to Anita. It helps to understand that Lou takes old friendships very seriously indeed; he and Anita still attend annual picnics of the neighborhood "social and athletic club" that he helped to found as a fifteen-year-old, and they spend a two- or three-day holiday every New Year's with seven couples (no divorces) they have known for twenty-five years. So he was not happy about Sydney, and whenever he thought about it, he talked about it—not to Sydney, but to Anita. "Then one day, about six months before I got sick, my wise wife said to me, 'Lou. Look. You've been friends for thirty-five years. Stop trying to change him. Either call him up and tell him how you feel or let it go.'

"I decided she was right. I said to myself, 'I'm over fifty—it's ridiculous.' So I called him up and we talked, and he said that's just the way he is. And I decided I'm going to stick with the friendship and work to make it better. Well, six months or so later, I had my problem, I was in the hospital the first time for about three weeks, and when I came home, I called Sydney up, I was very emotional, I called him up and said, 'You know, you so-and-so, you called me more times in three and a half weeks than you did in thirty years.' He made it his business to call me once or twice a day, every day." Lou paused at this point, and Anita starts to cry, which she says she never did while he was sick, and Lou shrugs and smiles and says, "So. *That's* a story."

He has one for each of his close friends, it seems. One man for whom he had done a "business turn" called and said, "I'll give you my trucks, my inventory." And he had throughout the perpetual attentions of his "very dear friend Marty," who makes the kinds of jokes about survival that Lou likes. Marty has had open-heart surgery twice and talks of his determination to "keep going back until they get it right." To Lou, he suggested, "Why don't you go to Atlantic City and draw a twenty-five thousand marker? They won't let you die."

In February 1981, Golbey judged that Lou's tumor had been reduced as much as was possible from the chemotherapy, and that it was time to open him up and take a look. "He had finished with his chemo," Anita recalls, "and as far as they could see, he was cancer-free. From all the other tests and the blood work, it looked good, but they gave him one last CAT scan, and when that came back, they said the lymph nodes were somewhat enlarged.

Which could mean that there was still a problem—or could also mean that he had just had large lymph glands all along."

"They couldn't see the mass," Lou says. "Either it had disappeared completely, or it was so small that you couldn't see it." Golbey explained that if anything was left behind, even microscopic disease, the same thing could happen again, and Lou could suffer a recurrence. "I had said to Golbey long before, knowing that this was an issue, 'Do I have to go in for surgery? Is there any way I can beat it?' I just wasn't ready for it. I wasn't happy having abdominal surgery. But he said, 'After all this work and effort, if we don't get it all, we'll have to go through it all again.' He made it quite clear that I didn't have much choice."

The man who would do the surgery was Willet Whitmore, "who Golbey told me was the best guy for the operation, and was in fact the chap who developed this kind of surgery. Once I knew that, I didn't really need a blow-by-blow description of surgery. I'm not the type—that kind of toughness I don't have.

"So the night before surgery, or what I thought was—the operation was postponed a day—one of the fellows came into the room about eight o'clock at night. Anita had just left, and he said, 'Are you aware of what is going to happen tomorrow morning?' I said, 'No, not fully,' and he said to me, 'No one explained it to you?' I said, 'There was no need for it. Whitmore is doing it, and I have complete confidence.' I was taking my usual *ha, ha, ha,* gallant stance—you know, 'I do this all the time, every weekend I go through surgery.' So he said, 'Well, let me just give you an idea of what to expect.' He started to talk, and I listened, and all of a sudden, he said, 'You know, *uh,* that chances are that after surgery—in the course of surgery, we have to locate, we have to do certain procedures, and you have very fine nerves that we can't see, they're that fine—and we have no choice when we go in there but to cut some of those nerves. And these nerves,' he explained, 'stimulate the muscles that provide you with ejaculation. Now, sexually there will be no change in you after surgery. You'll have the same emotional mood, or desire, everything will be the same, except you'll simply have no fluid.'"

Lou tells this story with his eyes widening and narrowing, his eyebrows climbing toward his brow and lowering darkly, a wry line at the corner of his mouth, and a bit of sighing for punctuation. He blinks and says, "I said to him, 'Gee, no one ever spoke to me about this,' and he said, 'I don't want you to get upset. It won't affect anything in the way you feel or act. It's just that those nerves having been cut, those muscles don't have the stimulation they need.'"

114

Lou shrugs, and says, "Well, again, hearing this, what other choice do you have? It's the only game in town. And he presented this as absolutely, positively sure to happen. Now it's about eight-thirty or a quarter to nine at night. Anita is gone. I was already psyched for the operation, and now I had to psych myself for this thing. I said to myself, 'I gotta think this thing out.' I said to the nurse, 'Don't give me anything now, if I want a sleeping pill, I'll call you. I don't want to be drugged, I don't want to be put asleep. I just want to get this through my head and make peace with it.' And so I came to the conclusion that (A) you got no choice; (B) it's not the worst thing in the world, you'll still have your sexual activity, you'll just have these changes, and then, having gone full circle with the whole thing, I thought, Hey, you're alive, baby, and you're clean, and this is the last step of the way. They're going to open you up and with God's help you're clean and it's going to be bye-bye hospital. And that was it."

Lou's ruminations were further tempered by the presence of his roommate, "a kid maybe twenty-one or twenty-two, who had just had abdominal surgery and had had one testicle removed. So when the doctor gave me the bomb, I looked over at this kid, and I was thinking of him at twenty-one and me at fifty-three. I would guess that sort of thing helps keep your head on balance. When you see somebody who's worse off, it's not that you're glad they're worse off, but it makes you feel better anyway—you know—things could be much worse."

As it turned out, the lymph nodes picked up by the CAT scan were clean on biopsy, and because some were close to vital organs, not as much cutting was done as anticipated. The result, Lou says, is that not all the expected nerves were cut. "So," he starts to laugh and looks at Anita, "I'm sort of at a halfway house. I'm not exactly the way I was and I'm not exactly the way I thought I'd be."

Which is fine with Anita—"since I wasn't hoping to have any more kids."

There was no sexual damage, but in the aftermath of the surgery, Lou worried about it anyway. Raising the general question had made him uneasy, and when he didn't feel his usual sexual interest—he "couldn't get that *click*," is how he puts it—he began to wonder. "At one point, I said to Anita, 'If this is it, honey, I'm sorry. Forgive me.'" But a couple of weeks after he was released and had made a full recovery, they went off to Florida to relax. And just as he would get his hair back, and his racquetball game, and his taste for hot dogs with mustard, his sex drive came back with a thrilling surge. Lou raises the subject delicately, hoping not to be thought crude, but wanting to express how good it made him feel, and how sweet a reward it was for them both.

In the ensuing months there have been regular checkups, on a schedule of decreasing frequency, and unfailingly reassuring reports. The Finkelsteins seldom think of the past unless an appointment with Golbey is scheduled or a bill from the hospital for blood work appears. They take a lot of vacations. They have been to California to see Lou's brother (with Marty and Estelle), to the Caribbean (with Sydney and Phyllis), and to Monte Carlo and Paris with a third couple. They threw a big family party to celebrate their granddaughter's birth and Lou's cure, and drank Dom Perignon and ate themselves happy. And they have managed some unhappy periods too—family crises haven't stopped occurring just because Lou got cured, and a few months after Lou's abdominal surgery, Anita's mother went into Memorial for a mastectomy.

Lou Finkelstein isn't going to live forever, of course; being cured of cancer doesn't guarantee anything but the opportunity to be run over by a truck, or develop heart disease, or eventually grow decrepit in old age like one's ancestors. But being cured has given him three years already, and the healthy expectation of many years to come, and it has sharpened his devotion to their enjoyment. "Philosophically, I was on this road before I got sick," he says, "but since then it's intensified. A lot of people have a lot more money than I do, but they can't bring themselves to take the time. I think success is the ability to do or to go when you want to do or to go. It's real freedom of choice. I said this to Anita when I didn't have a dime, and it's still true for me. I haven't got horses, and I haven't got women, and I don't shoot up. But I love to go, I love to travel, I love to see, to smell, to taste, to meet, to take part of, and part in." He nearly exhausts himself with the line of glorious loves. And then in an unconscious variation on a familiar metaphor for being dead, he nods his head sharply for emphasis, and says, "I'm still smelling the roses."

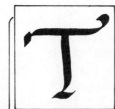erry O'Brien was sent home from Memorial only two days after her emergency admission in April, with instructions from Dr. Golbey to eat as much as she could of a soft diet, and to take Haley's MO as needed. The following Thursday, April 30, she returned for a checkup hopeful of getting chemotherapy, but her platelets were still low, and Golbey put it off another week. His record of the visit indicates that the complaints of the previous week had lessened, but that she now reported recurring pains in her right hip and at the base of her skull. Golbey arranged for her to see the radiologist the following week and noted that if her counts were improved he would start her on a new program of chemotherapy, a three-drug protocol used for breast cancer.

When she came in the following week, however, her counts were still too low. "Pain in neck worse," Golbey wrote in his neat hand on her chart. "Still weak in legs but gets around without great difficulty. CEA* [taken] 4/23/81 [two weeks earlier] is 510, marked increase from month prior."

And she felt as sick as the facts made her out to be. Also annoyed. Sitting waiting for treatment in the radiation area, she is in a first-rate snit that focuses pointedly on the radiologist Golbey had sent her to. "This place is *ridiculous*," she says, talking in a low voice, short of breath, exasperated and agitated. "Came in

---

*CEA is short for a CEA Assay, a test for carcinoembryonic antigen in the blood. A low CEA level indicates that treatment has had some effect, while a high-level CEA indicates continued malignancy or a recurrence of a tumor.

this morning—Golbey had told me I might be getting chemo and radiology—he brings this guy [the radiologist] in, he says, 'We want to give you five more treatments.'" She pauses, takes a breath, and says, "Which is fine with me, because my neck is killing me, and now I've got this pain around *here* again," she says, reaching around with her arms as she bends forward in her chair to indicate her right lower back. "But he can do it only at night!" she says with a look of disgust. "He says that that's the only time he can get the machines." Her glower turns to a sly smile. "I'm thinking, Haven't you got any *pull?* What do you mean you can't get the machines? The *other* doctors all need them in the morning? So I said to him, 'Doctor, I didn't mind coming in late the last time, because my husband happened to be in the hospital, but I can't come in every night.' He said, 'Maybe I can get you in this morning, then Wednesday, Thursday, and Friday night. And if you don't mind—'" Mrs. O'Brien rolls her eyes— "'Saturday morning.'" The idea strikes her as absurd. "I've got two girls going to the prom Friday night," she says. "I've got to be there to take their pictures."

She is called to be marked for treatment and returns after a few minutes wearing a blue smock over her slacks, which bag at the seat and hang low on her hips. (All her clothes are oversize now, accentuating her growing thinness; sometimes she pins herself in, but as often she does not, and tugs upward on pants that want to slip ever lower each week.) She makes a disgusted face and tosses her blue-and-green-striped sweater onto a pile that so far includes her voluminous tan raincoat, folded once and placed on the seat of a chair, her spring handbag, beige and lighter by a few ounces than her winter one, and a hardcover copy of *Free Fall in Crimson*, a John D. MacDonald thriller.

She lowers herself into her chair, grasping its arms as if to balance the pain. "O-o-oh," she says. "I'm becoming a real bitch. I'm tired of being sick." She squints as she points to the base of her neck, where a wobbly magenta stripe edges upward from the top of her wrapper. "The pain in my neck is shooting up to my ear," she says.

Coming in for her appointments is getting harder and harder all the time, she says, because she's so tired and uncomfortable. But at least it gets her off the couch at home. "You've *got* to fight this thing," she says, carefully turning her head. "The worst thing you can do is lie around all day. I do enough of that already."

She talks bluntly about whether the radiation or the chemotherapy, if she ever gets it, will help. Then she says, "It may not matter at this point." She reaches back with two hands and feels along the upper part of her spine. "The tumors are all along here," she says, pressing lightly and looking almost surprised to be able to feel them.

She alternates between moods of resignation and complaint today, sometimes mixing the two. It's as if she suddenly understands how legitimate a case she's got. "I'm just disgusted," she says. "I'm tired of being the nice girl. Ray says, 'You've really become a bitch!' I say, 'Why not? It's my turn.'" She laughs uncomfortably. Some compensation, her look says.

It is a long wait for treatment this morning. She clucks and looks around. "Isn't this for the birds?" Her resilience, like her appetite for life itself, is thinning. She mentions that another couple would like her and Ray to go to Florida with them again in June. She shrugs. "Ray would like it, but I'm really too tired. You get to the point where you don't want to go anywhere. Unless I'm coming in here, I don't get up now until twelve or one o'clock. I do a few chores and then I'm exhausted. It's a terrible feeling."

The only empty chairs remaining in the crowded waiting room this morning are directly opposite, across the opening to the outer hall. A young mother comes in with her two small children and settles them there. Mrs. O'Brien stiffens. The older of the two boys is perhaps six, with dark, burnished-brown skin and close-cut black hair that has been shaved carefully up and around his right ear, which faces us. The entire right side of his face is distended by a tumor that sits, swollen and hard, between his ear and his shoulder, a tumor as big in itself as his entire head. The boy's face when he slowly turns is placid and intelligent. He shifts his position every few minutes for comfort, but not with the jerky movements of an ordinary child. When he sits forward in his seat, his right shoulder sags downward from the tumor's weight and his arm hangs low as though being tugged from underneath. His little brother, no older than three, sits beside him happily, kicking his feet under the chair, chattering to himself as he dips his hand into a bag of Dipsy Doodles.

The older boy glances to his left from time to time, toward his quiet mother and his noisy brother, but mainly he stares in front of him. He strokes his tumor absently, occasionally shifts his body to take it gently in both hands. He traces with his finger the raised stitching scar that runs vertically beneath the ear. It is yellowish-pink, picked out sharply against the almost-black skin stretched so thin over the unnatural mass.

After a few seconds, he is not horrible, only mesmerizing; the tumor begins to seem less grotesque, more a part of him. He is so calm, so apparently at peace with this baggage that one is loath to pity him. He is no longer a terror, once again human. Yet, when Mrs. O'Brien has finished her treatment and is dressed and on her way out again, she speaks of the boy with sadness. His youth and suffering make her ache; she finds it impossible to reconcile the two. *Her* coming to the hospital doesn't depress her, she says. It's what she sees here that does her in.

She returns the following day almost two hours early and manages to get treated at a quarter to five. When her treatment is finished, she approaches the appointment clerk seated behind a small window in one of the waiting-room walls and tells him that she has to change the remainder of her appointment times and her Friday appointment to Monday. On each of the four appointment slips she holds in her hand, she has crossed out "6:15" and written in "4:30." When the clerk asks her who made the change, she answers blithely, "The doctor."

It is a needed triumph, like sneaking up to Ray's room in April without a proper pass. But when she leaves the radiation area, her strength dissolves. Her words come faintly and in single, breathy spurts, until she says, "I think I better not talk till I sit down." It is a long way for her to the first-floor lounge, where she settles to wait for Ray and Gene.

Seated for a few minutes, she recovers, and talks normally again. In fact, she is garrulous, going on about the dance that Carol and Nancy are to go to on Friday, the one she has just arranged to be home in time to take pictures for. She says that Nancy's dress is a "see-through number" requiring a special slip underneath, and that when they couldn't get the slip to hang right, she volunteered to sew it to the dress. "So that was my job on the way up here," she says, laughing. "And I can't sew. Oh God, the stitches came through in a couple of places—" She does a wild pantomine with her arms, face screwed into a knot of fake rage, of Nancy ripping the badly done garment apart.

She is more than usually excited about this event. She longs to have something to throw herself into, even a hated sewing job. Her children drive her crazy, she says, in the way that mothers who adore being needed and harassed do. That she is in fact easing out of their lives—both because they are growing up and because she is dying—is a reality that she would rather not dwell on. So she complains comically of their continued dependence, of how Chris, who is twenty-two and still living at home because he can't find an apartment in Manhattan, hasn't yet learned to shut the garage door, of how the girls need this or that, of Carol's driving, Sean's grades. None of her complaints seems genuine, nor does she seem the least bit annoyed by the faults she lists.

They are the character traits of lively children who make her laugh. Her face loses its tension as she talks of them. Chris, she says, drove down to Maryland over the weekend to visit Sean. "Isn't that sweet that he wants to see his brother?" she says, then reports what Sean did when Chris left to come home. "Sean is on a radio program at school; he announces, introduces songs and things, and when Chris was driving home, he could listen to Sean on the car radio for a certain number of miles, and all of a sudden, he hears Sean introducing a song—'This is dedicated to Christopher O'Brien driving north on Route 15.'" Their mother sinks back in her chair sighing. "Chris asked me, 'What would you have done if he'd done that to you?' I said I would just have pulled over to the side of the road and sat there and cried."

It is close to six o'clock now, and Mrs. O'Brien is beginning to wonder what's keeping Ray. "Maybe I should call him," she says, then covers her mouth with her hand and says, "Oh, Christ. I told him I'd call him when I was through." She struggles out of her chair, collects bag and book, and heads for the phone. She seems unnecessarily frazzled by her error, guilty almost, but calms down as soon as she has reached him. She says she'll be waiting in front, on York Avenue.

It is a beautiful day, still light, and sweet-smelling from the fruit trees that line the block. A week earlier they were all thick with pink blossoms, but now they are pale green, the petals all blown away. I mention how quickly they have changed, and Mrs. O'Brien looks up and says, "Oh, aren't they beautiful." Then she points farther down the street, to the small landscaped garden of Rockefeller University across York Avenue. The dogwood is in bloom behind a fence, and azaleas line the walk. "Those pinks," she calls them. She says she has never known for certain the names of most of the flowers and trees, but she loves them anyway. She is still moving like an old woman, a step and a breath at a time, but the spring invigorates her and she says suddenly. "Oh, I love the warm weather. The good Lord won't take me at least until October or November. It's too beautiful now." What about Christmas? She looks crossly at me and shakes her head. "Oh, no. I don't want to be around then. It's too cold."

On Wednesday, May 13, her radiation over, Mrs. O'Brien arrives for her weekly appointment with Golbey, and she is feeling worse than usual. "Putrid" is the word she chooses. Waiting to be called to the examining area, she says, "This has got to stop. This isn't living," and her answer to Golbey's first question, "How do you feel," is an uncamouflaged "Awful."

"What's the matter?" he asks her.

"I'm nauseous all the time. All day and all night."

Golbey asks whether it is since the radiation or earlier.

"I'm not sure," she says. She points to her right foot and tries to lift it off the floor. "The ankle's all swollen," she says, "and there's no feeling all along the right side, up to about here," she says, indicating the middle of her shin.

Golbey kneels down and feels along her foot. "It's pressure on a nerve," he tells her. He helps her over to the examining table and gives her a boost up. He examines her fully clothed . . . camel's-hair pants, white blouse beneath a camel's-hair, black-white-and-green-striped sweater. She is still dressing for cold weather in the middle of May. Her feet dangle above the floor. The right foot is shoeless; on the left is a very clean white canvas sneaker. Golbey feels slowly along her neck, down her back, under her arms. He listens to her lungs from the back. He lifts her head gently with his hands and asks, "Do you feel any pain?"

She rolls her eyes as far to the right as she can, trying to bring him into sight while locked in his grip, and says, "Ha, ha. Yes," as in, "Are you kidding?"

When he has finished, Golbey leaves to check her blood counts. Mrs. O'Brien slides herself off the examining table and moves stiffly toward a chair. "You know," she says, "coming in this morning, we stopped at an intersection downtown, and I saw this black traffic cop standing out in the middle directing people and I thought, I'd trade places with him this minute. I really would. I'm getting jealous of normal people."

When Golbey returns, he tells her that her blood counts, including her hemoglobin, are low, which helps to explain why she feels so bad. He explains, as he has before, how the cumulative effect of chemotherapy and radiation to the bones, where blood is manufactured, work to depress her counts. She nods. "So, no chemo, right?"

Golbey nods, then mentions the hormonal therapy he has been considering, one of several treatments for breast cancer and one that will not produce side effects of this nature.

"What would the effect be?" she asks.

"If it works, it could decrease the size of the tumors," Golbey tells her.

He raises the subject of her current condition. "Are you out of breath?" he asks.

"Oh, yes. That's the worst. Not being able to walk from one room to the next. Not being able to *talk*." Her voice rises along with her sense of incredulity.

"Well, a blood transfusion would help," Golbey says.

He starts to write the order, and Mrs. O'Brien watches silently for a minute before saying, "I'll never get chemo, will I?" Golbey looks up from the desk. "Oh, yes," he says, "You'll get some."

The visit seems to be taking place in overlapping stages. Golbey never hurries, and is solicitous in his care, frequently disappearing to make arrangements, returning always to clarify, his manner courteous. But today they joke very little with one another. Neither seems to have the heart for it, and suddenly Golbey's concern, his delicacy, seem weighted. The mood lifts when he asks her about her pain medication. It turns out that she has neglected to fill the prescription for Percocet that he gave her several weeks ago, preferring to tinker with combinations of Darvocet and Tylenol III, according to the level of pain and degree of nausea she is feeling on a given day. "I'm trying to be a doctor, which I'm not," she says, when she has explained what she's been doing.

"That's not being a doctor," Golbey says. "That's being a good patient. If you can track symptoms and date them, you help." She tells him she had a fever the night before. "You seem to react to many things with fever," Golbey says, and she laughs at that. "I thought about not coming in. I thought I'd call and say I was too sick. But then I thought, what better place to go than to see your doctor?" Golbey smiles at her and says, "I've always thought there was some inconsistency in patients being too sick to come to the hospital."

Though she has been given blood at Memorial many times, Mrs. O'Brien must be tested for the order, and one of the nurses comes by to see if she is ready. When she is gone, Golbey starts to make some notes on her chart. He writes for a while, then looks up and says, "It's starting to move."

When Mrs. O'Brien returns, he brightens. "Already? Your veins can't be all that bad."

"My veins are *fine*," she says archly. "It's the nurses in this hospital who are the problem." Immediately, she takes it back. "They're really very good," she says, quietly.

She sits down while Golbey completes her paperwork.

"I never know what's going to happen to me when I come in here," she says. "It's fun."

"You sit around all week thinking up new problems for us to deal with," Golbey says.

"That's right."

He describes what he's ordered for her today: Tamoxifen, an anti-estrogen, to be taken once a day, and Compazine, for nausea. He tells her to start with two tablets of Compazine every four hours, and when she begins to feel better, to cut back to one every four hours. Nausea generates nausea, Golbey explains, and what he hopes is that they can break the cycle long enough to get her eating again. She nods. She hopes so, too.

There is a long wait while her blood order is prepared, and Mrs. O'Brien says she'd like to go somewhere for a vanilla shake, all she has appetite for. There is an ice-cream parlor a block and a half away, but ten yards up 67th Street, she says she can't possibly make it. She clutches her chest and pants as we return to the hospital, where she collapses into a chair in the first-floor lounge. "I really need that blood," she says with a frightened laugh.

She is stunned by this latest evidence of her decline. She keeps on being surprised by the fact that her condition gets worse every week instead of better. "I was looking at some pictures from Raymond's wedding the other day," she says, "and I looked fine. I was running around doing everything. That was in October. Look how fast this happened," she says, ticking off the months. She shakes her head. "People who are young and poor worry about money. I never thought about what it meant to be well. Now I think they're crazy. I'd rather be poor."

Her blood order is supposed to be ready at eleven-thirty, but when we arrive at the transfusion room on the third floor, behind the surgery clinic, they say it will be another hour. Mrs. O'Brien doesn't look as if she'll last that long, but when she sits down in the empty waiting room, she picks up. She decides to call Susie at work and fishes her page number out of her handbag. "You can never get her at home," Mrs. O'Brien says proudly, Susie obviously being too valuable and hardworking. She crosses to the pay phone and in a short while is laughing and talking to her daughter. Of all the children, Susie is the one to whom she has spoken most openly about her illness, not just because Susie is a doctor, but because she is the eldest and they have been close a long time. The two of them see each other only sporadically, but they talk almost every day. That Susie is a doctor only complicates it more for Susie.

"I could say," she would reflect later, "that the day I heard she had bone metastases, I knew she was dying. When they caught it with surgery, I thought maybe everything would be okay, but once I knew she had metastases, I knew she had less than a year—I couldn't have specified exactly. But she and everyone else had more hope that something could be done." In the beginning, her mother would ask Susie what she thought about the treatment, or her chances, and though Susie would properly declare herself unfamiliar with the intricacies of oncology, she tried to respond in some way. "She would ask me if I thought she was dying—I'm not sure if she would actually say that, but she would say something like, 'Do you think this is going to work?' Or, 'What about this, what do you think?' Most of the time I would just say, 'Oh, I don't know'—hedging maybe, but—I tried not to be too hopeful. At the same time, I didn't want to say, 'Yeah, you're dying.'" Like her mother, whom she resembles less than she does her father, Susie squints when she's talking about something painful, though her words keep coming, and she doesn't shy from the truth. "I don't think I was hopeful at all," she says. "Probably I wasn't, because after a while she didn't ask me so much."

Returning from talking to Susie this afternoon, Mrs. O'Brien is up. "She's coming down to visit tonight," she says. "That Sue, you never know—some weeks she wants to come, some weeks she doesn't." She pauses and then adds. "She must be afraid I'm dying. Probably thinks I've got two weeks to live."

Mrs. O'Brien's blood order is ready just before twelve-thirty. The big room is nearly empty, with only one other patient getting blood. Someone has a radio turned on low. One nurse is on duty, and she quickly inserts an I.V. into Mrs. O'Brien's left forearm. These days, Mrs. O'Brien barely registers the needle going in. She turns her attention from the I.V. as soon as the blood starts flowing and starts to talk of other, more pleasant matters.

A friend who was widowed a couple of years ago is getting married again, she says somewhat conspiratorially, though the event is no secret. What's exciting is that it's a contemporary who is getting married, and it seems to make her feel very young again. She talks on about details of the wedding, and of the house the friend and her husband-to-be are redoing. Because she has been feeling so poorly, Mrs. O'Brien says, she hasn't been as involved with her friend as she'd like, but then the friend came over the other night, she says, and the two of them—Ray was out of town—gabbed for hours like a couple of teen-agers. "Oh, we had such fun," she says.

And so it goes for the rest of the afternoon. An hour or so after the blood began dripping into her vein, word comes over the radio that the Pope has been shot, but it seems so preposterous a piece of news that no one pays it much attention other than to cluck about a world gone mad. The second packet empties into her arm just before three-thirty, and she is up and out in minutes, briefly invigorated and eager to go home.

The following Saturday, there is another wedding to go to, one of Ray's brother's children. Despite her fortification in midweek, she spends most of her time at the reception sitting down, Mrs. O'Brien reports afterward. "If you can't walk, you can't get up and leave if you happen to sit down next to someone boring," she says, not altogether joking. "At one point," she says, giggling, "I got stuck with these two people at a table—they were driving me crazy but I couldn't get up—I had to get Sue to rescue me."

The story is told the following Tuesday, when she is back in for her weekly clinic appointment with Golbey. She has been waiting since a quarter to nine, and at ten-thirty, Mary Ann Barletta, Golbey's secretary, comes out to check on her. Mrs. O'Brien tells her in an uncharacteristically chilly voice that she's been waiting for almost two hours.

"Well," Mary Ann says, "they take the sick ones first."

Mrs. O'Brien looks up at her stone-faced, putting it on thick, and says, "Ah—ha, ha."

Mary Ann touches Mrs. O'Brien's shoulder and lowers her voice. "How you feelin'?" she says gently.

"Not so hot."

Golbey has been delayed because of a couple of emergencies, Mary Ann tells her. He should be ready for her soon.

Mrs. O'Brien stares straight down the corridor to the chart table outside the examining area, fixing her eyes on the spot for minutes at a time, interrupting herself in the middle of a sentence periodically to mutter, "What the hell is going on?" She is suffering today, and can't hide it, doesn't even try. She says she may get downtown to see her mother today if Golbey ever calls her. Kak and Brian are going to be there today, she says, "But I told them, 'Don't count on me.' . . . I never know what I'm going to be doing from one day to the next." She recalls how late she was here the week before, then suddenly wheels and says, "How can you stand coming here every day? Don't you get depressed?" Before I can answer, she says, kicking my chair lightly with her good foot and flicking her tongue mischievously, "I bet you feel good though, that you don't have it, don't you? It's like being the only healthy person in a leper colony." She is silent a minute, then adds, "I wouldn't come here if I didn't have to."

A little after eleven-thirty, Golbey intones her name over the microphone. She does her best to leap to her feet. "What do you know?" she says. Earlier thoughts of complaint dissolve en route, and she unburdens herself to Golbey with a single crack about his busy schedule. Golbey has her blood counts in hand and tells her that they are still low, despite the transfusion. Her condition confirms the same thing to his eye. She tells him dutifully that she has been taking the Compazine as directed, and that the nausea

126

has let up slightly, though her eating has not increased.

Golbey pulls the curtain to examine her. Their voices carry readily and their conversation suggests a routine meant for an audience.

"You've got black-and-blue marks on your legs," Golbey says.

"I always have," Mrs. O'Brien says. "I never know from what."

"Are there more than before?"

"No."

"It's a very feminine trait."

"That's why I have it."

When the exam is finished and Mrs. O'Brien is again seated in the straight-back chair that she favors, she tells Golbey about a new pain, just below the base of her neck, between her shoulder blades. Golbey asks when she first noticed it. She looks at him warily, then says, "When I got home last week, I leaned down to open a cabinet in the kitchen and suddenly felt it—I don't know whether it's psychosomatic or what."

Golbey gazes at her without speaking for a few seconds, then asks, "What are you taking for pain?" Astonishingly, he must ask this same question each week, because he can never be sure. But there is no hint of reproach in his voice. It's her pain.

"Darvocet," she says today.

"It's not working, is it?" Golbey says. "What were you taking before?"

"Tylenol III and codeine. But I stopped because I thought they were related to the nausea."

He nods and makes a note. He is sitting on the edge of the desk, facing her. "About your activities," he says. "I think it might be a good idea to take it easy for a while."

She defends weakly: "You can't lie there all the time."

"I'm not asking that," Golbey says. "I haven't been following you around, so I don't know exactly what you've been doing, but this isn't the time to push. I'd like you to cool it for just a little while, huh?"

She looks relieved. "I honestly agree with you," she says.

"It's like healing a broken leg," Golbey says.

"I think I have been pushing too hard," Mrs. O'Brien says.

They are talking in each other's air spaces, nodding agreement, when Golbey says, his voice calm, "Because if it continues, we'll have to put you in a collar." Mrs. O'Brien looks horrified. "One of those foam-rubber jobs," Golbey says. Again, she rushes to explain. "I was thinking, I'm so weak, I'd try to build up by doing more." Golbey repeats the warning gently, reiterating his point

127

about strain, and in the middle of his speech, she bobs her head quickly and says, "Thank you."

It's as if she has been waiting for this dispensation for weeks. Yet she would not ask for it. A week ago, she had been recounting with astonishment how it had taken her a couple of hours to iron a batch of Ray's handkerchiefs, as if there were no reason for her exhaustion. "I had let them go for a while," she said, "and there were about twenty-five of them, so I thought I'd get them out of the way. But I couldn't believe what was happening. I had to sit down after every one." Now that Golbey has helped her let go of her resistance, possibly she will no longer feel that she has to demonstrate her will to live with such tasks.

When Golbey raises the subject of chemotherapy, Mrs. O'Brien is instantly alert. She looks at him sideways and spreads her arms wide. "I want the strongest stuff you've got shooting into me," she says. That's not about to happen, he says softly, but since she has tolerated the Tamoxifen well, he wants to increase the dose to two tablets daily.

Golbey's last words to her this morning are, "If anything changes, if you feel worse, call me, day or night."

Mrs. O'Brien laughs. "Don't worry, Doctor," she says. "There's nothing I'd like better than to wake you up in the middle of the night to tell you I'm dying."

There is no question of what is happening now; only the details of how, and how soon, she will die remain uncertain.

Because her platelets are so low, Golbey explains later that day, she could bleed to death internally if one of her many tumors were to hit an artery. She could succumb to infection, since she has almost no immune defenses left. Against that, he says, the hospital is no protection and in fact, the longer she can stay out of the hospital, the better off she is in terms of avoiding infection. "And sometimes," Golbey says, "in cases like this, the *coup de grâce* is an invasion of the liver." The signs include nausea, loss of appetite, fatigue—all of which she has—but, although they watch her blood work every week for evidence of liver involvement, it has not yet shown up.

It is hard to say how long she can survive. With support—transfusions primarily—she could conceivably last several months. Or she could go any time soon. But clearly, the rewards of survival are lessening for her all the time, are they not? It would seem so, Golbey concedes, and he raises the subject of patient attitudes. Some of his patients collapse into a state of childish, or even infantile, dependence at this stage, he says. Others deny what is happening in bizarre ways. But Mrs. O'Brien is a remarkable woman. He has no doubt that she understands exactly what is happening to her, and that her way of facing it, day by day, still trying to hold on to her life, is an important choice. "In general," Golbey says, "it's my belief that people like Mrs. O'Brien do better—they don't necessarily live longer, but while they live they get more out of life."

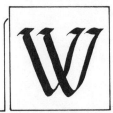hen Celine Fink was a girl—her last name was Dwyer then, and her father was a general practitioner and surgeon in Passaic, New Jersey—she wanted to be in the theater. She was beautiful enough, and she could dance, and though her parents weren't absolutely sure that it was respectable, they let her travel to New York from Passaic as a teen-ager, so that she could perform as an extra in Metropolitan Opera productions and take lessons at the School of American Ballet. At one point in high school, she was taking eleven lessons a week and loved it, but when she was about seventeen, she began to lose weight rapidly and became chronically exhausted. Her father at first thought she had heart trouble, but it turned out to be a thyroid condition, and after she spent six months at home in bed, her thyroid gland was removed. A thin, faint scar that circles her neck like a tribal marking is the only visible evidence of that period, but Celine remembers clearly, almost forty years later, how her mother could not understand why she didn't bounce right back after surgery. When she speaks of her mother's impatience, there is in Celine's voice both the hope of sympathy and the uneasiness that clings to ancient, unsettled wrongs. Being sick did not turn out well for Celine, and admitting to frailty, though she often feels exceedingly frail, costs her.

When you ask her these days how she is feeling, after three cancer operations, four courses of hormonal therapy or chemotherapy, several courses of radiation, and two years' reliance on a cane or a walker to get around, she still smiles a little apologetically before answering, particularly if she is feeling so poorly that she can actually bring herself to say "not too good." For a long time, she answered all queries about her pain or her mood with a hurried "fine," as if every questioner were her mother. And before her answer had time to settle, she would turn the question around. "How are *you?*" she would quickly ask, with a sincerity that was no less genuine for the fact that it got her off the hook. There is no doubt that Celine Fink is an exceptionally sweet-natured woman, honestly eager for news of other people's lives, but it is also true that for a long time she has been afraid that if she talks too much about her own troubles, she might be taken for a hypochondriac.

There is more to it than that, of course. Like everyone else who has cancer, Celine Fink does not want to be singled out, and she does not want to be left out. She does not want to be a cancer patient first, herself second. The first time around, though she was very depressed for a couple of months after her mastectomy in May 1979, it was not all that difficult to get to the point where she could believe that her trouble was behind her. Her experience was much more private than the articles in the newspapers and in the women's magazines would suggest. There was no Reach-to-Recovery volunteer at her side when she awoke after surgery, no exercise class for postmastectomies at the Y. Her surgeon, a local man who had been a friend of her father's, was "traditional," Celine says without irony, and he advised her not to drive for quite a while, not to hurry to get a prosthesis after surgery. Only after talking to a friend who knew someone who knew, did she get the information that she needed and a companion to help her shop for a proper prosthesis. Because she had always been a big-breasted woman, a couple of months into her recovery Celine decided that she wanted to have reduction surgery on her remaining breast, to lessen the imbalance. Her doctor was not especially encouraging, but Ray, her husband, championed her as he has done all along, and pursuing her own wishes helped restore her confidence.

The second time around, it was harder. Celine had been back at work for a year, in a part-time office job that she loved and that left her time for her husband and two sons, the younger of whom was then still at home, a senior in high school. She was as active as before her surgery; she sewed and saw friends, took aerobic dancing and rode her bike. She was still a pretty woman at fifty-two. Pictures taken of her and Ray on their honeymoon in 1954 show a strikingly beautiful young woman, Ava Gardner-like but sweet and open-faced, bosomy and slim-hipped, sexy and demure. Ray is her physical match, dark-haired, tan and trim, perfect white teeth smiling at the camera. They look so happy and nice it makes you ache. And the pictures that fill several albums covering the years since that honeymoon are of a piece with those first snapshots on a beach. Ray and Celine in their new house, a simple cottage on a street filled quickly with young couples like themselves and soon with their children. The Finks arrived on Patricia Place when David was one; Larry was born four years later. Celine had liked working before and in the early years of her marriage, but she liked raising her children best. Theirs was a close family, in which the parents' interests naturally became the children's. Both boys took to the theater as their mother had as a child, spending several seasons each as members of the children's chorus at the City Opera. With David the life took, and since graduating from NYU with a degree in the arts, he has worked under the name David Edwards, as an actor, extra, singer, dancer, and member of a cruise ship troupe. When the boys were growing up, the Finks spent most of their away-from-home vacations on short cruises, including one unusual one in the Caribbean, aboard the *Maxim Gorky*, a Russian luxury liner that plied the Caribbean for a few seasons. Larry was twelve at the time and was so smitten with things Russian that he eventually chose to study foreign policy. In 1980, the year his mother's cancer came back, he started his first year at Johns Hopkins University in Baltimore, studying government, diplomacy and Russian language.

The first time around, Celine had found her cancer herself, the lump that she had dreaded for years appearing one morning beneath her fingers. It surprised her by its shape: it was not the round knobby bump she imagined, but a little oblong stone that nevertheless was unmistakable in its meaning. But the second time around, she had no idea of what to look for and, despite having had cancer, no real expectation of its coming back. It had been over a year—almost a year and a half—and so, when she started having trouble with her ankle late in the summer of 1980, it seemed to have nothing to do with her breast. For a couple of months, she kept going as before, taking aspirin for the pain, and worrying about arthritis. She started an aerobic-dance class as planned and continued her normal activities, but the pain, which had been annoying at first, became agonizing. She talked with several doctors: her surgeon, who examined her other breast and gave her a prescription for a painkiller, but never did a bone scan; her general practitioner on several occasions; and eventually a rheumatologist, to whom her G.P. sent her on the assumption that the trouble might be arthritis. The rheumatologist took an X ray of the ankle and said it was broken. Then he took Ray aside and said he strongly suspected that there was a malignancy in the ankle.

By now it was late October. Up to that point, everything about Celine's care had been modest and low-key and local. Mastectomy was common enough, and it hadn't seemed urgent that they seek out a specialist. The ankle business galvanized Ray overnight, and he started asking around for recommendations. A friend insisted that a surgeon at Memorial named Joseph Lane was the man to go to, and, without an appointment, Ray simply showed up at Lane's office with Celine's X rays in hand and talked himself inside. He got Celine an appointment with Lane for early November; surgery to remove the tumor was scheduled for December 4. Despite the long buildup and the slow dawning of what the tumor meant, it all seemed to happen very fast at the end, and Celine held on hard to her earlier feelings of optimism. Though anxious about another piece of surgery, she entered Memorial with a cheerful attitude, acting as if—and persuaded of it for the moment—the surgery would settle things. So she was shocked by the attitude of one of the young interns or fellows— she isn't sure which—who reacted sharply to her smiles during an exam. "I don't know what you're so happy about," he snapped. "You may not realize it, but you're a very sick lady."

And so she was, though she did not want to believe it, and she fights the notion still, holding to the expectation of recovery, of restoration, of a return to things as they were before.

After the surgery came chemotherapy, or more precisely, hormonal therapy. While she was still in the hospital, Lane referred her to Thomas Hakes, a young Ob-Gyn specialist on the solid-tumor service, a former fellow who had been invited to join the staff several years earlier. Hakes started her off on the mildest of known treatments for breast cancer, Tamoxifen, which she would take in pill form for the next five months.

Celine took comfort from the fact that something was being done—the surgery and the medication reassured her, and she wanted to be reassured. She was also grateful not to be getting real chemotherapy. There were some side effects to be expected from Tamoxifen, but nothing on the violent order of what she had heard about chemotherapy, and in a way, the moderateness of her treatment was further reassurance that she was not deathly sick with cancer, not a hopeless case.

What was hard was the disability forced on her, so peculiar a manifestation of a cancer that was still called breast cancer. She wore a cast for six weeks, and when he removed it, Lane told her not to put any weight on the ankle for another six weeks. Unable to climb the stairs to the bedroom that she and Ray share, Celine spent almost three months confined to a bed or the couch downstairs. It was Christmastime, and the many neighbors to whom she had been close for years were generous with fruitcakes and casseroles and errands and Christmas cookies, all of which she was grateful for, all of which helped her to gain weight. Everybody fussed over her, all of them numb with what had happened to her. You could see it months later in the faces of friends who accompanied her on visits to the clinic, before Ray started taking one Monday a month off from his job, as Director of Elderly Services for Passaic County, to be there himself. Friends from the little winding street in Clifton and friends from girlhood, who would look sidewise at Celine with affection and worry, and shake their heads when she disappeared into the changing room outside X ray, or move awkwardly with her walker down the long corridor from the fourth-floor waiting room to the examining room where Hakes or one of the fellows would check her over.

Everybody knew that when it spread it was bad, and Celine knew, too, but remained hopeful. One thing that grew to bother her about her attitude was that she never asked questions. She would mention this often in the spring of 1981, as it wore on her that her ankle had not grown stronger, that her hip, where another tumor had been discovered, did not improve, as the pain in both spots waxed and waned and then grew stronger again, lapping up her reserves of optimism, making it tougher and tougher to keep from panicking. She would say in such moments, a worried, anxious look on her face, "I'd like to ask Hakes whether I'm getting any better," but she never quite put the question, and most Mondays she emerged from the clinic temporarily lifted by his gentleness, and with instructions to continue the Tamoxifen, only to get home and discover again that she still didn't really understand what was happening to her, that she hadn't asked him directly when her ankle was going to be able to take real weight again, or whether the Tamoxifen was working.

Sometimes she would tell herself that she would bring a list, but once she got into the examining room, she seemed to shift to the task of instinctively putting her doctors—Hakes and whatever fellow was working the service that Monday—at ease, and would forget to ask the specific questions that had been nagging at her since the last visit. To their questions, "How are you feeling?" "How is the pain?" she always answered shyly, apologetically, as if reluctant to deliver bad news.

Occasionally, without asking for it, she would come away with specific information, as Hakes had a habit of ending the sessions with a comment about next month's visit. Sometimes it would be that he wanted another X ray, X rays of the known tumor spots being the chief means of checking whether the treatment was working. Sometimes he would ask her to schedule a bone scan for the morning before her next afternoon appointment with him, periodic bone scans being the best way to detect new tumors before they grew large enough for her to be aware of their presence because of pain or a break. And sometimes, when Hakes had enough information to make a decision, he would simply tell her what was happening from the perspective of her X rays, blood counts, and known course of the disease.

Hakes always spoke in a low, uninflected voice, often with his eyes staring down at the floor, and only courteous glances upward punctuating his delivery. Prematurely white-haired, with a small goatee, Hakes looks like a young man got up in the antebellum costume of a Southern colonel, a style at some odds with his diffident personality—a style that Celine, who away from the examining room recovered her sense of humor rather quickly, captured in the title, "the friendly undertaker." In fact she seemed to bring out in Hakes a sort of numbed courtliness that was not apparent in his dealings with Johanne Johnson or other patients. He seemed at times almost frightened of her condition, and he was as careful with her as one is with a vase that's been broken and mended several times.

In March 1981 Hakes told Celine that he would decide by her next appointment, April 13, whether to switch her from Tamoxifen to a stronger treatment, indirectly confirming that she was not doing as well as he would have liked. Before then, she was to see Lane, and by the time of that appointment, April 1, the pain in her ankle and her hip had increased markedly. Reviewing the most recent X rays of her hip and comparing them with ones taken in December, Lane informed her that she had to keep her weight off it or "run the risk of a fracture into the pelvis." Celine had expected the radiation she had had in March to have made a big difference in the hip, and she seemed disappointed to hear Lane say that she needed to keep to the walker faithfully for at least another month, to give the hip time to mend.

But though she was worried about the hip, her chief concern on this visit to see Lane was the state of her ankle. Any pressure on it was excruciating, and it could take no weight at all. "When I put the covers on at night I can't stand it," she told Lane, who by then was in a half-kneeling position at the bottom of the examining table, turning Celine's ankle by single degrees to test it. Almost

135

before she finished describing it, he announced that she needed to wear a brace, and also a splint at night, to prevent torquing of the ankle while it had a chance to heal. If Hakes's manner is subdued, Lane is electrically charged, a little man wearing bright red socks and tie that day, spouting expert opinion with a confidence that only surgeons are reputed to possess. Ray Fink characterizes Lane, approvingly, as a "football coach," energetic, speedy, given to aphorism and slogans rather than long explanation.

After cautioning Celine about the importance of giving both the hip and ankle as much rest as possible, Lane tells her brightly, "People in New Jersey are tough." At which peak point of understanding Celine bursts forth with a relieved "It's not all in my mind, then?" and when Lane shakes his head to confirm the genuineness of her ailments, she summons the nerve to mention a separate and secret dread she's been harboring, that a bump on her head first noticed a few weeks back is another tumor. This possibility will soon be dispelled by X rays, and Ray tells her now to stop counting the bumps on her head, but the problem for Celine is one that is common to many patients: How do you know what is serious and what isn't? What symptoms can be ignored, and what symptoms signal a new disaster? She is caught among doubts, hoping not to be thought silly, but afraid that what has happened not once, but twice, could happen again.

There is reciprocity for several services between Memorial and New York Hospital across the street, and it is to New York that the Finks are directed so that Celine can be measured for her brace and splint. Ray wheels her up and down sidewalks the three blocks from Memorial's clinic to the Orthopedic Appliance department at New York, a little shop in the basement which has the air of an old-fashioned shoemaker's.

The proprietor is a boxy fellow named Sol, whom Celine recognizes from a visit here years before, when she drove a neighbor's daughter in from New Jersey to be fitted for a brace. Sol has the manner of a good-humored garage mechanic, the kind who can make you believe that a cracked block can be put right in no time. He takes a look at Celine's doubtful face and blond hair (lightened as her dark hair began to gray in recent years) and says to her, "What are you doing here? You're just a girl." Celine says later that the procedure reminded her of visits to shoe stores as a child, in the days when it was routine for salesmen to X-ray children's feet for a fitting.

But as she settles into the wheelchair again for the ride back to the car, the dimensions of this setback sink in. "I'd been using my cane most of the time lately instead of the walker," she says, "determined not to pamper myself. And I was feeling ready to start exercising again." The brace and the splint are proof of the handicap that she has been trying to ignore. Dejected, she tells the story of a recent visit to a restaurant with her mother, who is now eighty-seven and fond of asking strangers to guess her age, knowing that the estimates will be decades lower. As mother and daughter entered the restaurant together, each moving along with the help of a cane, Mrs. Dwyer remarked that there were two invalids in the group—which infuriated Celine, who could only answer angrily, "I don't see two invalids."

To sustain hope and sanity, a cancer patient must to some extent practice denial. For some the denial is most powerful at the outset, a great "no" pronounced at diagnosis and given up only gradually as the truth becomes more credible, if not more palatable. For others the denial is fragmentary and cyclical, forming a necessary scrim through which seep enough facts to keep one attuned to reality: one has cancer, but it is under control, going away, being taken care of. Or, one has cancer, but it shouldn't make any difference in how one's life is conducted. Or one has cancer, but one is still healthy—only the cancer separates one from the great body of healthy people.

In some patients denial is made up quite simply of hope alone, and Celine Fink's denial has been like that. Not complicated, but held to, tenaciously and fervently. It is bolstered by a certain defiance of her history as she perceives it—she is determined to bounce back this time, to demonstrate that she is not sickly, but strong, that she is not really compliant, or capable of being cowed, that she will fight. Its flip side is despair and depression and fantasies of bumps on the head turning to tumors, the ordinary alarms of every cancer patient. But though she chides herself for requiring babying and longs to be able to do everything for herself again, she has proved tougher and more realistic than even her doctors expected, and no one in his right mind would ever take her for a hypochondriac, or for anything other than a sturdy woman with a big disease.

One by one, many of the things that have most frightened her about having cancer have occurred. The lump she had waited for all her adult life appeared, and she surprised herself by her lack of hesitation in deciding what to do. She neither panicked nor hid her discovery, and though she put off seeing her doctor for a couple of weeks, it was because she and Ray were about to leave on a long-awaited vacation, and she did not want to give it up. She never considered not having surgery; in fact, she was in a hurry to have it over with. "I'm the same way about having a tooth pulled," she said once.

She remained afraid of surgery, and yet, when it came time for the ankle tumor to be removed, she got through that too. She talked often in the next year of how much she dreaded being thought handicapped, and of the real limits imposed by her disablement, but she managed to resume at least a portion of her normal activities, and prodded by Ray and her sons, she did several of the things she swore she'd never do, like going to Lincoln Center in a wheelchair or attending a big political dinner wearing a long gown and the dull-tan oxfords that go with her five-pound ankle brace. Before getting chemotherapy, she was frightened of losing her hair, and like many patients who have not suffered it, she flinched in sympathy and nervousness from the sight of the many bald heads, wigs and knotted head scarves in the clinic or radiation waiting rooms. And yet when her time came, she managed that too.

Ray came with her for her April 15 appointment with Hakes. The last few days had been among the worst she had known, forcing an apologetic "not so good" from her on the first inquiry. Since the Friday before, she had been in terrible pain. Both legs hurt, from the hip down, and she had spent the weekend in bed, unable to find a comfortable position, and with the painkiller unable to blot out the pain as long as Celine, who remained as suspicious of it as Terry O'Brien had been, was unwilling to increase her dose beyond the original recommendation of one every four hours.

Waiting for Hakes in the early afternoon (they had left Clifton at nine-thirty that morning, in order to pick up the brace and splint ordered two weeks before), both Finks seem slightly on edge. Because of Hakes's mention at the previous appointment that he would make a decision by today on whether to continue the Tamoxifen, they have arrived at the clinic expecting that a change will in fact be made, and they are hopeful that today's visit will inaugurate some new and more clear-cut phase of her treatment. Ray is as usual more sanguine than his wife, and he talks without accusation of the doctors' "trying different things, like an engineer," in the effort to hit on the proper drug. He works at his optimism, taking the long and generous view of most people and of events, at the same time as he tries to package for his wife any good news about her situation. When she says disparagingly of herself, "I'm becoming a bore, all I do is talk about my illness," he tells her that it is not so. And when she goes on to say, "Also, my world is so small, all I do is sit and watch television," he corrects her a second time. "You read, you're interested," he tells her. "Don't be so hard on yourself."

When Ray talks this way, Celine listens to him as if holding her breath, as if wishing she could say, "Stop trying to cheer me up," yet she often says that his countering of her fears is basic to her ability to keep going. Her sons push her along in their respective ways too, David teasing, entertaining, accompanying her to clinic when he is between jobs, bringing one of his acts to her hospital room at the time of her ankle surgery. Larry lugs Russian texts with him when he drives her to clinic on visits home from school, and substitutes for her or Ray as escort for his grandmother, who cannot drive and is fond of frequent shopping expeditions. All this increases Celine's guilt at having been so foolish as to contract cancer. "I feel like such a burden on my family," she says today, as she does so often. "I used to do everything for everyone else. Now I can't do anything for anybody."

Her losses are big in that way, and one of her friends says quietly one day, spontaneously vouching for Celine's former whirlwind pace and high spirits, "You should have known her before. . . .

"I feel so sorry for her sometimes," the friend says. "I go over in the morning, and she's so depressed. If I were in her place, I would probably die of depression. It takes a lot to get her depressed. She has such great hopes. She's such a fighter." And another friend remarks with sympathy that Celine's illness has come at a bad time, with her boys suddenly grown and her active role in their lives inevitably diminishing. But it is hard to conceive of a good time for cancer, of a convenient or plausible time, of an acceptable one. Her sense of being rendered useless after a lifetime of value to others is shocking, but so would it have been five years ago, and so would it be ten years from now.

At three o'clock, the Finks are called to the examining area, where, after examining Celine and reviewing her blood counts, Hakes tells them that he wants to stop the Tamoxifen, have all her areas of pain X-rayed again, and then see her again in two weeks. Although the Tamoxifen seemed to work for a while, Hakes says it does not appear to be helping any longer, and to Ray's question, whether it could have contributed to her sudden increase in pain, Hakes answers that at times, if a medication is not helping, it can hurt. But it is his opinion that the main cause of her pain remains the breast cancer, and he says he suspects that she is not taking enough Percocet to "keep ahead of the pain." Throughout this discussion Celine listens quietly, taking it in but not asking any questions. Neither does Ray press for an interpretation of

Hakes's new orders, and only after they leave the examining area does either of them express the nervousness that the interview has instilled. "It gets me scared when he starts poking around everywhere," Celine says with an uneasy laugh, and while she is having her blood taken for the second time, an unusual occurrence, Ray says of the whole series of decisions just made, "That makes *me* nervous." Hakes's attitude today may have further intensified their alarm, however unintentionally. He was extremely subdued during the exam and unusually solicitous afterward. As Ray wheeled Celine slowly down the narrow corridor to the billing desk, Hakes walked alongside, making small talk in a low voice, and before parting, took her hand in his and twice squeezed it hard, exactly the sort of gesture one makes when there seems nothing more to say.

By the twenty-seventh, the date of Celine's next appointment, she is feeling better and is in less pain. She has increased her Percocet to one every three hours, as Hakes suggested, and is feeling altogether more in control as a result. She is calm, and when she raises the fact that she never asks questions, it is not in the helpless tone of similar comments earlier. She is matter-of-fact about her neglect of her own interests and goes on to speculate more generally on the origins of her cancer, a subject few cancer patients speak of openly, however much it may gnaw at them privately. "I do wonder what causes it," she says thoughtfully, and adds without melodrama, "I wonder whether I'll live long enough to find out how I got it."

Three doctors come and go during Celine's examination: Hakes, an oncology fellow names Tauseef Ahmed, whom Celine knows from earlier visits, and a visiting oncologist from Latin America. Hakes is clearly juggling an overload of patients today, and so Ahmed acts as Celine's primary doctor, conducting her physical and explaining in detail the treatment decision Hakes announced to the Finks before going off to see another patient. He wants to start her on chemotherapy, which comes as no real surprise, since his office had called and asked Celine to have a heart scan done locally the week before. Celine has heard that people her age are generally given a cardiac check before starting chemotherapy, and so she and Ray simply nod when Hakes tells them his decision.

The X rays taken two weeks earlier display the expected lesions, Ahmed explains, including on the skull, but not on the spine. The disease has continued to progress, though slowly, and that is why Hakes is going for the stronger drugs. Ahmed, a tall, dark young man who speaks perfect English with an unfamiliar but entirely understandable inflection, then explains to the Finks what the protocol will be, assuming that Celine chooses to undertake it. It is based on two antitumor drugs, Adriamycin, which Ahmed described as "the single most active agent against breast cancer," and Mitomycin, also active, but not as effective alone. In combination, the drugs have a good record: both are conventional, with known side effects and have been used for several years to treat several different forms of cancer.

Explaining all this, Ahmed is serious, efficient and courteous, pausing periodically to give the Finks as chance to ask questions. They do not, and he continues formally. "However," he says, "this protocol has certain problems which I will tell you about. One is that it can make you nauseated. Another is hair loss." Very soberly, but without really stopping now, almost as if he has memorized this part, having worked out the least upsetting way to put it and not wanting to alter the words, he says, "I suggest that you buy a hair piece right away. There are some good ones on the market, and with the Adria, your hair will probably start to come out exactly two weeks to the day after treatment." That Celine is not devastated as this bad news comes tumbling out is owing partly to Ahmed's calm, partly to the fact that it is what she has expected to hear all along. And then he moves on to the possibility that the Adriamycin will lower Celine's white count, which would make her more vulnerable to infection, and to its possible effect, at a certain high dose, on her heart's functioning. Mitomycin's side effects are fewer and less alarming, primarily lowered platelets.

When he is done, Ahmed hands Celine a sheet that describes the full protocol and explains all the side effects in writing. She and Ray look at it, not quite capable of a careful reading at the moment, and Ahmed tells them that the only thing left to be arranged is whether she will be randomly assigned to the monthly or the weekly group, the patients being treated with this protocol having been divided into two units for research purposes. Except to express her hope that she draws the monthly schedule, which she does, Celine has no comment. She looks up at Ray, who is similarly incapable of thinking what to ask just now, and says to him, "I don't really have any choice, do I?"

A few moments later, Celine, thinking perhaps of how she will soon be sick to her stomach, raises the subject of the water shortage in New Jersey. A dry winter and spring have resulted in water rationing in their area, and in order to avoid a fine, she would like a letter from the hospital certifying her special need. She tells Ahmed that she thinks an extra ten gallons a day would

141

be enough, but he is aroused by the issue and bounces off the chair to say, "Let's make it fifty!" As he starts to write out a letter for her to present to her local water board, Hakes returns and the session grows lively, the tension forgotten as everyone joins in. "I want to get better," Celine says trustingly, hopefully, to Hakes, who says he hopes this treatment will help, and the sooner it's started, the better. He mentions the hair loss, telling her that she should "plan on it, and that in terms of the treatment relieving bone pain, don't look for it too soon. Maybe a month or so."

Meanwhile, Ahmed has finished the water document, to his great satisfaction. He flourishes it above the desk and gallantly hands it to Celine, determined that she should not be so humble about her just rights. "Read it over, please," he tells her, "and see if you think it's adequate, or if," he finishes with flying eyebrows and shoulder thrown back, "you need me to go over and punch someone in the nose!"

The atmosphere has lightened with Ahmed's performance, and the Finks, more relaxed now, manage to ask a couple of questions. Ray wants to know more about the anticipated nausea, and Ahmed says it could be rough but that he will prescribe Compazine, which sometimes helps. Ray asks about the serious risks, and Ahmed says that the monitoring is quite close—Celine will have blood tests every week in New Jersey to keep track of her counts—and the fact that she has not had any previous chemotherapy makes her a better risk.

As they leave the clinic, following Celine's injection, which takes only a few minutes, Ray says, "So, he gave you the least first."

The effects of the chemotherapy did not begin until late that night. To Celine they seemed overwhelming, an uncontrollable nausea that persisted for hours, along with shaking, trembling and an intolerable agitation. "I just didn't know what to do with my body," she said afterward. Despite the warnings from Ahmed and Hakes, neither she nor Ray could quite believe that the violence of her reaction was acceptable. On Tuesday, she reached Hakes on the phone and asked him what she should do. He told her to just stay with it and it would pass. And it did, eventually, though it was hard to believe it ever would. By the middle of the day, the vomiting was over, and by late Wednesday afternoon, she had begun to feel close to normal, with her sense of humor returning. At nine-thirty that morning, she said, two neighbors appeared at the door with gifts of food, a quiche Lorraine and chocolate-chip cookies. "It was very sweet of them," Celine said, and she laughed. "Ray said they must be from the most distant part of the neighborhood."

Shocking as the chemotherapy-induced vomiting was—and Adriamycin is among the harshest of the drugs used in cancer treatment—Celine had now lived through one more event that she had dreaded. Within the week she would go to a dinner dance with Ray, wearing the unhappy brace and foregoing the dancing that she so loved, and in that too she would manage better than she had imagined she might. At her next checkup with Lane, in early May, she hears reassuring words about her ankle ("You can jump up and down on it, if you like," Lane told her) and more cautionary ones about her hip. Lane urges her to protect it carefully, and then performs some fancy footwork to demonstrate the correct way to walk, always starting out with the right foot first. Celine watches with the eye of a longtime dance student, and repeats his motions in pantomime behind her walker, nodding and trying not to laugh out loud. Despite her recent enforced fast, she is still heavier than she was before getting sick, which compounds the difficulty of her already restricted movement, but her arms are strong and she swings the walker easily before her as she goes.

A few days later, her hair begins to fall out, exactly as predicted. It is upsetting, but it turns out to be not the last straw at all, not the end of the world, and when she comes in for her next appointment, in late May, wearing a short wig, she is more concerned with the questions of whether she is getting better and how she can deal with her frustration at being inactive than with the prospect of getting another dose of chemo.

Waiting to see Hakes, she says how much she hates having to ask other people to do things for her, to which Ray says, "I tell her all the time, don't say, 'Would you do me a favor,' just say, 'Do this, get me this.' We know it's necessary. But she thinks it has to be in terms of a favor." Which is true. Just as she cannot get used to being handicapped and berates herself for the limitations her cancer has brought about, she cannot accept the fact that her situation demands this reversal of roles. That Ray and her boys find it acceptable that they wait on her and fetch things she cannot get for herself is of little avail right now. Every "favor" they perform reminds her of what she cannot do for herself; it is impossible to say whether her guilt or her frustration causes her more anguish, but when she permits herself to think ahead, it is the uncertainty that hangs over her that is the most troublesome. What she wants to know more than anything is that this is all only temporary, that there will be a restoration, a certain recovery of mobility and independence. It is a notion that she has held to against the evidence for months, and only now that she has been switched to a second treatment and can report that she feels no lessening of pain has she allowed herself to formulate the question that she has so far avoided asking: "How come the doctor doesn't tell me I'm going to get better?"

Today when Hakes first asks how she feels, she answers, "Pretty good," and smiles up at him from her wheelchair, only to be called on it by Ray. "Tell him the truth," he says, and she laughs and says, good-humoredly, "I didn't say wonderful, I just said okay."

There is a new fellow today, who asks her how she has been feeling lately. Celine seems reluctant to spill out her list of pain complaints, as if it might upset him, and so he has to inquire about areas of the body one at a time. Ray interrupts to say to his wife, "You're making the doctor be a detective," and she speeds up her account, telling him that her ribs hurt, and that the arch of her left foot hurts, and, of course, her hip. The arch is a new area of complaint, and the fellow says he thinks it should be X-rayed. When Hakes reappears, summoned by the fellow, it is to see about the foot, and Celine says apologetically to him, "I hate to be a hypochondriac."

Hakes ignores the remark, and asks her how she has been getting around. "Better than last winter," she says, but she leaves it to Ray to tell Hakes that she is terribly concerned about her inactivity. "She equates activity with health," Ray says, "and she is always talking about all the things we did last summer." Celine looks mildly flustered, and also as if she wishes she were able to explain in particular the urgency of her desire to be up and around. As Ray goes on, in what he means to be an assuaging, helpful way, saying,"Look at the runner who ran across the country on one leg and who died later. There's a certain denial at work," she looks at him as if to say, "Exactly. And why not?"

The struggle goes on all summer long and into the fall. There are two more treatments of Adriamycin and Mitomycin, the last falling on Celine's fifty-third birthday, on June 22. When she comes in that day, Celine is feeling understandably low, but instead of being angry at having to get chemotherapy on her birthday, she feels guilty about her continuing illness. It is a guilt mixed with shame, as if she had done something unpleasant to herself by getting cancer. She mentions having lunch with a group of fellow workers from her former job, and though everything she has said about them and their continuing connection with her over the last six months suggests otherwise, she concludes that she is an object of pity to them. Ray contradicts her passionately. "I think they admire you," he says, and though it is obvious that they have had this or a similar conversation before, Celine looks surprised.

She does not, as Ray tells her frequently, give herself credit. When Hakes asks her during her exam what she's been doing at home, she answers, "A little sewing." From the other side of the curtain Ray adds, "Also, in the cellar." There is a pause, and Hakes asks, "What's in the cellar?" "The laundry," Celine answers, as if expecting a rebuke. But Hakes simply says, "That's okay, just be careful." Encouraged, Ray says he wants to take Celine on a trip somewhere to give her a break, perhaps to Cape May or Honolulu, where David is winding up a three-month tour on a cruise ship. From Celine's side of the curtain comes a slightly exasperated but gentle refusal. "I don't see how I'm going to get around on a vacation trip." The sparring continues a few more beats. When he has finished with his exam, Hakes inquires about her appetite and energy level and watches carefully as Celine steps without the aid of her walker from the examining table to a chair. She tells him that her appetite is good, her energy not so good, and Ray says he'd like to get her into a swimming pool for the exercise she so misses. "I can't go into a pool," Celine says, gesturing at her ankle brace and walker. But Hakes says mildly, "That might not be a bad idea."

Cornered by boosters, she can only laugh and deflect them good-naturedly with a shake of her head. She has not yet accepted that this is the way it is going to be for a while, or perhaps forever, and so, unlike her husband and her doctor, she is not ready to "adjust."

When Celine goes in for her injection, Ray speaks sympathetically of her attitude. "You do feel guilty when you're handicapped," he says. "The social mores of this country make it very hard to be less than perfect, to be sick or frail for any length of time. You begin to think you've lost your value." Though he wants Celine to acknowledge her situation, make the necessary adjustments, and stop feeling guilty, he admits that it is pointless to blame someone for the attitude she brings to a crisis like cancer. "Who knows what shapes us, what the influences are that frame our reactions to something like this?" Because of his work, he is accustomed to the idiosyncrasies of the aged, and respectful of them, and that modifies his frustration with his wife, who has been prematurely handed several of the aged's trickiest problems all at once and who continues to insist, timidly, almost secretly,

145

but also doggedly, on having her old life back in full, not some piece of it only.

Many oncologists talk of the usefulness of patient anger; anger can wonderfully focus the will, just as a resistance to defining oneself as ill can increase one's sense of power, despite all the evidence pointing the other way. Though conditioned to please and to accept, Celine Fink would not let go. It was not her habit to be angry, or oppositional, but she refused to be cheered out of her private sense of outrage at what had happened, and she would not, for most of the first year of her disablement, accept what had happened to her. That was her way of getting back, of resisting, of expressing her fury. She did not rage or lash out, but she was not about to "be a good girl" about this thing.

As the summer of 1981 wore on she felt no better. In July, Hakes told her he wanted to discontinue the chemotherapy program begun three months earlier. Her ankle and hip continued to show new damage, and it was decided that she should have more radiation for pain relief and in the hope of curbing the existing tumors, before starting out on yet a third form of chemo or hormonal therapy. The young radiologist who examines Celine and schedules her treatments pleases her enormously by telling her, "You're too young to be a cripple."

It's the sort of boost she needs. "It's a constant battle to keep her morale up," Ray says the morning of Celine's last radiation treatment. "What happens is she wakes up in the morning— sometimes she actually forgets she has cancer, and then she wakes up to a new day and it hits her all over again. She's begun to count the days. It's eight months, now it's nine months. She worries about the drain on me. But I go to work, think about other things. It's the only thing she thinks about."

In the radiation waiting room, Celine and Ray sit side by side opposite the appointment window before she is called. She has changed into a blue wrapper and leans forward on the lower bar of her walker, which is drawn in close about her chair like a cage so as not to block the way to the treatment rooms. Looking to the left as she talks, Celine suddenly whitens and interrupts herself with a veiled shudder. Too kind to let anything more obvious show on her face, she lowers her voice and says very softly, "I'll never feel sorry for myself again." A moment later, she is called for her treatment, and a figure appears to Ray's and my left, to fill an empty seat. I look up, the way one does instinctively on a bus, to acknowledge a stranger's arrival, and then quickly looked away, seared by an image of a dozen odd-sized lumps, purple, red, pale tan, darker brown, that combine to make up the violently disfigured face of another woman in a blue wrapper. This is the face that made Celine ashamed of her own sorrow. It is the worst I have yet seen—or not seen, for my reaction is so quick, so self-protective, that I am almost afraid I have imagined worse than is there. But the reactions of others in the room tell me I have not. Every pair of eyes takes care not to settle there; in this roomful of affluent patients, citizens with sound insurance policies and still intact faces vibrate the most basic shared dreads—of disfigurement, pain and death.

I am heartless in my terror for long minutes, wishing nothing for my neighbor but that she had worn a veil to hide herself from me. She is not like the little boy I saw with Mrs. O'Brien. He was beautiful, despite the tumor that weighed him down; his skin was smooth and familiar, his eyes, nose and mouth were still the eyes, nose and mouth of a small boy. He was sad, but not alien. This woman is both. Though I am too frightened to check, I am certain somehow that the very features of her face have been transformed by disease, and her nightmare quality expands mercilessly in my imagination in the ten minutes we wait for Celine to emerge. Ray is careful with his eyes too, keeping them downcast, but like his wife, he is too considerate to let anything show on his face, just in case the woman should look his way.

When Celine is ready to go, we flee the waiting room with relief, as one would the vicinity of a snake charmer's unattended basket. The effect of this sighting on Celine is bracing; as she works her way down the corridor, she repeats, "That poor woman," and, "I'll never feel sorry for myself again." And at the restaurant in the theater district where the Finks have decided to celebrate Celine's final radiation treatment, her underlying sympathy and identification with the disfigured woman become clear. What they share is a deep sense of isolation, the knowledge that they are cut off from other people in a big way, in a way that is not easily circumvented by the most devoted friends or loving family. Earlier in the day, Celine had talked about trying to accept the possibility that she might remain handicapped, considering for the first time the idea of adjusting, rather than fighting. "I think if I knew that it was permanent, I'd have adapted by now. We'd make the necessary adjustments around the house, we would have the car fixed for me to drive more easily." All along she felt it was so important to believe that it would pass. Now she is not so sure, and she wonders whether her resistance is cutting her off from things. Similarly, she has begun to think about finding a group of women to join in order to be able to talk about her situation. The hospital, amazingly, does not sponsor such a group for breast-cancer outpatients among its more than forty-five therapy groups of various kinds, and so she will have to find something in New Jersey if she can. Again, it is the sense of being cut off that upsets her and that has grown to be such a big part of her illness.

At lunch, Celine is suddenly overcome with feeling as she speaks of it. "It's hard to talk about how I really feel, even to my close friends," she says, tearful and glancing sideways at Ray. "We go out to lunch and everyone treats me like there's nothing wrong, but when it's over, they go home to their lives and I go home to mine." Her voice is very thin and girlish, but she is getting it out at last, her habitual brave smile failing to mask her pain; Ray tries to comfort her with reasonable words about state of mind, and of how illness is a part of life like anything else, but she talks right through, not hearing him, her own voice like a narrator's making sense of flashing scenes on a screen: "I'm never not thinking about it, it never goes away. Either the pain reminds me of it or the fact that I can't get up and go where I want, or the guilt. It never goes away."

She has finally said it, hit on what allies her to the woman with the pulpy face, and what separates her from her friends and family. Ray, as he has said himself, can go to work and get lost in the problems of other people or the bureaucracy, her boys have their worlds to disappear into, her friends have their own houses, their own troubles. Everyone has somewhere to go to get away from Celine's cancer except Celine. It is always with her, in the dull aches and sharp pains, in the several kinds of pills, in the stool softeners, and the high toilet seat, in the braces and the dull-beige oxfords, in the walker, in the cane, in the wig, in the prosthesis, and in the endless, solicitous "How are you?"s of all who love her. It simply won't go away, and she cannot escape it. *It* is the thing that isolates, the thing that separates, what Sal Giovia was referring to when he said angrily of the world in general, "They say they know what you're going through, but they don't know. They can't."

Relief, when it comes, comes with feeling better, with distraction, with a return to work, with a clean X ray or bone-marrow, or the word *remission* if one is lucky. At the end of August, Celine was handed temporary relief in the surreal form of an eighty-nine-year-old aunt, her mother's older sister, who needed to be taken in. The aunt had lived alone and without disaster in Florida until recently, but now she could no longer, and in the middle of August, Ray flew down to check on her and—as he expected he would have to—bring her back to New Jersey to stay with them.

Though they were not sure how they would manage, there was no question of putting her in a nursing home unless things became very bad, and Ray knew as well as anyone in the state of New Jersey what services were available for the elderly that would make home care possible. There would be visiting nurses, and a woman to come in and help with the housework in the small and already tidy house. Still Celine was anxious at first, less about the effect on her own health and sanity than about her ability to help her aunt when she needed help. "She's so glad to be here," Celine reported a few days later, "she's so grateful for anything we do for her. I'm really touched." All her reports on the aunt are of endearing rather than irritating episodes, and where nothing else has succeeded in taking her mind off her cancer since her surgery almost a year before, the arrival of Aunt May has.

Luckily, the timing is good. Celine's pain has let up for the first time in months, most likely the result of the radiation. And at her next appointment with Hakes, she learns that he wants to try a third program of treatment, a drug called aminoglutethimide, once used for the treatment of epilepsy but discarded because it was too toxic, and now being used again under different conditions to treat various adrenal disorders. In recent months its benefit to some women with advanced breast cancer has been demonstrated, and Hakes wants to try it with Celine. Because it depresses certain of the adrenal hormones, it is to be taken in conjunction with cortisone acetate, which is the likelier of the two drugs to result in side effects, specifically weight gain. Hearing this, Celine, who looks better today than she has looked in months, trimmer, and more supple, able to move around without her walker much of the time, laughs and says, "Oh, great, I'll have to stop eating completely." And when Hakes stops by to speak to her before she leaves and asks whether she understands what they are trying to do, she smiles at him and says, "Yes. I'm going to get fat." He laughs at that and says it may not happen, then goes over the fine points of the medication, stressing the importance of maintaining the body's natural level of cortisone. "If you get a cold, take more. The body usually produces more cortisone under stress, and you won't be producing your own." Hearing this, Ray says blank-faced to Hakes, "We have no stress," and Celine gaily tells him about the aunt's arrival. Hakes looks at her in astonishment, and says, "Maybe you ought to start with three."

Though Aunt May has in fact distracted Celine, after a month the burden begins to tell. The demands of senility are exhausting, and, despite the help they have lined up, Celine is beginning to feel a little desperate, which works to push her out of the house. She has been feeling better physically, with only her ankle acting up, and in late September she reports with great excitement that she drove herself to the store for the first time in nine months. "Ray was worried, but I said, 'I bet I can.' First I drove around the block, then I went to the supermarket. I parked in the handicapped zone and took a basket. A clerk came up to me and said, 'Miss, this is for the handicapped.' I said, 'I am,' and I showed him my cane." There is no reluctance in sounding the word, its sting buried in the victory of the outing. She is suddenly filled with energy again, talking of painting the house, of a trip to Florida in October, of going back to work one day a week. "It feels so good to think about something else," she says. "For so long I've thought about nothing but myself."

The trip to Florida comes off, and the return to work, and for a time—too brief, of course, but long by recent standards—things are looking up. Toward the end of November, Aunt May suddenly worsens, and the Finks have to put her in a home after all, where she dies a few days later. A couple of days after that, Celine, who had been waltzing about with only her cane most of the time, driving to work and the store, cooking for the family, and having "such a good time," is stopped cold when her tumor-weakened ankle collapses beneath her.

The cast in which the ankle is set takes three days to dry, requiring Celine to stay put for that time, and when she sees Dr. Lane in early December, she learns that there are new tumors on her hip. She asks him if that means that the cancer is spreading, and he tells her not to worry about it. But she cannot help but worry. Hakes is "casual" when she queries him, and she begins to feel a distance opening up between her and her doctors. When she sees Lane a few days before Christmas, to have the cast off, he startles her by telling her that he thinks she needs surgery on her hip. "He said it so quickly, I don't know if he'd really thought about it. He was fooling around that day, joking so much that I didn't like it. He said I have two bad legs—I started out with a bad left and now I've got a bad right as well. It's nice when they joke with you, but this was too much."

Things are looking bad all over at the moment. Celine has finally made a connection with another patient, a telephone "pal" arranged with the help of one of the social workers at Memorial. This new contact is a woman who, like Celine, has breast cancer, but Celine is flattened when she learns that the woman's cancer has spread to the bone, the lungs and the liver. "I guess I was looking for someone with a happy ending," she confesses. "This woman is worse off than I am."

Worse news is that Ray's job is in danger; the local November elections have brought in a new state administration and a new group of selectmen in Passaic County, one of whom is threatening to fire Ray and several other people. It is a political mess and may cost Ray the job he has liked best and held for six years. Further, the Finks are concerned that if Ray does lose his job, they will also lose their Major Medical coverage, which would be devastating financially. On top of it all, David has contracted hepatitis, but that, at least, is the kind of medical calamity that is manageable, Celine says, happy to be describing a finite crisis.

Her January 4 appointment with Hakes is unexpectedly encouraging. The fellow working with Hakes, a young woman named Gail Stanton, had been there at her previous visit as well. Celine asks her about the meaning of her ankle's collapse, and Dr. Stanton says they don't believe it's related to active disease. They've had a report from Dr. Lane, and everyone is persuaded that it was a weight-bearing problem. Celine asks about the total hip-replacement that Lane mentioned, but Stanton and, later, Hakes think it may not be necessary. At her last visit, Celine had volunteered the fact that she had a lump behind her right ear, something she had been keeping to herself for six months. Stanton had been able to put her mind at rest, but she remembers how frightened Celine had been and asks her now whether she has any other secrets she would like to unload. Celine says no, and later, when I ask her why she didn't tell anybody about the lump for so long, she is embarrassed. "Oh, I don't know," she says. "Did you think the worst?" I ask her, and she says softly, "Yes."

Despite the last month and a half's trouble, she looks better today than usual—her cheeks are rosy, her hair, which has come back curly, is a glowing white, that very fresh white of the prematurely gray middle-aged. Hakes compliments her on her appearance and asks her whether she has been getting around. She says that she and Ray went to see *Reds;* she calls the four-hour film a "two-Percocet movie."

But in the next couple of months, her mood and her hip go quickly downhill. Ray does lose his job as they feared, and though they are able to continue their Major Medical, the uncertainty of it all and her increasing confinement because of her hip depress Celine so much that she begins to take medication for it. By April, her hip is nearly locked in place; though Lane has been talking about a hip replacement since December, when Hakes reviewed her February bone scan he assured her that there was no worsening. Clearly there had been some mistake, Celine felt. "He said it must be muscle strain, but I kept saying it hurt too much." The pain had never been worse, and by May her mobility was virtually nonexistent. "I couldn't go to the bathroom. I could only get into bed by doing arabesques."

In early May, her two doctors get together at last, and the hip replacement is agreed upon. This time, Celine looks to surgery with relief. She checks into Memorial on a Sunday, May 16, and on Thursday the twentieth, Lane gives her a new hip. He has warned her that recovery will be slow because of all the steroids she has been getting, but two days before surgery she mentions that she has neglected to ask what the prognosis is. "I guess I should have asked," she says. "What I want to know is, will I walk well?"

It is a week and a half before she is out of bed for a trial. A gigantic black stitching seam runs down her right side, from above the hip joint halfway down her thigh; inside, her new hip starts to mend. Celine has been picking up information about hip replacements in pieces—a word from a friend, a few questions answered by Lane in his early-morning visits—but she is going mainly on faith, not quite certain of all the details yet. In the days immediately following surgery, the pain is excruciating, and at the highest permissible dose of painkiller she is not comfortable. Forced to lie flat on her back, she finds everything soon itches and aches, and her insides are locked. Painkiller is a certain con-stipator, and Celine has been barely mobile for a couple of months. But somehow she is cheerful in her misery, grateful for the distraction of visitors and especially for the tenderness of a couple of the nurses on the floor.

After a few days, the hip stops hurting, but the night after she first takes to her feet on crutches, her right knee explodes with pain, a whole new source of it, which Lane explains as a probable strain, this being the first time in months that it has taken any weight. Still, it is shocking. There is so much pain. By slow stages it lets up, and two weeks after the operation, she is approaching comfort again. The nurses help her out of bed every day, and a physical therapist appears to instruct her in simple exercises to help her regain mobility. Contraptions appear: above her bed since she first came in has swung a triangle bar to allow her to lift herself off the bed. Now she is presented with a frame to place over her ankle at night, to keep the weight of the covers off it, and a peculiar gadget that is supposed to help get her stockings or socks on while she still cannot bend her leg. Celine demonstrates this awkward invention successfully after several tries, pleased by its ingenuity and the modest independence in dressing it will provide.

A month after admission, she returns home. Ray speaks of the timing of his continued unemployment as a blessing in disguise, as Celine needs complete attention for several weeks. In early July, they return to see Lane, who is pleased with Celine's progress. She is mobile, if still stiff, and the huge incision has healed quickly. He removes the giant stitches, somehow missing four, as Celine later discovers; these she pulls out at home with a pair of tweezers.

By the middle of July she was again walking without cane or walker around the house. Her gait was jerky and tiring, the hip still not flexible, but it was so much improved that she was persuaded that it could only get better. Her ankle, she understood would not, but the face she made to indicate that this was so also indicated that it was not as worrisome as it had been.

"I feel better," she said, smiling a smile of gratitude that seemed directed indiscriminately at the world, and she was soon talking of other subjects.

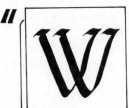"rite this down," Golbey instructs, standing beside the bed in Mrs. O'Brien's hospital room, the sixth she has occupied at Memorial in two years. "I told her to call me whenever she felt bad. She started feeling bad early last night while folding a towel, and she waited until four this morning—no five-thirty," he says, correcting himself, "when I was awake anyway—to call me."

"See?" Mrs. O'Brien hoots. "I didn't wake you up."

"That wasn't the point," Golbey says.

It is midafternoon, Friday, May 22, the start of the three-day Memorial weekend, being celebrated early this year, and the two of them bicker gently, like a married couple staging a quarrel for onlookers, about why she insisted on waiting so long before calling, "I told you to call," Golbey repeats several times. "I know you did," she says, "but I wanted to be sure. I'm an idiot," she says. "I always think I'm imagining things—I don't know whether to take it seriously."

The events of the last twenty-four hours have been rendered nearly comic by her account, and by the fact that she is now safe in the hospital and giddy with oxygen supplied by a tank. She inhales dramatically and gratefully through a pair of flexible, flesh-colored plastic tubes that are loosely anchored in her nostrils. But earlier this morning, and all through the night, she had been sure she was going to die. "I said to Ray last night, 'Something is wrong, I cannot breathe.'" Today she cannot explain what she was waiting for, nor why she kept modifying her complaint whenever Ray or one of the children would say, "Then call Golbey."

It was a case of repeated alarms and repeated retreats. Early in the evening, she recalled, "I'm sitting there at the table with Sean, who's just come home from school, poor kid, and he's eating this huge sub sandwich, and I'm thinking—I can't even breathe, and I'm thinking—Don't be a horse's ass—which is the last thing I should be thinking about myself."

She went to bed early, but hardly slept, awakening short of breath all through the night, until she finally called Golbey, who told her to come in as soon as she could. Still, she would not act on the emergency, and instead of having Ray or one of the boys drive her in immediately, she let the morning unfold as it usually did, taking a shower, packing her things, getting dressed. When Gene arrived around seven, she and Ray, Sean and Chris loaded up and rode into New York together.

Right up to the last minute, she couldn't make up her mind whether she was in real trouble or not. "I'm lying there with my head propped up on the pillow, and I'm thinking, It's a quarter to six, I'm not going to make it to a quarter to nine," (the time she figured she would arrive at the hospital). Yet she also thought there was a chance that Golbey would look at her and send her right home. She tells him this now, and he shakes his head in disbelief. "Anyone who calls me at five in the morning—" "Five-thirty," she says "—to tell me she's dying and then thinks she's going home the same day is crazier than I thought."

It was almost nine by the time she arrived in Bedholding. "The girls downstairs asked me, 'What took you so long?' I didn't want to tell them the story of my life, so I said we got stuck in traffic."

Secure in her breathing now—she hugs the oxygen tube close beneath the bedcover—she asks Golbey to explain what happened. He tells her that her blood counts are way down, causing the breathing difficulty. "Blood is manufactured in the bones," he tells her, "and right now, your bones are taken up with other activities. You're not making enough blood." He does not specify what activities occupy her bones, but she says to him shrewdly, "Am I right that I'm having a bone-marrow?"

"Yes," he answers.

She groans. "I remember the last one," she says. "It was the worst pain I ever had in my whole life. It was horrible."

Golbey tries to reassure her. "It is frightening," he says, "but it's no worse than a root canal. And we're better than a dentist. We can do it while you're asleep. We'll sneak up on you."

"No thanks," she says. "I want to be awake."

They talk of other things for a while, and then she brings up the bone-marrow again. She rolls her head back on the pillow in response to one of Golbey's reassurances. "I'd rather have a baby," she says. "I'd rather be dead."

In midafternoon, Mrs. O'Brien begins getting what are called packed cells, concentrated red blood cells drawn from whole blood, and meant to improve her flow of oxygen. Transfusions have become commonplace, and the line leading from her body to a pack overhead seems as much a part of her get-up as her glasses. Her hand moves instinctively and often to her face, where she feels for the oxygen rig. "I love it," she says fiercely, "I never want to take it off. You don't know what it's like not to be able to breathe. I've never been more scared in my life. I was petrified. I was in a panic. I wondered, Is this the way I'm going to go?" Her small mouth is pursed over her tipped teeth in a little half moon of doubt. "What's next?"

Over the long weekend, she has many visitors from Colts Neck. Ray brings Nancy and Carol in. A young doctor gives her the bone-marrow, and she reports that it was much easier than the first. She can't understand why she was so upset the first time, except that this time the doctor explained everything before he did the procedure. But, despite her good report and the blood support that she has been getting for several days, by the end of the weekend it is clear that something important has changed for her. She is no longer in charge. Her nerves are shot and she can't sleep. Most of the day, she roams the halls until she is too tired to stand up, then gets back into bed until she can't stand it anymore. She can't sit still, and as she watches this happening she comes close to panicking.

When Golbey arrives to see her Tuesday afternoon, after the long weekend, which he had off, she is briefly at rest in the armchair underneath the big window.

"Where have you been?" she asks him, with raised eyebrow, her arms squeezing the wooden arms of the chair. "I've been sticking pins in dolls."

"I felt it," Golbey says.

She lifts her eyes toward the ceiling, then looks at him. "I need a tranquilizer," she says. "I'm like this—" she holds her hands high in front of her to show him how they tremble. As she says this, tears start to well up. She is embarrassed, and says to her roommate, "See, now I'm going to cry because my doctor's here." She fights the tears, and they subside. She turns to Golbey again. "So, you had a nice weekend," she says sarcastically.

"I did?" Golbey replies, amused.

"And now I'm going to have a liver scan. Great."

She tells him that her gums have been bleeding over the weekend. They had started bleeding on and off a couple of weeks ago, and she had been thinking of going to the dentist, she says, but now the nurses tell her it is due to her low platelet count. She looks to Golbey for confirmation.

He nods. "A dentist would say it's not a dental problem, and he would be right." He tells her that he will make sure she has some soft brushes, and she says the nurses already have provided them.

"I really missed you the whole four days," she says, stressing what she considers his long absence.

"I'm sorry," Golbey says.

She smacks the arm of her chair. "See? He apologizes!"

She goes on, while Golbey sits calmly at the foot of her empty bed and listens with a patient smile. "I know," she says, "you have your underdogs do all the work." She hears her mistake and laughs. "I mean underlings," she says, then abruptly changes tone. "What *is* this?" she asks him urgently. "I can't sit still. Is this something new? I've never been like this."

Golbey tells her that he will prescribe something for her, and he tries to reassure her that her nervousness is temporary, a possible effect of the pain medication.

"What *about* pain?" he asks.

"Pain?" she answers casually. "I've got it." She describes a new source, in her side, and Golbey says that it is probably tension.

"But why this nerve business now?" she asks. "I never had it in the hospital before. I don't know why I should feel so bad about being here. Not being home to find out the freezer is broken, the air conditioner is out—is that why I feel so bad I'm here?"

Golbey says he is ordering more platelets for her, and she asks when she can go home. "I'd like to have you not bleeding first," he says.

"That could take forever," she says.

"Well, then, we'll send you home sooner."

She waves her hand at him. "You're impossible."

When Golbey has gone, Mrs. O'Brien repeats her litany of shot nerves. "I can't sleep. I can't sit. I can't think."

Her roommate, Rita, a white-blond in her seventies, nods and says with sympathy, "She's a nervous wreck."

Room 426 is one of the four largest double rooms on the floor, a south-facing corner room designed as a private suite but never used as one because the patient load so exceeded the expectations of the planners by the time the new building was finished. A second, smaller window faces east, and, since Rita and Terry never pull the curtain between them, the space has a friendly, open aspect.

The two women have been roommates for several days, and they have fallen into a simple, wise-cracking friendship. While Rita affects an expression of peaceful indifference, reclining against the bed pillows in her satiny negligee and robe, one tanned, shapely leg rising from the depths to confirm her excellent muscle tone, Terry invites her visitors to guess Rita's age within a decade. They are equally tickled by the diplomatic estimates coughed up by flustered O'Briens and friends. No one comes near seventy, though whatever age Rita is, it has nothing to do with youth but rather genes and careful preservation. "Can you believe this one?" Terry says of Rita proudly. And Rita, as solid and self-sufficient as a Cadillac with a full tank, coos, "Oh, Terry." Mutually solicitous, each seems to know when to talk, when to fall silent, and each seems to believe that the other has drawn the crueler sentence.

Now Rita can see that Terry is bursting, and she says, "Two weeks in this place! I'm gonna have some bill. But what's money, hey, Ter?"

"That's right," Mrs. O'Brien answers.

"So I *don't* have anything left to will to anybody. I spend it all on myself."

"Let 'em get their own," Terry says.

Rita smiles. "I'm feeling more relaxed now, Terry."

"Well, you're all done, that's why," Terry says.

Rita corrects her. "I'm getting chemo tomorrow."

"That's right."

"But then I'm going home, I think."

"You are?"

Rita nods. "Gonna miss me, Ter?"

"Sure," Terry says, then turning from Rita she adds, "This is the one who didn't even want to come in. Look at her!"

The phone rings. It is one of her children. "Hello, brat," she says, smiling. "Who is this? Carol or Nancy? How are you, honey?"

There follows a long confused conversation about how the daughter in question cannot get her money out of a savings account without her mother's signature. Exasperated, Mrs. O'Brien finally says, "Get your father to give you the money and I'll straighten it out when I get home." Pause. "I'm *sorry*." She starts to steam. "There's no other way to do it." She sighs, puts her hand over the mouthpiece and says, "O-o-o-h, they're really worried about me. Now they're fighting." She speaks into the phone again, sounding impatient. "You obviously don't know what you're doing," she says sharply. A moment later she is soothing. "That's a good girl. Right, you've got it, right." She is silent, with a concerned look on her face as her daughter tells her something further. "Call the police?" she asks doubtfully. "Going fifty-three in a forty-mile zone? Listen, have you got any good news? It all sounds bad from here." The conversation ends a few seconds later, with a fulsome, "I love you, too."

She hangs up the phone, slides off the bed and announces, "Jesus, Mary and Joseph, I'm going to get a tranquilizer."

When she returns, still fretting, Rita tries to reassure her. "Your feelings change every day, Terry. I felt awful yesterday, remember, and now I'm much better."

Mrs. O'Brien waves the advice away. "That was yesterday," she says. "Sure. Today you're fine, tomorrow you're dead."

The following day is a little better. She has had visitors from Colts Neck, she reports, but had a hard time paying attention to them. Speaking of Golbey, she says, "He thought I would be able to sit and relax in here. Not this time."

Her only distraction today is Rita, who is in a state over the chemotherapy she is about to receive. When she asks Terry if it hurts, her voice is cracking like a child's.

"It's nothing, really, Rita," Terry says, "like giving blood." Rita shivers in the sun that bathes her bed. Mrs. O'Brien talks about how scared she was the week before at the prospect of a bone-marrow, and how it had turned out to be not half as bad as she had imagined. Rita keeps on trembling, until Terry says she can't stand it, and goes to find the "chemo girl." She finds a nurse in the hall, relays the message, and returns to talk to Rita some more. "It's nothing, really," she repeats. "I always come alone for my treatments," she says.

After a while, she tires of the direct appeal and picks up a Rubik's cube someone has given her. She starts to play with it, absently at first, then with concentration. "If I get this, you got to smile," she says to Rita, then twists furiously at the multicolored block, gritting her teeth and bearing down comically, as if strength would do the trick. "Get over here, you son-of-a-bitch," she mutters, succeeding in arranging no more than a single row. She exhales and laughs. "This is how to drive people in Sloan-Kettering crazy," she says, and places the cube on the window ledge with a sigh.

She changes the subject quickly, as much to relieve her own

tension as to distract Rita, who stares at her like a worried dog, all her nerve flown. Mrs. O'Brien says that when Ray called earlier in the day, he reported that he "loves what the decorator wants to do"—explaining to Rita that Ray had had to meet the man alone last night because she was in here. She is full of other domestic details more believable than the image of Ray O'Brien swooning over wallpaper choices. She jokes about messages from her daughters at home. "Hem my clothes before you die!"

While she is talking, Rita suddenly starts to weep. "I'm a terrible coward, I know," she says when Terry tries to comfort her. "No you're not, Rita," Terry says, "you're just scared." She stares helplessly at Rita, then her face hardens. "Why does God *do* this?" she says, furious, her voice low. "You're seventy-six years old, you've led a good life, and He says, 'Plop. Here. It's your turn.'"

The I.V. nurse arrives and Terry gets up from her chair. "Can I help?" she asks. "I've had chemo." Rita says eagerly, "Yes, please," and the nurse nods. Terry pulls a straight chair over between the two beds and takes Rita's right hand, while the nurse finds a vein in the opposite arm. When the nurse is about to insert the needle, she says to Rita, "Do you want to look away?" Rita's eyes bulge, and she says, "Yes," and turns toward Terry. "I'm afraid I'm going to vomit," she says.

"You're not going to vomit," Terry says calmly.

"You're so good to me," Rita says, then winces as the needle goes in, and is surprised that merciless pain doesn't follow.

Just then Golbey enters the room, accompanied by a young fellow named Steven Berman,* whom Mrs. O'Brien had met for the first time the week before. She looks up from her post at Rita's side and says coolly, "Is there anything I can do for you?"

"I see you've found employment," Golbey says.

Mrs. O'Brien moves from between the beds to the other side of the room as soon as Rita's chemo is finished. Golbey reports that the liver scan done the day before was fine, but that her platelets are still low. She nods. "What else is new?"

"What we need now," Golbey says, "is the passage of time. In the meantime, go up on the Tamoxifen. I'd like you to go to four a day for a couple of weeks."

"What about oxygen?" she asks. "I'm afraid of that happening again."

Golbey tells her that if she is worried, she can get a supply of

---

*Pseudonym.

miniature oxygen bottles to keep at home. She asks whether he thinks it will happen again. "Or would you rather not say?" she adds. "It could," Golbey says. "Right now, though, your blood count is great. If it starts coming down again, we'll give you more blood." As he prepares to leave, he assures her that, other than the platelets, everything is for the moment under control. "That's great," she says, "because I would never want to come into the hospital again not breathing." When Golbey has gone, leaving a residue of gravity behind, Terry turns to Rita and says, "It's always frightening when they take you too seriously. The best thing is when they say, 'You little bitch.' But when even Ray starts with, 'Now take care of yourself,' I start to fade. At least when they yell at you, you can yell back."

When she leaves the next day around noon, it is with the cancer multiplying in her bone marrow, in a race with the healthy cells still there. She sleeps through the afternoon and all night, barely opening her eyes to greet Ray when he comes home. By coincidence, Ray has kept a long-standing appointment with their lawyer that Thursday, to update their wills, a chore he attends to periodically. Speaking of it the following day, he acknowledges its fresh meaning this year. It is clear to O'Brien that something big has changed for his wife this last week, both in terms of her confidence and her physical condition. He talks about how powerfully she has held to the conviction that something would eventually go right in her treatment, how if she could just persist in living, her life would not end.

"She never gave up," he says. "Maybe until now. I don't know. This tranquilizer business upsets me. I've never seen her like this. I don't know whether it was the trouble breathing, or the pain, or what, but I think something has changed, frightening her. I think she woke up in the middle of the night last Thursday and thought she was going to suffocate."

He is speculating, he knows. He can't be certain. "She's a very proud woman," he says. "It's hard to know what goes through her mind. She holds back, even from me." There is a limit, he indicates, a border of long standing that he cannot cross. She is so used to protecting him and the children that she doesn't know how to stop.

O'Brien draws a sharper picture of many things than his wife does. Certainly his reading of his children's attitudes toward their mother's condition is more explicitly formulated than hers, though it is hard, he concedes, to tell what they really think. "The two younger girls don't confide in me," he says. "If it's something important, they tell me, but otherwise they confide in their mother. The older ones are more outspoken," he says, with a laugh that connotes understatement. Of Nancy and Carol, fifteen and seventeen, O'Brien says, "whether they realize that their mother is almost certainly going to die, I don't know." Sean, on the other hand, simply "doesn't believe it. He believes in miracles," his father says fondly.

The three older children do not. Raymond comes to visit his mother when she is in the hospital, and often on weekends, with his new wife, but he says very little. Chris, who is still living at home, sees his mother declining day by day and can barely bring himself to come to the hospital, though he does. His mother has mentioned with sympathy how painful it is for him, and reminded of this now, his father nods and recalls his own visits to *his* father's hospital room, in the old Memorial. "It was very depressing."

Of all the children, Sue is the most able to speak directly about what is happening. "Sue says forget the chemo," O'Brien says, "leave her in peace." He looks both intrigued and mildly alarmed as he reports this. "Doctors have to be a little cynical," he says, "but it shocked me. Though I don't know," he adds. "She may be right."

One of the difficulties he's having is figuring out just what is happening. There is the obvious, and then there is the residual hope that he keeps discovering whenever he begins to think there is no reason for any. It is hard to get a definitive answer from Golbey, he says, and there is the added problem of his own reluctance to pursue one. "I realize I treat Golbey differently than I do other people," he says. "Ordinarily, I would screw somebody to the wall if he didn't give me a straight answer, but with him I hold back. Businessmen are constantly putting their necks on the line. They have to deal in probabilities. They're forced to. But I'm planning to call him again today, and I'm sure he'll tell me he doesn't know. I feel like saying, 'Who the hell are you not to give me an answer?' Yet, I'm sympathetic. I like him personally, and he's been very good with Terry. Plus, they're breaking new ground, and people do react totally differently to these things. So how can they say?"

Hard as it is for him to let go of the idea that something can be done, he has finally allowed himself to read Golbey's responses as adding up to exactly that. "I just have the feeling he's never going to give her any more chemo. Maybe I'm just discouraged, but the way things are going, I don't expect she'll live to Labor Day. Maybe," he tries again, but his voice lacks conviction, "maybe if she got strong enough and they hit on something with

162

the chemo—" He tries another time. "The thing I'm afraid of is that she's too weak now; she won't ever be able to stand the chemo."

Before lunch, O'Brien had been to a noon Mass at a church across the street from the bank, a habit seldom found among middle-aged bank executives, even Catholic ones. But although there are things Ray O'Brien can take or leave about his church, he is essentially devout, and his religion means a lot to him. He is hoping that it is going to help him now. "Both of us believe in our religion," he says. "I *think* that makes a difference." He squints and resettles his gold-rimmed glasses on his nose.

"Also," he says, pursuing what he must think are optimistic thoughts, "as you get a little older, you get a little less afraid of the unknown—" He cuts himself short with a shudder. "How can *I* say that," he says, frowning. "*She's* the one."

There is really no way out, no comfort to be found. He would so like to believe that because it is inevitable it is also somehow tolerable. It is not.

He is silent for a while, and then starts to talk of his wife as he thinks of her, not wasting daily, not in pain, but as the tough and continually surprising woman he has known for thirty-three years. He speaks in a burst of affection, as if to shore up his memory with her virtues in advance. "She's done what she wanted to do," he says proudly. "Her family is her life and she's been a wonderful mother. She's a *professional* mother," he says, invoking the adjective with respect. "It's the one thing that really mattered to her. She's not a competitive woman. She's not trying to have a better dinner party than you or be the best-dressed woman at some event. Consequently, she doesn't have any enemies."

Over the weekend, Ray O'Brien will explain to his two younger daughters that from now on they will have to take turns staying with their mother whenever he and their brothers are at work. She is too weak to be left alone, and he doesn't want her to ever wake up and not be able to breathe without someone there to help her.

Also on the weekend her gums begin to bleed again and she complains that the Percocet is not helping. She switches to the Dilaudid that Golbey prescribed, and she gets some relief, but at the price of a terrifying side effect: her words won't come out right. She mixes up her children's names and can't say what she means. The first few times it happens, she is able to laugh at it, but when it doesn't go away, she is badly frightened.

Her next scheduled appointment with Golbey is for Tuesday,

June 2. She wakes early that morning after a bad night, gets up, showers, dresses, and then lies down on a couch downstairs until it is time to leave for the city. Nancy has been appointed to accompany her mother to the clinic; it is Carol's last day at school before her graduation, and everyone agrees that she should not miss it.

This morning there is no wait. Mrs. O'Brien and Nancy have not yet sat down when Golbey calls them at nine-fifteen. As soon as Golbey sees Mrs. O'Brien, he asks whether she wants to be admitted. She says she'd rather be home, even though she feels terrible, because she couldn't sleep the last time she was in the hospital. But she is very upset by her mental confusion, she tells him, and wants to know what can be done. "What good is the medication doing?" she asks. "The pain is shooting across my back, down my legs." Her lips are thinly crusted with blood that she repeatedly licks off or dabs at with a tissue. Her body is stiff and she moves as little as possible, slowly, and with Nancy's help.

Golbey tries to explain the complications of pain medication, of how difficult it is to hit the right dose of the right drug, of providing relief without knocking her out or making her miserable in a new way. Morphine, for example, used for what Golbey calls "intractable pain," is generally reserved for bedridden patients because, among other things, it can cause severe constipation and nausea. Because it needs to be given by injection, it is also impractical for outpatient use. Dilaudid, what Mrs. O'Brien is taking now, is a morphine derivative that can be taken orally and is somewhat less hard on the system. But anything potent enough to give her relief is likely to cause some degree of drowsiness and confusion. Golbey tells her that she does not sound as confused as she thinks she does, but Mrs. O'Brien is not persuaded. This is what she has been trying to avoid all these months. She tries to joke about it but has a hard time. For what must be the first time in her life, she is afraid of her own speech, for fear of what she might say without meaning to.

There is no question of her getting chemotherapy today, but Golbey orders two units of packed cells to relieve her breathing difficulty. He tells her to continue the Tamoxifen, and he adds another drug to go with the pain medication, in the hope of reducing the pain medication's side effects.

She is barely hanging on today, brittle, tentative, scarily thin. Her face is tiny and drawn, and her head trembles on her neck like a flower too heavy for its broken stem. She seems held together by the clothes she wears, winter clothes in June, a gray cardigan over a blue knit shirt, dark-blue slacks. The sneakers have been replaced by beige slippers.

164

Nancy boosts her mother onto the bed in the transfusion room, and, settled there, Mrs. O'Brien recovers for a moment, seeming almost lively as she tells of the start of her speech trouble over the weekend. She struggles to enunciate, as if that were the problem, but it is not so much a slurring of speech as a literal slowing, the words coming out in syllables, as if she is falling alseep. Her eyes, in fact, close from time to time, and if she is sitting upright, she begins to sway from side to side. Then suddenly she will catch herself and start to speak again. "I can *tell*, I can *tell*," she repeats. "I can make myself say it right," she says. "But sometimes I start to fall asleep, and then I say things that don't make sense."

She winks and looks at Nancy. "Nancy was dying to come with me today," she says. Nancy ducks her head and lifts it again quickly. "I didn't care," she says, meaning "I didn't mind." Except for smiles, which come and go when her mother says something funny, Nancy's face is expressionless, suggesting a firmly checked terror at her surroundings and her mother's condition. She is a pretty girl with thick, shiny, dark hair that swings past her cheeks when she moves. She looks more like her father than like her mother, with thick eyebrows and blue eyes, and she blushes whenever her mother calls attention to her.

"Isn't this better than going to school?" Mrs. O'Brien says at one point. Nancy seems unsure of what to say, then goes for honesty, the family habit, and says cautiously, "No-o-o-o, because it's the seniors' last day." Mrs. O'Brien says, "But you want to help your old mother, don't you?" Nancy shrugs uncomfortably and nods, Yes. It's an awful moment for a fifteen-year-old to live through, and the months of protection that Mrs. O'Brien has insisted on for Nancy and Carol suddenly seem simultaneously foolish and wise.

When Nancy goes off to get some lunch, Mrs. O'Brien seems relieved, as if her daughter's continued appetite were some guarantor that she will come through this all right. "She sees enough," Mrs. O'Brien says. "She doesn't talk about it. She hears the word *cancer* of course—I say it all the time." She considers a moment, then says, "I think she'll take it very well." She fades in and out as her mind wanders. When she is coherent, she seems a frail woman in her late fifties, terribly tired and sick; when the words don't come and her eyes go glassy and flat, she is an old woman, senile, floating out of reach. She catches herself repeatedly and is furious, struggling to regain control, screwing her face tight with concentration, muttering "damn" under her breath. Occasionally she sighs and shifts her position, and at one point she blurts out, "The *pain*. Is this the way I'm going to die? I'd like a little less." She's still not asking for a lot.

Earlier she sipped from a can of Sustecal that she had brought with her, a protein supplement that Susie has been giving her for several weeks, and which is about all she can get down, and then from a vanilla malted that Nancy bought in the coffee shop. Now she slips in and out of awareness as the thick red packet empties into her arm but stirs awake when her daughter returns from lunch, and she asks for help in sitting up. Nancy grabs her mother's hands and forearms firmly and pulls her steadily into a sitting position, lowering her legs over the side of the bed.

"Hand me my pocketbook, will you, Nancy?" Mrs. O'Brien asks. She takes a compact and a tissue from her bag, inspects her lips, now dry-caked with blood from her gums. She smiles narrowly, facetiously in the mirror, and groans at the sight of her pink teeth. She sips water from a paper cup, wipes her lips and teeth clean, then powders her mouth carefully, as if applying lipstick. She hands all her things back to Nancy and lowers herself back onto the bed.

Midway through her first packet of cells, Golbey appears in the transfusion room. He is about to leave on a five-day lecture trip, and it is clear that he thinks it is a bad time to be leaving this patient. He did not really have to come down just now to see her, so his presence alone has an edge to it, which he tries to soften with advice about pain medication. He tells her to stick with the Dilaudid–Tylenol III combination every four hours. "If you need to, you can cheat on that a little," he says. "It won't hurt. And take a Valium at bedtime if you're not sleeping."

The two of them choose their words carefully, avoiding the possibility that is foremost in both their minds. When Golbey finally moves toward the door, Mrs. O'Brien smiles at him and calls, "Goodbye, Doctor. Lord Have Mercy."

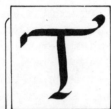he first phase of treatment for acute lymphocytic leukemia, called induction, lasts approximately thirty-three days. Remission may take place within a few days of the start of treatment or not at all, though that is rare. Jimmy Polack was brought into remission thirteen days after beginning chemotherapy, while Sal Giovia, who was much sicker at the outset was brought in after nineteen days. Both boys were released from Memorial within a month of admission and received their last combined doses of induction-phase chemotherapy in the clinic, as outpatients.

Having started treatment almost a month before Karyn Angell, they were ready, after a two-week break, to begin the second phase, called consolidation, before she had completed her first. Karyn felt the contrast between her experience and the boys' intensely. Not only did her slower recovery mean that she had to stay in the hospital longer, it had possible long-term implications as well, since there appeared to be a statistical correlation between the speed with which a patient comes into remission and the remission's length. By that measure, Karyn stood a fractionally greater chance of suffering a relapse within the first five years following remission, assuming that it occurred, and awareness of this made the last couple of weeks' wait for remission especially tough. Yet, however frightening, the long-range implication of her slow response was more easily pushed aside than the day-to-day frustration of being confined to the hospital and the knowledge that she still had close to a year of intermittent inpatient treatment ahead of her.

As part of the clinical testing of L-17M, Karyn, Sal and Jimmy had been randomly assigned on admission to one of two versions—one long, one short—of the consolidation phase of treatment. The purpose of the trial was to see whether the modification being tested, the short version, would further reduce the incidence of early relapse in patients who achieved remission. The over-all results Memorial had been getting with the L-17M program were appreciably better than with previous protocols, but there remained a period of particular danger of relapse— within the first six months—that they hoped to correct with a consolidation course that, though abbreviated, was more intense.

The original L-17M consolidation sequence called for six separate courses of chemotherapy, entailing six separate hospital stays of roughly a week each, broken by rest periods of twenty-one days and followed by two weeks of outpatient treatment. By the most optimistic estimate, this phase of treatment would last close to five months. Realistically, it could be expected to last considerably longer. Even if nothing else went wrong—and the possibilities for disaster were many—the risk of infection following each course of treatment, when counts were at their lowest, meant that the actual number of hospitalizations on the long arm of consolidation would be closer to ten or twelve. Each extra stay could delay the next treatment by several days (hospitalizations for fever usually last seven to ten days), so that the actual total would be more like six or seven months.

The modification being tested, however, called for only two week-long courses of inpatient treatment, with a hiatus of three to four weeks and two weeks of outpatient treatment following. Assuming two hospitalizations for fever, one could still be done with the short consolidation in a couple of months and, barring disaster, certainly within three.

If the short arm of the protocol had not already been designed, surely someone in Hematology would have thought it up to accommodate Sal. Coaxing him through six to twelve hospitalizations might well have finished off his vigorous parents; what it would have done to Sal is unimaginable, but as it turned out, he drew the short protocol on admission.

Karyn and Jimmy drew the long arm of L-17M, turns of fate that the rules decree should be left undisturbed. In Karyn's case it was, and she remained assigned to the long consolidation, but when Dr. Gee thought about the effect it would have on Jimmy— adding as many as three or four months to his stay in New York—he raised with the Polacks the possibility of switching him to the short protocol. The abbreviated consolidation phase had been designed to correct some weaknesses in the current treatment but did not represent a radical departure from it, and there was every reason to believe that it would be just as effective, if not more so—the determination of its possible superiority being the point of the trial. In Jimmy's case, the additional advantage was clear, at least to him and to Dr. Gee: the sooner he got back to normal life and his own friends, the better off he would be, emotionally and medically.

The Polacks had come to New York prepared to stay as long as necessary, and Morris Polack had a particular faith in Dr. Gee that made him glad they had come. Yet he too knew that Jimmy would be better off at home, as long as it was safe. In New York, Jimmy had his grandparents' deference, unprecedented indulgence, his choice of restaurants to eat in (and when he wasn't sick or recovering from being sick, he was a ravenous, adventurous eater, eager to try everything New York offered), his own room and bathroom (Valerie slept in the living room), and the knowledge that his three companions would have traded places with him in an instant if it had been within their power. Still, it was a cage, as everyone in it with him knew. Reassured by Dr. Gee, the Polacks agreed to the change and Jimmy started counting backward to the day when he could start home.

With some conniving, Philomena Casey, the woman in charge of scheduling leukemia patients for inpatient treatments, arranged for Jimmy and Sal—who had spent New Year's Eve together drinking champagne in the hospital—to start consolidation on the same day, February 9, 1981, in adjoining single rooms on the twelfth floor. February 9 was a Monday, but to insure that they actually got their rooms, both boys were officially admitted over the weekend, then went home on overnight passes. When they returned Monday morning, they slipped away from their families and took a tour of the hospital that led them straight into the path of the president of the hospital, who reacted with professional calm to the sight of these two semihysterical bald teenagers exploring their temporary home. Jimmy at the moment was wearing a Christmas wreath picked up in the lounge, and Sal was passing himself off as a doctor. Words were exchanged, and snorts of muffled laughter, and then the two candidates for chemotherapy retreated to their rooms.

Sal's parents have gone off on an errand in the city, to return later in the afternoon, but at mid-day Jimmy's room is occupied by Mrs. Polack and Valerie, who have only the barest dampening effect on his mood. He reels off the schedule of treatment that will rule his life in the coming months—"I'm in all week this week, then a month off, another week in, then a month, then two weeks of Monday, Wednesday and Friday, then the same thing again." He smiles. "Then back to Seattle."

He jokes with the nurse who comes in to take his blood pressure and temperature. Mrs. Polack and Valerie, who dresses always in black, as if trying not to call attention to herself, look on. They watch him fearfully, as if at any moment he might evaporate. Valerie tries to keep her solicitude in check and from time to time breaks her pensive expression with smiles as she watches Jimmy. Her mother can't, and wears a permanently fretful look on her handsome face. She makes small noises with her teeth as she listens to him tease the nurse. "Our mood swings with his," Valerie says, nodding her head toward Jimmy. "But when you get too optimistic, you become insensitive in his eyes."

Mrs. Polack's mask of grief never softens as she adds, "We all hope he comes out of it, but once you have this thing, you're labeled." She squints in emphasis as Valerie interrupts her softly. "It depends on who your friends are," she says.

Though he can hear every word, Jimmy elects not to comment. Instead, he says to the nurse, "What if I get seasick and have to blow chips?"

"Talk English," she answers, amused.

As Sal is being prepared next door, the nurse notices a faint red rash on his body. When asked, he says it itches a little. Also, yes, he's been around other kids lately. He stopped by his high school the other day to see friends. And he's been to discos. A frantic scene follows. The rash looks to the nurse like scabies, a minor infection to ordinary people, but a potential plague on the floor, where most patients are being treated with chemotherapy and are, like Jimmy and Sal when their counts are low, terribly vulnerable.

Hearing this and picking up the general alarm—more nurses rush to his room from the station down the hall—Sal's face freezes and then cracks as he gives way to the kind of embarrassed hysteria that usually overtakes a person in church or in a hushed concert hall. "We've been all through the hospital!" he shouts, unable to keep a straight face. Emerging from his room next door, Jimmy says, "He was up on the twenty-first floor. The president of the hospital shook his hand." The two friends spin madly around the little anteroom between their respective rooms and the hall, banging against the walls and laughing. "I've got *scabies*," Sal says, lifting his eyebrows like Groucho Marx. "I've got *leprosy!*" Jimmy howls.

The nurses finally separate them again, return each to his room and post a sign on Sal's door pending determination of whether he's really got scabies. When the Giovias arrive shortly after, they are told they must wear masks and gowns into the room. They shake their heads and wave at the Polacks through the open door to Jimmy's room, then suit up. They look weary, like the parents of a colicky baby. Two months into this thing, there is little that surprises them. Rose Ann rolls her huge, mascaraed eyes as she ties the mask over her face. Sal senior blows air through his teeth. They peek into Sal's room through a crack in the door, then disappear behind it.

By evening, the alarm is over. Sal does not have scabies; he has not brought the hospital to its knees. He and Jimmy are started on medication. During this stay, they will receive three different drugs more or less simultaneously, starting with the antitumor antibiotic Daunomycin in an intravenous feed over three days. Ara-C is given in an I.V. push the first day, then by continuous infusion for the five days following. A total of ten doses of 6-Thioguanine will be given as well, two a day, starting with the infusion of Ara-C.

Within a few hours, Jimmy and Sal are both thoroughly, violently sick. Jimmy later reports that he lost track of his own vomiting after the fifth time, of Sal's after "about the fifteenth." Mr. Polack, who routinely disregards the posted visiting hours and can be found in Jimmy's room anytime between six in the morning and midnight, often playing a quiet game of chess with his grandson, teases Sal a couple of days later about his behavior. "You were cursing the other night, Sal," he says. "You're a Catholic," he says, winking, hoping for a reaction, "but you curse." Too weak to make a response worthy of his reputation, Sal waves and says something in a low voice about God having to understand.

Tuesday is a lost day for both boys. Exhausted by sickness, they sleep on and off into Wednesday. By midafternoon that day, Sal, still plugged up to his I.V. pole, is alert, restless and irritable. Though he is flat on his back and supposedly enervated by drugs, his motor races. His fingers play up and down the tubes that hang from his pole overhead, or nervously switch stations on the miniature television set that extends from the wall on its own retractable boom. He pulls the screen to within an inch of his face and stares at it without interest, yet intently, as if scanning the flickering lines. It is something to look at, its chief virtue being that it projects something other than what is going on in this room.

His mother returns from the lounge down the hall, where she has been having a cigarette. Since Sal got sick, she has lost ten pounds and started smoking again, and though she is always quick to make a joke out of the calamities that seem to increase with each day, her thin, pretty face is showing wear, the bags under her big eyes sagging lower and lower beneath her makeup. At times she seems held together by her sense of humor alone, and now as she sits down next to Sal's bed, he turns to her without warning and says, "You know, I might not have hair for three years." Rose Ann looks startled. Sal turns his head from her sharply and stares overhead, his fingers playing the I.V. tube frantically. "Why didn't you tell me?" he asks her accusingly. "You shoulda told me," he says, slurring his words. He says he has just asked one of the nurses and been told that there's a chance he could keep on losing his hair with every couple of cycles of treatment.

"Sal," his mother says, "we told you we didn't know—that's what they told us. It could happen, but it might not." He turns his head away again. "I told people June," he says.

He stares at the ceiling for a minute or so, then shrugs. "I can take it, it don't matter," he says. "But you should have told me."

Mr. Polack appears at the door. Jimmy is asleep, and, as he often does, he turns to Sal, toward whom he feels obviously paternal affection and a fair amount of shocked amusement. Mr. Polack is a collector of horror stories about leukemia, as if only by knowing the worst that could happen can he coach Jimmy clear through to safety. Now he starts to tell Sal about a girl he has heard of who felt so good after two years of remission that she quit chemotherapy, only to relapse. Sal sighs. "I'm not a moron," he says.

When Polack has returned to Jimmy's room, Sal turns to his mother with the manner of someone setting the record straight once and for all. "I don't plan on quitting, but it's all got to be according to what I want. The treatment of the disease, everything." He points next door. "If you're too protected, you give up."

Sal's strategy against leukemia is to resist, and it is manifest in every movement of his wiry body. In the enormity and openness of the Polacks' alarm over Jimmy—and over Sal, for whom Valerie and Mrs. Polack share an affection, and about whom they worry too—is a suggestion that the opponent may be too powerful after all. Sal doesn't want to hear it, nor does he want to have to listen to them exhorting Jimmy to be a good boy.

On Thursday, Sal senior takes his wife's place in the room. He makes and receives business calls, trying to keep his livelihood in order in the middle of chaos. There are casting calls for commercials, the possibility of a movie role, and weekends at Gross-inger's to be arranged. Sal needles him about talking on the phone all the time, and Sal senior retaliates with a Borscht Belt line or two about paying the bills. He remarks on how different Sal's mood is this time around. "Last time he was running around, cheering people up. This week it's harder. The drugs are rougher." He is sympathetic, and Sal notices.

Gesturing toward Jimmy's room, Sal junior says, "She [meaning Mrs. Polack] thinks we're sick, we're gonna die."

"So, what do you think?" his father asks.

Sal laughs. "I think I'm sick, I'm sick." He pushes the subject along. "Some jerk at school asked me how long I'm gonna live," he says. "I told him ninety. Another friend, he saw the story about me in the paper and says to me, 'I don't like what they're printing about you.' That I have leukemia," Sal says. "I told him, 'It's true.'" He pauses a moment, then with a disbelieving shake of the head relates a third reaction. "Another friend said to me, 'Sal, I *knew* you.'"

Hearing these remarks, his father wants to say how terrifically Sal has handled the sometimes difficult responses he gets from people. "My friends who are comics say he cheered them up when they called." Sal, with a satisfied nod, concedes that this is true. Another time he will remark on his presence in the hospital, "Other people get upset, but I'm here to joke around," but he's got the down side on his mind right now and is not ready to let it go. "Some people think I'm doing this for attention," he says. "As if I have a choice." His exasperation grows, and he slaps the tiny television lightly. "Some people call up to tell me how sick *they* are."

Sal senior says it's hard to find a balance. A lot of people are concerned, and they all have their own ideas of how to show it. "Some are overprotective. Others try to make light of it, not knowing what to say. If we say he's doing great, they say, 'See—we told you you were worried for nothing.'"

"People want to come over and visit. But by the time we get home at night we're exhausted. It's usually not till nine or ten. I've been up since six this morning," he says, and he looks it. There are dark circles under his dark eyes, weariness in the way he sits and in his voice. At midnight, one can drive the sixty miles from Manhattan to Smithtown in an hour. Between 7 A.M. and 7 P.M. it can rarely be done in less than two hours, and one bad tie-up can make it three. It is Sal junior's turn to sympathize. He looks at his father and says, "People say, 'We know what you're going through.' How do they know? They don't."

"Remember how you felt last time," his father says to him, "tired of putting up a front? Your mother and I got to that point this time."

Sal stares at the television. "I wish people didn't know, period. In the beginning, I wanted it, but then it got to be too much."

Earlier, Rose Ann Giovia had talked about how ironic it was that her husband had done benefits for people in trouble all his life. Now he brings it up, mentioning one he had done for a neighbor's wife who had cancer. "I felt bad and wanted to help, so I said, 'If you're not too proud—' Then when this happened—" he pauses, and a remnant of the incredulousness that must have overwhelmed him when Sal was diagnosed is reflected a moment in his face. "I remember running outside on the lawn one night, I was feeling really crazy, and I was shaking my fist at the sky and screaming at the top of my lungs, 'You owe me! You owe me!'"

His eyes wide, Sal junior says, "And I bet somebody across the street said, 'How much?'" The two of them laugh at Sal's line, but it is obvious that this is the first Sal has heard of the scene on the lawn and he is thrilled by it. He asks his father, "Did you really do that?" His father nods. "I kept asking, What did he ever do to anybody? I'd think about the past, about times I'd hit or scold him—I'm a typical Italian father—I'd ask myself, Why did I do it? Lose my temper? Be hard on him? I finally realized I did it because I'm a father."

This quiets Sal. He understands the code his father has just described, and approves. Like their new intimacy, so unlooked for, it is something bigger and more important than their differences, or even the punishing quality of life right this minute. Though things remain very bumpy—and will get much worse, with explosions of anger, impatience, sentiment, and even piety on occasion, punctuating their days—for now, the Giovias believe that in this crisis they have been restored to one another.

The effect of Jimmy's illness on the Polacks is different. They are deeply shocked, not by the appearance of trouble, for they have had plenty of that, but by its striking them this way. It is like a kidnapping. Their security as a family has been breached, their most precious member singled out, and they are having a terrible time with it. The incongruity of the young being struck down while the old thrive is part of it. Mr. Polack will turn seventy-six in August; his wife, who looks perhaps sixty, is just a few years younger. But Jimmy represents more than youth to the Polacks. He is their future, their fulfillment and, in their old age, their hope.

Morris Polack was fourteen when he left Russia with his two

brothers in 1919. They made their way through Romania, stowed away on a ship, and ended up in Belgium. They got on a second ship, which took them to Algiers, and a third, which brought them to Halifax, Nova Scotia. A Canadian friend had obtained papers for them, and with those they rode out to Vancouver by boxcar. Two years later, with two dollars among them, the Polack boys arrived in Seattle.

They began working furiously and by 1924 were all tithing. In 1927, when he was twenty-two, Morris bought a poultry farm, and "by twenty-five," he remembers with exact pride, he "was the biggest producer in three states." He eventually got out of the farming end of chickens, and Acme Poultry is now a packing and distributing business with 150 employees, among them a handful of Polacks. It is a prosperous company, one that has allowed the Polacks both to live well themselves and to pursue a habit of generosity to which Morris is addicted. This Jewish patriarch from Odessa, who through some odd synchronicity of geography and physiognomy, has come in his old age to look like one of the surviving Indian chiefs of the Northwest—a blocky body and square head, with straight lined features and squinting eyes that could have been lifted from a Kikuit carving—is a man who presses favors and gifts on others in a fervor of charity. He cannot help himself; it makes him feel so good. "I love to give people things," he said one day, and it was clear that he was not talking about getting credit but about pleasure. "And you know what? I always have enough left for myself."

Not all is benevolence. This urgency to bestow clearly has a connection with power, and Polack is unmistakably a fellow who is capable of rearranging large chunks of the world to get what he wants. His favorite stories are parables of adversity overcome, and the dominant theme of his life appears to have been not hard work or cleverness, of which there had to have been plenty, but rather tenacity, a stubbornness that simply overwhelms opponents and obstacles of all kinds.

When he was forty-two, he lectured Jimmy one day, his life was threatened as Jimmy's is now, but from a massive tumor in his head. He packed his bags, left wife and children and business behind, and took himself to the Mayo Clinic. Eleven months and three days later, he returned to Seattle cured, with a metal plate in his forehead. He taps against the lined flesh now. "You can beat the game if you try," he tells Jimmy. "All that is required is that you know what you want. And I wanted to live."

This message is what he feels he must get across. Jimmy's periodic depression and his lack of interest in his future alarm his grandfather, who dreads Jimmy's giving way. The expectations that attach to this boy, his male heir, are considerable, and Jimmy has never for a moment been unaware of them. He is son and grandson to the Polacks, though in an irony seldom referred to, he has none of their blood in him. His mother, Marlene, was adopted; Valerie, Jimmy's aunt, was born soon after. And when Marlene had Jimmy, very young, after marrying and then divorcing a man her parents did not approve of, it was easy for them to draw Jimmy to themselves. Already in their fifties, they raised him from infancy, while his mother remarried and eventually had two more children, a girl two years younger than Jimmy, a boy five years later.

When Jimmy was fourteen, a year past his *bar mitzvah* and old enough to understand—"I wanted him to know, and to want it," his grandfather said—the Polacks formally adopted him as they had earlier adopted his mother. So, in a sense, he was twice chosen, twice blessed, twice indebted.

"When I was a lot younger," Jimmy recalls, "I was rebellious, just like my mother. But I was a male, and so it was different. It was all right, get it out of my system. I'm the one who's supposed to take care of everyone. That's been pounded into my head since I was old enough to speak English. *You're* gonna take care of the charities, *you're* gonna run the business."

The sense of duty never lifted. When he was in high school, Jimmy started working for the business, loading turkeys onto trucks, later driving those trucks to make deliveries. He liked the physical work, liked the long drives, the practical details of getting a chicken to a customer. He worked hard and was the good son—smart, good-natured, loving, and respectful—that his grandfather had always hoped for. He also enjoyed considerable privilege and personal freedom, living a life of semi-independence while still in his grandparents' house. Like Sal, he was more interested in his friends than in school and had no sense that he had to do well academically to make good in life. His grandfather would teach him what he needed to know and indeed had begun to tutor him in the public life of a generous man.

Morris took Jimmy to fund-raising events, banquets, award ceremonies. The summer before Jimmy got sick, the two of them traveled to Israel, Egypt and Greece together. It was Jimmy's first trip to Israel, Morris's twenty-sixth. Mr. Polack first visited the country, for which he has been a sturdy fund-raiser and contributor, in 1949. He says he once mentioned to Golda Meir that he dreamed of living there for a year someday, but she scolded him, "Not even for a day." It was better that he keep on mailing checks from Seattle. In bringing Jimmy, he was vouching for the continuation of that support, and so Jimmy was taken around to ministry offices, introduced, photographed smiling, getting a feel for what it meant to be a friend of Israel.

This year, 1981, the year Jimmy was spending in treatment in New York, was to have been the year in which he started working in the office instead of on the loading docks. He was to have settled down in school long enough to master the necessary business courses and then prepare to assume by stages the several roles already written for him.

Now all that is in jeopardy, along with Jimmy's life. The Polacks had no difficulty in sorting out which was more important. The family was ready to leave Seattle the third morning after Jimmy was diagnosed, not knowing when they would be back. The problem is what to do while they wait to see if he lives. All along, they have believed they could do everything for him. Now they must live with the knowledge that they can do almost nothing but wait. So they sit in one room after another, hospital room, apartment, clinic, restaurant, watching Jimmy in hope and dread and, as the days pass, increasing bewilderment.

By the end of Jimmy's and Sal's first week of consolidation, they are able to get out of bed and stand up. The treatment has given Sal a sweet tooth, and he has been hounding his parents to bring him treats. Yesterday it was Fruit Loops, which his father eventually bought at a market on First Avenue. Today Sal appears in Jimmy's room wearing his usual costume, sweat pants and a printed tee shirt, and pushing his pole in front of him. "Got any Oreos?" he asks, a friendly leer on his face. Mr. Polack offers him a tin of butter cookies. Sal shakes his head. "Nah, those ain't any good." Morris is not offended, but Jimmy takes the opportunity to remark on Sal's accent, which comes and goes according to his meaning and mood.

"I never heard anybody talk the way you do," Jimmy says to Sal in his own drawn-out slightly flat, western voice. Sal is nonplussed. "Whaddaya mean? Everybody in New York talks like this." He surveys the room, but there is not another genuine New York squawk to be found. While they discuss the origins of Sal's blend of Brooklyn and Long Island speech, Karyn and her mother appear—to speak in lightly inflected, regionless tones—and the talk turns to counts. Karyn's are still hugging the floor, preventing her from going home, and Mrs. Angell says to the Polacks that she has tried to reassure herself by remembering something she has read, that patients with the lowest counts early on do best. "I find myself doing this more and more," she says, "homing in on what is most hopeful."

Sal asks Jimmy what his counts are today, and when Jimmy says he doesn't know, Sal says he's sure *his* counts are higher. "I bet you five bucks," he says. "We'll wait and see," Jimmy says. "No," Sal says, "Find out now. Call down to the desk and ask." Jimmy tries to put him off, but Sal insists and finally picks up the intercom mike and buzzes the nurses' station. In a somewhat stilted voice, free of accent, he says, "This is James Polack speaking. Would you please tell me what my counts are?" Jimmy stares at him, amused, and just before hanging up, Sal smiles and says into the mike, with a look at Jimmy, "On the double." When he hangs up, he says to Jimmy, "That's the only way to get things done around here."

Over the weekend, Jimmy and Sal are released, to begin a rest period of three to four weeks before the next round. Healthy, and with no signs of leukemia in their marrow when they came in, as a result of the treatment they have just received they are now about to enter a period of danger nearly comparable to when they were first diagnosed. Over the next nine days, their blood counts will steadily drop, until they are so low that they will almost inevitably contract fevers and have to return to the hospital.

This is one of the predictable costs of chemotherapy, and one that closely parallels the final stages of the disease itself. When leukemia proceeds unchecked, irregular—that is, cancerous— cells in the blood eventually kill off all the body's healthy blood cells. (Actually, a patient would die well before this point of cell "extinction," most likely from hemorrhage or infection.) Although they go at the job differently, the drugs used to treat leukemia also kill off healthy cells in the process of eradicating any leukemic cells left in the system. The difference between the disease and the treatment is a matter of both degree and control. Dosages are finely adjusted to body weight and mass, blood counts are continually monitored to ensure that the patient is not given more than he can tolerate. The process is highly refined, and the results usually predictable, but there remain risks that cannot be alleviated, only guarded against.

In the course of treatment, patients' counts follow something of a planned parabola several times over, being driven down by drugs, rising again as healthy cells renew. The staff at Memorial is far more relaxed about this pattern than are most patients, who understandably blanch at the news that approximately nine days after certain treatments they will have white counts as low as 200 or even 100, and hence no immunity from anything. "You could get an infection from the bacteria on your own *skin,"* is how Karyn Angell puts it, getting it exactly right. And if it were left untreated, die from it.

Despite this danger, the precautions observed are fairly modest. Patients are encouraged to take their temperatures daily, for an early warning of fever, but what really decides the matter is one's white count. When a patient's polys—the most mature form of white cell—drop below 500, it is time to come in.

The day the boys are released marks the start of Karyn's second full month in the hospital, and she does not fail to notice. Physically, she looks rosily fit, though she complains, like Jimmy, that all her muscle tone is gone, and she laments the lethargy that has taken over. It gets harder each day to push to exercise, to get up and walk laps around the building's core. Bald, bored, and stir-crazy, she is like an inmate to whom parole has been denied on a technicality. She has had her last dose of Vincristine and has begun to taper off Prednisone, which does not help her mood. She is edgy and occasionally petulant with her mother, who remarks casually on the change and its cause, then lets it drop. Karyn is scheduled for just one more spinal, and if her counts would come up there would be nothing to keep her in the hospital another day. She could receive her last medication, a combined dose of Cytoxan and Adriamycin as an outpatient, as Jimmy and Sal did. But on February 14 she is not yet in remission, her white count is still 300, and Dr. Gee wants to see it climb almost to 1,000 before he sends her home.

Karyn reads the sluggishness of her bone marrow as frustrating but not serious, and she concentrates on outlasting her growing impatience by means of soap operas, a lately acquired vice, food, and sleep. But for her mother, the start of Karyn's second month triggers newly bleak visions. For the first time, she considers the possibility, unlikely though it remains, that Karyn could in fact fail to come into remission altogether. Letting in that one thought opens the way to a whole range of terrifying considerations that she has up to this point successfully suppressed. That things might not pick up, that Karyn could prove to be among the 10 percent of patients with ALL who never achieve remission, was something she had never permitted herself to think. But if it were true, then it meant that what they faced in the next couple of years was not the serious trouble they had braced themselves for, but certain disaster.

This dread possibility hits Dee Angell on a Saturday morning, seated at the counter in her kitchen, and it shakes her to her core. Her husband is still in Europe, her three younger girls are tiptoeing around trying not to see how scared their strong mother is, and the exhaustion of the last weeks overtakes her like a wave. Recalling the moment a few days later, she says that it was the first time since Karyn's diagnosis that she had let herself think the worst, and that the emotional catharsis it brought on was exactly what she needed. The tension of sustaining a wholly optimistic outlook had been too much for her; besides, it was time to begin to think realistically about what could happen, not just what they hoped would happen.

Standing in the hospital corridor, out of Karyn's hearing, she speaks in a calm voice, her eyes dry, and tells how the experience of the weekend has changed her thinking. "If we are going to lose her in a couple of years," she says quietly, "if this is the reality, then things change radically. We'll have to rethink our futures, all of us. For one thing, if she is going to die, I don't want her to think she has to go to college. Maybe she'll want to spend her time some other way. We can't afford to send her around the world just because she has leukemia, but maybe we can spend the money that would have gone to her education on something that makes more sense to her, if this is what's going to happen."

And there are other considerations. This afternoon, she says, Karyn spoke for the first time of her wish to have a child, and of how pleased she would be to add a fifth generation to the four now alive: both her maternal grandmother and her great-grand-mother are alive, and neither shows signs of disappearing. It is Karyn's survival, and, because of the possible effects of chemo-therapy, her fertility, that are suddenly in question. Dee is moved by this confidence, which also reminds her that her daughter is a virgin. She says now, "She isn't going to want to stay one for-ever."

The degree to which life's most ordinary expectations can be wrenched loose by this disease is slowly coming clear. Having made the leap from single-minded optimism, Dee Angell is let-ting herself be washed by all kinds of questions that she cannot answer, and that she knows Karyn is not yet ready for. For now, Dee sees her and her husband's joint role as an entirely support-ive one, to buoy up their daughter's hopes whatever their private apprehensions. This is not the time to raise their fears with Ka-ryn, Dee believes, although she is confident that Karyn herself will in time begin to play with some of the fearful feelings that must be there.

It is a remarkable assessment, even, or perhaps especially, for a mother to make of a daughter, and it reflects an amazing duality of perception on Dee Angell's part. Clearly she is able to see her daughter as a distinct personality, someone whose identity has taken shape, if not fully, then very nearly so, and whose wishes must be respected. She treats Karyn like an adult, and her presence in the room is never fussy or coercive. Yet she is tender and sympathetic, and lets the adult Karyn slip away when necessary, pampering the much younger Karyn who materializes periodically. The two of them agree on their differences in temperament, Dee being the more openly tenacious and aggressive, Karyn the calm observer hoping to avoid a fuss and still get her way.

But what astonishes about the mother is what astonishes about the daughter, a streak—or rather a backbone—of realism that directs their emotions but does not still them. Later in the year, Dee Angell will remark that the concept of fairness does not figure in her scheme of life (except when it comes to distributing privileges or chores among her daughters; on that all the Angell girls testify to a meticulous even-handedness observed by both parents), and perhaps it is her sense that the world begins off-balance that accounts for this quality of calm in the face of potential loss.

By Karyn's sixth Wednesday on the sixth floor of Memorial, her white count has risen to 700. Four attempts to take a bone-marrow sample for testing produce nothing but a back that is still sore the next day and a rare acknowledgment from Karyn that she has about had it.

"I don't know why I'm so upset," she says, as if she hasn't sufficient cause for complaint. "But right now it feels like time passes so slowly. The problem is waiting only to get out and being told repeatedly that you can't. The thing that really bothers me is that I have no control. I can't eat a certain thing, I can't exercise, I can't sleep to make my white counts come up. I can't do anything to help and neither can anyone else."

The days are mild for February, with sunny mornings and sudden afternoon downpours mimicking spring. After five weeks in the hospital (and three before that, at home) in bathrobes and slippers, Karyn can think of nothing that would please her more than to be able to "take a walk outside every day, in my own clothes." Beyond that goal lie more ambitious ones, notions of exercise to get back into shape, an independent study project for school (nothing to do with leukemia), visits with friends.

On Thursday, her white count is 900, and in the late afternoon, she and her mother are told that she will be able to go home the next day. This strikes everyone as a felicitous piece of timing, since Dave Angell is due back from Belgium sometime Friday afternoon.

Early Friday morning, Dee and her mother drive in from Westport with an empty suitcase for Karyn's things. Kim, Janet, and Jennifer have prepared the house for a welcome-home party, expecting Karyn to be there when they return from school. Dave Angell has been alerted and will call from the airport to make sure where everyone is before starting home.

Shortly before her mother and grandmother arrive, Karyn receives a final check from Dr. Small, who, like everyone else involved, is excited that Karyn is going home. She checks the chart to make sure that everything is in order and sees a notation on a lab report that had not been there the night before. It's a report on a blood culture taken nine days earlier, and it is positive, for a strep infection. This is one of the predictable, small-potato disasters that plague leukemia patients, but it comes at an awful time. A series of brief and excited conferences between Dr. Gee and his staff and what Karyn calls "the infectious disease people" ends with a ruling that Karyn must stay another week. It is too dangerous for her to go home.

Hearing this when she arrives, Dee Angell is for the first time really furious. She is so upset that hours later she still cannot sit still in her chair, and she keeps crossing and recrossing her legs in a bristling outrage. She is spitting out words like "incompetence" and "stupidity" in a thin, cracking voice. Her target is the lab, a faceless outpost of the institution that has, amazingly, taken this long to finally let them down. Until this moment, everyone involved in Karyn's care has been so unfailingly competent, correct and solicitous that identifying a culprit has been impossible. There has never been anyone to blame for Karyn's illness, and nowhere for Dee Angell to take her terror or her rage. Now she, like Karyn, suddenly knows she has had it with leukemia, and with holding herself together. This is as good a moment as any to blow up.

While her mother fumes, Karyn lies flat on her back and stares disbelievingly at the curtain at the foot of the bed. All her things were ready to be packed, she was ready to go. The disappointment is almost unbearable, and, for the moment, unexpressible. Later, when her mother and grandmother go off to the coffee shop, she tries to talk, alternating between politely put explanations of what caused the problem—the strep most likely developed from the mouth sores that she had a couple of weeks ago—and bursts of muted anger.

182

"This is going to make it six weeks," she says. The sudden reversal is worse than if she had never been told that she was going home. For the first time she seems close to defeat, helpless, and there is a painfully mechanical quality to her protest. Even as she says, "I'm really mad," her tone is flat and her anger checked. "I would really like to scream," she says finally, "but I'm never alone. And I feel like there isn't any place here I can go to be alone."

The phone rings and it is Dave Angell calling from the airport. Karyn is charged with energy suddenly and struggles to sit higher in the bed without dropping the receiver as she tries to tell him everything in a single spurt. "You would not *believe* what happened today," she tells him, adding for unnecessary clarity, "I'm still here."

She proceeds to tell him the story of the mixup, recovering the natural outraged tone of a seventeen-year-old. Afterward, she no longer seems helpless. Sitting cross-legged on the bed, she says, and this time with juice in her voice, "It's the first time I've been really mad." Then she adds, already starting to take the long view, now that she has cleared the decks, "Although that's silly, I know, because there's nobody to be mad *at*. That's the problem with this whole disease."

She talks about how much easier it would be if there were someone to blame, some appropriate target for her feelings. Fatalism, as her mother made clear a short while earlier, has its shortcomings, too. Karyn says that she has tried hard not to internalize these feelings; if it's no one person's fault, then it's certainly not hers. Soon she is speculating philosophically on how much better it is that the infection was caught now rather than later. If she had gone home and had to come right back with a fever, she'd feel even worse than she does right now.

As it happens, she is very sick on Saturday and later says she is very glad she stayed. Her father comes in to spend the day with her, but she has a high fever and is awake only five hours. She sleeps through a good part of the next week as well, as much from a desire to escape as from fatigue.

By Wednesday, her white count is 1,600, her platelets are at 227,000, and it seems certain that she will go home by the weekend. But Karyn remains skeptical. "That's what they *say*," she says, staring at the covers. Her face is taut these days, and the easy smile doesn't materialize automatically anymore. She reaches her peak of animation talking about food. After weeks of saying that the hospital food wasn't bad—or that it actually was good—she has begun to knock it. "It's a good thing to complain about when you're looking for something," she says.

In the late afternoon, Dr. Small stops by. She is a tall young woman, with a thin, expressive face and an intense manner. Seemingly the quickest and most assured of the fellows who care for Karyn and the boys this year, she is also very much their favorite, and although she will soon rotate out of Hematology, she will continue to visit them whenever they are in the hospital, a gesture that makes them all feel special. Now she pauses beside Karyn's bed and asks her how she is doing. Karyn says that she has been feeling sorry for herself, and when Dr. Small gently asks, "Why?" Karyn's eyes fill with tears. Dr. Small sits down, and the two of them talk privately for a quarter of an hour. Afterward, Karyn is visibly cheered; her tolerance, which has been worn so thin this week, seems good for another few days.

The next day, Thursday, forty-three days after Karyn first became his patient, Dr. Gee takes a sample of bone marrow from her back. He studies it himself, as he does all his patients' marrows when the reading is critical, and that night tells Karyn and her parents that she is in remission.

The Angells are euphoric. "I can't tell you the relief we felt," Dee Angell said a few days later. "It was the first time since this thing started that we've felt at all safe."

This time Karyn would really be going home, though she remained superstitiously wary until she was actually out the door. The night before leaving, her parents suggested that they take some of her things home with them, to make it simpler the next day, but she would not let them. "She was so afraid something would go wrong," her mother said.

Nothing did. By midafternoon Friday, Karyn was in Westport, settling into the room her sisters had prepared for her. Everyone was pleased by how well she looked, but no one failed to notice that she could not make it up the stairs by herself. Dee Angell had remarked on the difference between being the only leukemia patient in a small hospital and one of many in a large cancer center. The gap between a hospital and a house is much greater. However remote from "real" life, a hospital existence has a clarity that amounts to a context; its structure and its purpose are overt, as is (although it may often feel otherwise) the patient's importance.

The context of a house is the family that lives in it. And although Karyn's personal value to her family had never been more explicit than it was now, for the first time in her life, her role within the family was not clear. She was the big sister who could do anything, except that now she could do very little. She had been the most independent, had flown the farthest from the nest, and now she was back, hobbled, confined, dependent—still Karyn, but with many of her most easily described characteristics neutralized. She had always been the comforter, the confidante, the example, "so good," as Kim said. Was she now to be comforted? Or left alone? Babied or teased, sympathized with, idolized anew, or treated as an invalid? Was she one?

She returned to a house in which everyone else had something interesting or consuming to do, as had always been true for her. But what she might do in the uncertain weeks between treatments that stretched from now through August was a mystery. For Karyn, life in Westport, where she had never lived, and where she knew no one but her family, was still literally unimaginable. She couldn't have found her way to the post office her first weeks home, did not even have a driver's license, a prerequisite of suburban survival.

Dr. Gee and his staff are with good reason strong believers in the therapeutic value of a speedy return to normal life. But normal life for Karyn meant school and the friends she had made there, and there was no way for her to return to that world until her consolidation was over.

The best she could hope for, Karyn thought, would be a part-time job with a flexible employer, and possibly a course or two at one of the local colleges. "I've got to do something," she said, "or I'll go bonkers." Speculating on the immediate future just before she left the hospital, she said she imagined that there would be times when she would be very tired, and also "times when I'll want to be alone, to think things out. I think I'm going to feel the change in my life more when I get out than I do here," she said. "They say this is the hardest part, but I think I'm going to have trouble when I get home."

Jimmy Polack and Sal Giovia managed to stay out of the hospital exactly one week before succumbing to fevers. They came in late on a Sunday night, within hours of each other. Sal's white count was 200 at admission—or, as he put it a few days later (claiming it was 100), "Any lower and you wouldn't be seeing me."

By midweek he is receiving visitors. Two girls from Smithtown—"just friends"—elbow each other and titter at Sal's ghoulish remarks. A clutch of older female relatives hover outside his room, as if afraid of intruding. His side of the double room, shared not with Jimmy, who is down the hall, but with an older man, is crowded with a balloon bouquet that another patient on the floor has refused to accept. Sal is in a joking mood, good-humored, cheerful. He outlasted Jimmy by a couple of hours, or a little longer than the length of the ride in from Smithtown. He interrupts himself when talking to the girls about Dr. Gee to ask me if he is Chinese or Japanese. Told that Gee is Chinese, he asks, "Well, then, how come he doesn't have an accent?"

"I didn't feel at all good about coming back," Jimmy had said a couple of days earlier, smiling a drawn-out, knowing smile, "but I bet they had a hard time getting *him* in." Knowing that this fever was inevitable, he is more or less resigned to waiting it out, and he adopts a gently ironic tone as he talks about treatment. "You know what the worst thing is about this disease?" he asks. "The side effects of the drugs. But what can you do about it? Suppose the doctor says, 'Yeah, they're gonna make you sterile, impotent, illiterate, and whatever.' What good does it do you to know it? What kind of choice do you have?

"What I noticed about me and Sal," he continues, referring to their return this week, "is disappointment. Sal screams and yells. I just get depressed. I don't know how I'd feel if I were seventeen," he says. "A lot of these older people give up. They sit in the lounge and they smoke, can you believe it? But they figure they're gonna kick anyway. You can get to a point where life isn't worth it. When it gets really bad . . ." He draws a line across his throat with his finger.

His grandfather sits in a straight chair across from Jimmy, listening to this talk with arms folded high on his big chest. "Jimmy!" he shouts when the talk veers too close to death. Jimmy glances at his grandfather and continues talking in a calm voice. "But I have a lot of things I want to do yet," he says. It is a gift to the older man, a reassurance that is also this moment's truth.

He soon becomes silly, telling of a trip he made to the X-ray area today. "I saw this guy, he had hair on his head, but he looked worse than a refugee, or a boat person. He was so emaciated you could see his spine. You could have put your hand around his neck," he says, with grisly amusement. Though Jimmy counts himself one of the freaks now, he has not lost his adolescent eye.

Later in the afternoon, Valerie and Mrs. Polack arrive. There is rarely a moment when one of the Polacks is not with him, and when Jimmy, ostensibly speaking of the terribly sick older patients he has seen in the hospital says, "With a lot of these people, you almost think their relatives want them to live more than they do," *his* relatives hear it and shudder.

Although they have been living with Jimmy's illness for almost two months now, they have never seen him as sick as he was earlier this week, trembling from fever when he came in Sunday night, requiring both whole blood and platelets. Jimmy shrugs off the danger, then jokes about how the doctors and nurses are so careful to warn patients ahead of time of what's going to happen to them. "It's great," he says, "sometimes they tell you three days in advance—'remember, you're going to have a bone-marrow Thursday'—so you dread it for three days."

Valerie says how tough it is to watch Jimmy get sick and not panic but that "Dr. Gee told us that we will learn to trust him, that when he says everything is fine, it is." Her mother's face is stiff with doubt. "Sometimes I think the doctors don't want to tell—" she begins, but Jimmy cuts her off. "Yeah, he's bullshitting me, Grandma," Jimmy says. "I'm going to die within a few days." He is sitting up in bed, looking burly and a long way from expiring. A bit later, he mentions having visited the Museum of Natural History, across Central Park from the Polacks' apartment, the day before he got his fever. "I think that's when he caught cold," his grandmother says. "He was wearing just a thin jacket."

"That's ri-dic-u-lous," Jimmy says. He turns to her and says "I caught it from you." Mrs. Polack takes the jibe gracefully, and says with a shrug, "I don't have anything."

Earlier in the day, Jimmy's I.V. had infiltrated, raising a pale-blue bump on the inner side of his arm, and it is still sore. A new needle must be inserted, and soon a nervous young I.V. specialist appears. Some are more relaxed about their work than others, but this young man meets no one's eyes as he concentrates on his job. He feels up and down Jimmy's arm with both hands, as if frisking for weapons, pressing Jimmy's veins lightly as he searches for a likely spot. He pulls a length of pale-pink rubber tubing from his kit and ties it tightly above Jimmy's left elbow to bring up the vein below. Jimmy's eyes bulge at the sight of this makeshift tourniquet, and later he jokes, "Why didn't he use piano wire?" The specialist asks Jimmy whether he has had chemotherapy in this arm previously. "Yes," Jimmy says. "Is that good, bad or indifferent?" The nurse says it just means that the vein may appear bigger than it really is. He makes quick strokes with his middle finger to bring the vein up, then pierces the skin with the needle he has prepared. Jimmy winces. They both stare at the needle in silence, waiting to see if it's in properly. Jimmy knows it's not before the nurse does. "It's infiltrating," he says flatly, and the needle is withdrawn.

The specialist searches for a second spot, and chooses Jimmy's right hand. Greg Mahoney, a high-school friend of Jimmy's on furlough from an Air Force base in Virginia, watches this scene, into which he has just walked, with controlled edginess. The needle enters the top of Jimmy's hand between the second and third knuckles and holds. Jimmy looks up at Greg and says, "Hey, you want to play bloody knuckles?" then asks the nurse why that spot is so painful. "Do you have more nerves in your hand or something?" The nurse, who seems eager to finish taping Jimmy's hand so that the needle will not be jerked loose, exhales, "Yeah."

When he has gone, Jimmy holds up his hand, to which stiff boards have been taped sandwich-style, and rates the specialist's performance. "For some reason," he says, "women with small hands do it better. These big guys just jam it in." He makes a sadistic face. "I could never stick a needle in anyone's *hand*."

The usual stay for a fever is a week to ten days. At admission, Jimmy's white count was 500, but today, three days later, it is down to 400. It must rise to 1,000 before he can get out, but he's not worried. His platelets are climbing rapidly, he says, which means that his bone marrow is developing. "I'm getting out tomorrow," he says. "Really, I'm known for miracles."

By Sunday, the eighth day, the miracle materializes, and Jimmy goes home. That is, he leaves Memorial for the apartment on Eighty-fifth Street, knowing that he will be back in in two more weeks. By his count, he has another fifty-nine days to go before he can really go home.

For the last several years, the first Monday night of every month has been the occasion of a meeting to which Dr. Gee has invited all his patients, their families and friends in turn. Notices go out the week before to patients who haven't appeared in a while, and anyone who is an inpatient is automatically invited. Attendance varies; sometimes the conference room, on the first floor of the York Avenue building, is crowded, and the self-introductions that start the meeting take so long that the names of the first people to speak are forgotten by the time the last have given theirs. Other nights, patients are outnumbered by hospital staff—two social workers as a rule and occasionally more, Dr. Gee, Kathy Dietz, the current Hematology fellow many months, several of the nurses who regularly work the Hematology clinic.

The tone of these evenings varies as well. Some nights the talk has the inevitable quality of a well-made play, or movie: it is seamless and urgent, and needs little shaping. Other nights, nothing sparks, and the polite prodding of the social workers casts a dull pall on the proceedings.

Monday, March 2, is Sal's last day in the hospital for fever, and, as it coincides with a meeting night, Dr. Gee suggests to the Giovias that they plan to stay late when they come to pick Sal up. Sal is not wild about this, and says he would rather start home, but his parents want to stay.

They badly need to talk and when invited to open the discussion by telling how they learned that Sal had leukemia, they both start at once. RoseAnn is so flustered that she gets the date of his diagnosis wrong. Just as her husband says December 19, she blurts out November 21. She hears herself say it, registers what Sal senior has said, and slaps herself on the cheek with the heel of her hand. She laughs, settles down, and she and her husband take turns filling in the details, Young Sal eyes his parents carefully as they talk about him. Rose Ann tells of taking him back and forth to the doctor for blood tests for almost a year but never learning anything that would have alerted them to what was coming. Sal senior gestures toward his son. "He doesn't drink, he doesn't smoke, he doesn't do drugs. There wasn't anything to look for.

"I'm an old-fashioned father," he tells the group, which tonight includes five other patients and a half dozen relatives. "When he didn't want to get up in the morning because he was so tired, I used to yell at him, 'You're going to school! No, you can't stay home.'" Giovia shakes his head sadly. "He was always tired." His son has never looked as angelic as during this public clearing of his name as a would-be truant.

Across the small circle sits a boy one year older than Sal. He is bald, lean and defensive, a two-year veteran of leukemia and something of a minor legend around the hospital. Billy* has suffered almost every side effect known to ALL patients. He has been in and out of the hospital with fevers, he has had a stroke, tracheotomy, and a long list of lesser complications. And he is still bald, a fact that Sal does not miss. Nor, despite Dr. Gee's soft-voiced assurances that Billy has continued to thrive despite setbacks, are the Giovias heartened. They ask Gee whether Billy's experience is typical. Gee says no patient's experience is typical, that everyone has a hard time in his own way. "It's not easy to be a patient," Gee says. Sal senior laughs and looks at his son. "He shows us that sometimes. He says, 'Get me outa here.'"

Sal nods and speaks up. "I tell them to get me out of here," he says with dignity. "I think I'm entitled to say that." Arms folded across his chest, he arches his spine against the back of the

---

*Pseudonym.

molded plastic chair. "I didn't expect to get the fever," he says, "They hook you up. It doesn't make you feel good. I know it has to be, but I still don't like it."

Referring to the medical complications, especially the fevers, Rose Ann asks Dr. Gee, "Will this go on for two years?" She glances at Billy, and her husband adds, "I thought the most dangerous time was the first six months." Billy interjects, "That's what they told me," and everyone laughs. Gee confirms that the first six months are the most dangerous in terms of possible relapse and side effects, but that problems can occur at any time, which is why patients must be closely monitored.

The discussion circles back to the difficulties of diagnosis, when Richard, a patient in his fifties who has the same disease as Sal and Billy, tells the Giovias that he too had had a blood test six months before diagnosis that failed to warn of the disease. Sal's father seizes on this and asks again what they could have done to have had Sal diagnosed sooner. The muscles in his face are rigid with tension. This is a big issue for him. Gee reassures him quickly that there is nothing they could have done beyond what they did that would have helped. "There's no reason for you to feel guilt," he tells him, and Giovia sags back in his chair.

The talk turns to emotions. Rose Ann says that the toughest thing for her has been the feeling of helplessness that comes with knowing you have no control over what happens. Her husband says, "She's numb. She tells me every night, 'Hon, I can't break out what I feel.'"

Richard says, in the softest voice, "I can't figure out who to be angry at, who to yell at." Sal laughs. "I yell at everybody," he says. "My dog, my brother, my friends." As he talks, he grows more serious. "They're overprotective," he says. "I tell them, 'Let's not talk about what I've got.' Sometimes I just go in my room."

Rose Ann says, "When he's up, it's great. When he's down, we're down."

One of the social workers says to Sal, "That puts quite a burden on you, Sal, doesn't it?"

He looks surprised. He smiles at her. "Sort of," he says. "I don't see why I can't be down when I don't feel good."

Billy says, "I try to keep it separate from the rest of my life. But when the phone rings and it's one of my mother's friends, it's Twenty Questions."

Sal senior asks Billy how his parents handle his illness. Billy looks theatrically pained. "I come in," he says, sighing, "they want my counts every day." He pauses for effect. "I make 'em up."

Giovia sighs. "We're like that, too." Rose Ann groans. "I ask him, 'How do you feel?' What a stupid question!" Everyone laughs. Sal, excited now, adds another complaint. "The other thing is, on the phone, I sound down, they ask me, 'What's the matter?' The *hospital*, that's the matter."

A woman in her thirties, a recently diagnosed inpatient who has come to the meeting in a bathrobe and towing her I.V. pole, confirms Sal's point. "We even have *patients* going around upstairs saying, 'Don't be depressed.'"

The talk wanders over other subjects for a few minutes, until Sal senior brings it around one more time, his voice tentative but his need persistent, to the question of guilt. He asks if any of the others, patients or family members, feels guilt because someone in the family has cancer.

"I feel absolutely no guilt," says the woman with the I.V. "Nor do my parents. Disease is part of life," she says deliberately. "Until it comes into your life, you don't recognize it, but it's as much a part of your life as your car, or the house you live in. It's part of the human condition."

Giovia nods at her then says to the group, "What I'm trying to find out is about the relationships people had when they were younger. I mean, was the mother around a lot, or the father? 'Cause *I* feel guilty," he blurts out.

Richard's wife, a social worker at another hospital, says, "I don't think anyone has that kind of power."

Giovia glances at her, nods, and keeps on. "I'm an entertainer," he says. "I travel a lot. Before Sal got sick, I said to my wife, 'Now that Sal's grown up—'" He lowers his head into his hand and begins to weep. Rose Ann places her hand on his back and her big eyes too fill with tears. Dr. Gee leans forward. "Children grow up very fast, don't they?" he says. "That's something I've learned from all of you, and it's why my family still comes first."

One of the social workers says to Gee, "But your work permits you that luxury." He nods. "That's right," he says. Giovia looks up and says, as if bargaining for absolution, "Mine doesn't. I have to travel to support my family."

The rest of the group reassures him that the two things—Sal's illness and his father's absence when he was a child—are not connected. The woman with the I.V. asks whether he knows the song "Cat's Cradle" by Harry Chapin. Giovia says, yes, excitedly.

"I know Chapin," he says, and he explains to the group that the song is about a man who is too busy to spend time with his child when the child is young, and then discovers in old age that his son is too busy to spend time with him. "I think that's what you're afraid has happened," the young woman says. Giovia nods and turns to Gee and mentions an earlier conversation the two of them had had. "How did you see so quickly that I was having a problem with feeling guilty?" Gee laughs and says, "I pick up a lot in twenty-six seconds."

Shortly before the meeting ends, a second inpatient, who has not talked much up till now, tells the story of her diagnosis. When she has finished, Sal senior continues the story he had begun earlier, of how Sal came to learn that he had leukemia. "Sal has a habit of picking up the extension phone at home after someone else has answered," Giovia begins, "because he thinks it's going to be for him—and it usually is." Sal's eyes are fixed on his father, his lips pressed together as if he is suppressing a smile. He listens to the familiar details of that first day, of how he overheard the doctor, of how he ran around the house screaming, "I'm going to die, I'm going to die." And when his father finishes, he picks up the story without missing a beat—"Then a priest came to see me," he says, and he pauses, his instinct as sure as his father's.

Someone asks, "Did you think . . ." and Sal smiles playfully and says, "Yeah." Everyone laughs. "But the priest told me, 'This ain't your last blessing.'"

"Did you believe him?" Sal is asked.

"Yeah," he says. He looks quickly to his parents. He shrugs. "I'm still here."

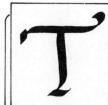The last of the packed cells Terry O'Brien received as an outpatient on June 2 emptied into her veins at around four in the afternoon. By six she was home in bed, as profoundly asleep as her husband had ever seen her.

By the middle of the next day, June 3, she was back at Memorial, seeking emergency admittance in Bedholding, complaining of chest pain and shortness of breath.

Her brother Brian brought her in. He had come down to Colts Neck to spend a few days with her and had been there only a few hours when she began to panic, saying that she couldn't breathe properly, finally asking him to drive her to the hospital. Ray O'Brien was at that moment having his stomach ulcer checked and did not learn that Terry had gone back in until he came home early from work. But Brian was able to reach Sean and Chris, who came by to see their mother before returning home for the night. She was in Room 426 again, in the same bed, in fact, less than a week after vacating it.

Dr. Berman, the fellow in whose care Golbey has left her while he was gone, tells Mr. O'Brien that evening that he is not at all surprised to see her back. "The cancer is in her bone marrow," Mr. O'Brien reports, "and she's not producing any blood. The only way they are keeping her going is by tranfusion." In theory, the transfusion she received the day before should have held her longer than this, but the fact that it did not suggests that the cancer is moving incredibly fast. "I don't know what to think," O'Brien says of this latest change. "I'm getting to be kind of numb. But, given the circumstances, she may be better off in the hospital than at home. At least they can control the pain there."

As an inpatient, Mrs. O'Brien is given Levo-Dromoran again for her pain, hooked up to oxygen, and given additional blood support. She absorbs these comforts as a parched garden soaks up the rain, and manages to sleep through the night.

The Levo-Dromoran is given every four hours. The most powerful of the narcotics she has had up until now, it also provides the best pain relief she has had so far, but there are problems. Like many powerful pain medications, it depresses the respiratory system, and Mrs. O'Brien is already having trouble breathing. Sometime after her midmorning dose on Thursday, she lapses into what the notation on her chart afterward describes as an "episode of lethargy." To a nonmedical observer who sees her just before noon, she looks comatose: her bony head thrown back on the pillow, her arms flat and bruised at her sides; her body absolutely still but for the faint movement of her face and chest in profile. The room is otherwise empty, and there is no one to notice her condition until one of the nurses checks on her and discovers that her breathing and pulse are extremely slow.

The nurse summons the intern assigned to the floor, and seconds later the two of them are standing on either side of Mrs. O'Brien, grasping her hands, bending low over the sides of the bed to shout into her ears: "Theresa, Theresa, can you hear me?"

Mrs. O'Brien does not stir, and their agitation grows. "What *month* is it?" the intern shouts, slapping Mrs. O'Brien's hand hard with her own. Mrs. O'Brien answers in a distant, drugged voice, "August," and the intern, trying to bring her awake, says, "No, it's May." Then, horrified by her mistake, she shouts, "June." Mrs. O'Brien's eyes open and she looks furiously at the young doctor. "What are you trying to *do* to me?" she asks, and then closes her eyes again.

She drifts off a second time, there is more shouting, and finally the intern administers a shot of a drug called Narcan, a powerful counteractive to narcotics. Within seconds, all the painkiller in Mrs. O'Brien's body is neutralized, and she bolts upright on the bed, clutching her chest, a wild look in her eyes. All the months of dulled pain implode in a staggering wash. It is the pain of dread, the pain that has hovered just behind the curtain of medication all these months. She looks around her and cries, "What did you *do* to me?"

Seeing the effect of the Narcan, the intern quickly injects Mrs. O'Brien with another dose of painkiller, which begins to take effect almost immediately. Mrs. O'Brien lies back, limp, rigid, and then rubbery in turn after this wrenching from one state of consciousness to another. In seconds, Dr. Berman and another two nurses have arrived. One of the nurses hooks Mrs. O'Brien to a portable electrocardiogram, while the intern explains to Berman what happened.

Mrs. O'Brien is just visible from the foot of her bed, a tiny, frail but resolute figure surrounded by busy, tense bodies still vibrating from the crisis. She is fully conscious now and badly shaken. "They almost killed me, didn't they," she will say the next day. "I really thought this was it."

But for now, she does not let on. She is fond of this young intern, who is about Susie's age, and understands that it was a mistake. She jokes with the nurses about what she thinks she said when she was out, and they laugh with relief at her recovery. She sits up in bed for a while, disarrayed, like the victim of a mugging, but still very much there. Her dignity has stretched to accommodate all sorts of things these last months, and it does not collapse now. Yet she is nearly transparent from shock. She wears a pale, embroidered nightgown, and no wig this day. Her hair has come back in, thin and frizzy and grayed, and she does not care. Her sister Kak arrives, and when Terry dozes off, mentions that when she came to visit last night, Terry's roommate (who has been elsewhere this morning) asked her whether she was Terry's daughter. "You know what she's got for months and months and months," Kak says, "but you don't believe it. It has to come to this." She says she called their brother, Jimmy, in Chicago after leaving here last night. "I told him, if there is a God up there, then He needs a psychiatrist. To let an eighty-three-year-old woman sit in a nursing home strong as an ox forever, and take the daughter . . ."

When Terry is lucid, she draws her sister to her with a look. They have not been close for years, and Terry has declined all Kak's overtures in recent months, preferring to "lie here on my couch" than be ministered to. Now something has changed. They no longer irritate each other. Kak is prepared to do whatever is asked, and Terry has finally begun to ask. She would like her back rubbed, she says, and Kak goes down to the gift shop and buys a perfumed powder to sprinkle on her sister's back. She massages her tenderly, as a mother would her sick child, and Terry submits. They talk in spurts of growing up in the Bronx, and often of their mother. Terry tells her sister about the scare this morning and laughs recalling that she said to one of the nurses, "Stop chewing that gum!" It is a fantasy, part of what ran through her mind in the half-light of her "lethargy," but she thinks she said it and she says to Kak, "Mom would have said that."

When she mixes up her words—it is happening periodically again—Kak gently corrects her, and instead of getting angry, Terry nods and says, "Do that please." When Kak takes the job too seriously, exaggerating her own pronunciation at one point as if speaking to a deaf person who was reading lips, Terry makes a face and snaps, "I didn't say move your mouth around like that, for Christ's sake."

When Te—as Kak and Brian and Jimmy call her ordinarily, and as Ray does these last days—falls off to sleep, Kak stares at her and cries. She talks about how emotionally strong her younger sister is—earlier in the year, she had said she didn't think she would want to know if she had lung cancer, she didn't think she could face it as well. The sight and the facts of Terry's decline stun her. "An orthopedist friend sat me down and told me what to expect," she says. " 'Figure out how many bones you have in your body,' " she says, quoting the friend, " 'and just hope it goes quickly.' "

While Terry sleeps, Kak reminisces about how her sister always knew what she wanted in life, about how tenacious a child she had been. "She always was a terror," Kak says. Remembering how her sister dealt with Ray back then, she laughs. "He was so big and tall and handsome, and he adored her. But he had a temper. Even his mother said to her, 'Don't marry him, he's got such a temper.' But Te said, 'It doesn't worry me.' "

Te wakes and wants to sit up again. Kak helps her to slide her legs over the side of the bed, and the movement seems to recall for her the scene this morning. She shakes her head. "That was a stupid thing they did," she says. "I was *petrified*." She is completely lucid, entirely herself. The missed synapses that so bewilder her start again around dinnertime.

By then the room has filled with her men. Ray and Chris are dressed in darkest bankers' blue, their white shirts still bright at the end of a hot day. Sean is looser, gangly and comic in his movements, wearing a checked shirt that works its way out of his corduroys every few minutes. He has his mother's newly bony face and none of the O'Brien sleekness. Chris is beautiful, sloe-eyed, opaque, and gentle. Brian Sweeney is there, too, a ruddy healthy male blend of his two sisters. He had lugged his movie projector from Connecticut to Colts Neck, intending to show Terry movies of Raymond's wedding, and has now brought his equipment to the hospital so as not to disappoint himself or her.

The screen is set up in front of the window, blocking the view of the Fifty-ninth Street Bridge and the tramway from Manhattan to Roosevelt Island in the East River. It is the sort of chaotic scene that Terry O'Brien loves, but though she is at its center, she is only intermittently joined to it today. She looks less strained than she did earlier, but her mind is wandering and she has begun to hallucinate. For the first time, she does not catch herself losing touch. Chris and Sean sit on either side of her on the bed, urging her to eat. Chris looks stricken, his blue eyes ready to water. All the men but Sean seem badly strained, wounded. Ray seems about to burst with pain. His eyes are almost always on his wife, he laughs hard at her jokes, which remain funny, and fusses with her things, trying to make her comfortable.

Only Sean seems able to engage with his mother as if nothing were wrong. "Come on, Ma, eat your peaches," he says, holding a slippery spoonful of canned gold fruit to her crusted lips. She shakes her head, and he says, feigning disappointment, "But you *always* eat your peaches."

Brian runs the movie, and everyone but Terry watches eagerly, calling out at the sight of various members of the family, hooting at goofy camera-conscious smiles. When Terry appears at the top of some stairs, her mouth wide open, Ray says quietly, "She was at her heaviest then."

In the middle of the movie, Terry points to her tray and announces, "I see bugs." Her sons help her inspect the tray, but find no bugs, and she gives up. When the movie is over, she looks up and says loudly, "Thanks, Brian."

Close to eight o'clock, the men get ready to leave, and they approach her one by one to kiss her goodnight. She reaches absent-mindedly for each one, receives their kisses and pats them on the arm or cheek. Sean is last. When he pulls away after kissing her, he drops his voice very low, bends at the waist, and says, "Bye, bye, honey." His mother's eyes are half shut, she seems on the verge of sleep, but when he is almost to the door, she tosses her head back, winks at him, and, her voice low and throaty in imitation of his, says, "Bye, baby."

She is transformed again the next day, lucid, sharp, in control. Ray, Chris and Sean are there again, and when Don Cameron, a close friend of the O'Briens, stops by to visit late in the day, her tongue is working at top speed; there are no missed words, no slurring, only an occasional pause, as if she has lost her train of thought. Until recently, Cameron could be counted as something of a good omen, a man who was treated here for Hodgkin's disease twelve years earlier and never had a recurrence. (His sister-in-law, Jean Campbell, is the coordinator of the fellowship program at Memorial and was counted by Terry as yet another familiar presence.) But Hodgkin's is not lung cancer, and whatever personal value his survival has had for her up to now, it is no longer meaningful. When he says to her, after recalling his experience, "Only the good die young, Terry, right? We're too rotten to die," she answers in an uncharacteristically small voice, "I'm not rotten."

She asks someone the date, and then realizes that tomorrow is Carol's high-school graduation. She looks very sad, and says fretfully. "She's graduating tomorrow and where am I? I haven't even gotten her a present." A moment later, she has forgotten, or blocked, what she can do nothing about, and talks entertainingly about her childhood. "I'll never forget how Kak used to hate having me in the room with her," she says without preface, the thought brought on perhaps by their revived intimacy this week. She grows giddy with recollections of forty years ago, and then turns her attention to Cameron, a small, benign figure who leans against the window ledge, arms crossed on his chest. With Kak's help, Terry has spruced herself up today; she wears a pale-aqua bed jacket over a pretty orange nightgown and has covered her hair with a bandanna. She fiddles with the ribbon on her nightgown and teases Cameron. "The first time he's been in a hospital room with a woman wearing a nightgown—poor guy doesn't know what to do." Cameron gives her a blank stare, then says, "Should I ask them to leave?" His wit makes her laugh.

For days she has held everyone's attention. It is not just that her family and friends must come to her, that logistics place her at the center. She has become fascinating in a new way, like the madwoman in the square. It is painful to watch what is happening, and impossible to look away. The only relief is to be elsewhere, yet they return, faithful and devoted, no one but Sean hopeful any longer.

Susie O'Brien comes when her schedule allows, usually late in the day, when the others have gone. Sometimes she brings Leo, her boyfriend and, like her a doctor, and Mrs. O'Brien, who is very fond of Leo, threatens him with the removal of her wig on the days when she manages to wear it.

Friday, the fifth of June, is her last good day. Over the weekend, she is more confused than coherent. Since the episode with Levo-Dromoran, she has been back on Dilaudid and Tylenol III, and though her disorientation has intensified, it is no longer due to the medication alone; the cancer is doing its part. She continues to receive platelets and packed cells, and on Sunday she is moved down the hall, to be closer to the transfusion room, for the convenience of the nurses.

On Monday, the eighth, she hovers between a sort of dizzy derangement and an intermittent coherence, in which reality bears down hard when it registers at all.

When Dr. Berman comes by late Monday afternoon, she is lying on her left side in the bed staring out at the hall. He pulls a chair close to the bed and faces her.

"What's up?" she asks, a question she has begun to put to all visitors, with varying expectations. Berman tells her that the pathologist has compared the cancer cells taken from her recent bone-marrow with those taken from her lung at the time of her operation two years earlier and is convinced they are the same. "Okay," she says, in a dull, gravelly voice. Berman goes on tentatively, trying to be thorough but reluctant to be cruel, explaining that there is no longer any point in the hormonal therapy. It's lung they are dealing with, without question. She nods. "Now I get it," she says.

"How is the pain today?" Berman asks.

"The same," she answers.

"Where?" Berman asks.

"Same place. In the hip," she says, reaching around carefully, "and down here," she says, stroking her leg. She hesitates, then says, "It's worse than ever. I can't get up and walk around by myself. I have to get someone to pick me up, walk me to the bathroom, help me to the toilet, help me back."

Berman suggests she try using the commode. She smiles. "Yes, well, I keep forgetting to do that," she says.

Berman says they are still hoping to give her better pain relief. They have thought of radiation, but are worried about the effect on her blood, already so poor. She asks what's causing the problem, and he says it could be one of several things, repeating the litany that she has heard so often from him and from Golbey: the effects of drugs she has had along the way, radiation, or simply, obviously, the cancer. Mrs. O'Brien takes this in like a slow student, with less than her usual comprehension. She seems at first confused, then about to weep. She controls herself with effort and says to Berman impatiently, "What the hell is it?"—meaning, "What is going on? What is happening to me?"

Berman is taken by surprise. "The pain?" he asks.

"You guess," she says crossly.

"I don't guess," he says slowly, comprehending. "I know. It's the cancer."

Mrs. O'Brien jerks her head against the pillow.

"So, in other words, it's worse," she says.

Berman nods.

"Do those things get better?" she asks, her voice straining, her body tensing forward, curling tighter on the bed.

"Some do, some don't," he says.

"*Ever?*" she cries. She has heard only the "some don't" and knows it applies to her.

Berman is silent, unable to say more.

"Oh, beautiful," she sighs, sinking back on the bed.

She requires no more from him. She sees the train bearing down, hears the whistle blowing, and she knows. There is no longer any hope of getting round it, nowhere for her to go now but into death. She sucks in air with the jerky gasp of a weeping child and then is silent for a long while.

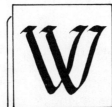hether one has the best prognosis or the most dismal, cancer, like life itself, constitutes an indeterminate sentence. It follows a sequence that cannot be hurried, though it can be stalled, and despite the "averaging" statistics that patients look to for what comfort they can get, it insists on being peculiar to each of its victims. The rules that we like to count on in ordinary life don't apply. "You teach your kids that acts have consequences," Dee Angell said shortly after the first anniversary of Karyn's diagnosis, "but this exists outside that frame of reference. With this, you put in your time, but you don't ever get to check it off. It isn't ever settled."

For the first six weeks of her illness, Karyn Angell lived for two things: remission and getting out of the hospital. Though she entertained fantasies of life beyond those paired goals, they were, by her usual standards, thin and imprecise, constricted by the uncertainties of her disease and by the unpredictability of her future. On achieving remission and winning her freedom, she replaced that first set of goals with another: to get back in shape and to complete the second phase of her treatment in time to return to school in the fall. Implicit in them both was the hope of being restored to normal, of working her way, a hurdle at a time, toward life as it was before.

The identical impulse was at work in Sal Giovia, in Jimmy Polack, in Johanne Johnson, and in Howard Mindus; ahead of each lay a prescribed course of treatment, of predictable content but unknown difficulty; at the end, safety awaited, or so it was important to believe. What one needed to concentrate on were the milestones in between, a simple enough task to contemplate while reading over one's protocol, but essentially a task that could not be credibly imagined ahead of time.

One of the problems in being treated for cancer, particularly when the treatment is harsh or especially long, is keeping the alternative in mind, and the stakes. In the beginning, it is easy enough. However reluctant one may be to undertake the treatment, its connection with one's survival is clear, and at that stage, as Howard said, "It's not something you can walk away from." Over time, several things happen. The patient's tolerance and endurance erode, and if he is feeling well, the treatment begins to seem like the enemy instead of the disease.

Looking back on the roughest and most volatile year of his life, a newly sobered Sal Giovia—by then still only eighteen—would say, "Every time you interviewed me, I said something different. The truth is, I didn't know what I thought." And Karyn, who seemed the calmest of all for months on end, would write a series of letters and reflections that chronicled the same internal confusion. "I feel so much like a collection of parts that weren't made to go together but are being changed and molded so they *can* fit together and work efficiently," she wrote in August 1981, as she approached the end of the second phase of her treatment. "Kind of like a secondhand '69 MG with a '73 Mustang engine and a '76 Honda clutch. I think if I can figure out how all the pieces fit together and form that whole, I can start to be whole again, too." And in early February 1982, back at school for five months and driving herself to a nearby hospital for her maintenance treatments (and occasionally still for fever), she would write, "I can't believe it's been over a year. I keep thinking back to the same time last year. I was so scared and felt so ignorant and out of control . . . I feel like I'm fighting me for myself. I feel as though the leukemia invaded my body and took it over for a time. Now it's a contest: between me and it for me. Every little thing that I can make happen—every time I succeed or accomplish something in spite of it—I'm taking a little more of me back."

Johanne Johnson's voice broke light and playful suddenly in the middle of an account of trouble that was nothing if it was not big and serious. As if she could not bear to repeat one more time the terrible details that described her situation at the start of 1982, she simply stopped, shifted tone with a laugh, and said, "Ah, who knows what's going to happen? All I know is that at midnight on New Year's Eve I was singing and dancing and having a great time, and the superstition is that whatever you're doing at midnight you'll be doing all year."

It was supposed to have been all behind her by then. She had put in her time certainly, and she had come close to believing that it had worked.

Since surprising everyone by surviving an operation that her doctors were reluctant to undertake two years before, Johanne had been through a lot. She was far from cured by surgery: her ovarian cancer was Stage III, meaning that it was well advanced, though confined to the abdominal cavity. Sixteen pounds of tumor had been removed but more than microscopic malignancy remained. In order to spare her a colostomy, her surgeons at Lincoln had left behind a small mass in the rectum, and to destroy it and any additional, undetected, cancerous cells, a potent, year-long regimen of chemotherapy was recommended. Though she weighed seventy-five pounds after surgery and could not take any food by mouth for the first fifteen days, Johanne was judged fit for her first treatment by mid-April 1980, less than a month after her operation. It was memorable. The drug was cis-platinum, the same drug that would flatten Lou Finkelstein and help to cure his seminoma and that would be considered too rough for Terry O'Brien. The first dose, which Johanne received as an inpatient (as she would subsequent doses of this particular drug, first at Lincoln, than at Memorial), knocked her out for days. After the nausea came exhaustion and aches and pains that faded terribly slowly. Without a doubt, it was the kind of chemo that makes one believe in its power to overwhelm a tumor.

In fact, the treatment for ovarian cancer is one of the most effective around, making the disease itself a Catch-22 cancer of the first order. If it were caught early enough, as cervical cancer usually is, almost no one would die from ovarian cancer, but because of its location and the absence of symptoms in the early stages, it is rarely detected until it has spread. Untreated, it is usually fatal within ten months; in 1983, there have been about 18,000 new cases and 11,500 deaths. Not that it was ever possible to attach precise odds to Johanne's life—her chances were good *if* the treatment worked, *if* the cancer did not come back.

In the fall of 1980, after three treatments at Lincoln, Johanne switched to Memorial and became a patient of Tom Hakes, the Ob-Gyn specialist who also treated Celine Fink. Her first inpatient chemo at Memorial was in October, her second over the Christmas holiday. The December treatment was the last of the cis-platinum and was followed by three outpatient doses of Cytoxan and Adriamycin, two widely used cancer drugs, for a total of eleven treatments. There were to have been thirteen in all, but in April Johanne balked and said she would have no more.

Her refusal was not lightly decided. "When it first happened,"

Johanne says of getting cancer, "I thought, I'll just let it consume me." But in the months after her operation, she worked hard to rebuild her life and her strength. To make up for what she had lost of her second semester in nursing school, she started summer school, but had to drop out. Undaunted, she started again in the fall, and this time she did better than she expected. She put on thirty-five pounds in a year, despite chemo. Her son, Michael, was a spur to recovery, and so was the feeling that she had to be strong for her family. "Going through the motions of life helped," she said, "but there were reminders. The scars from the needles, the burned veins, the missing hair." The first time her hair fell out, two weeks after her first treatment, Johanne laughed. But then it started to grow back in, and when it fell out a second time, "I cried like a baby. I was upset for three weeks. My friends wouldn't talk to me about it anymore." Everyone advised her to relax and buy a hairpiece, but she would not. "To have worn a wig would have been an out-and-out admission of what had happened."

Throughout that first year, Johanne struggled with her own reluctance to acknowledge what had happened, and her fury that it had. She was simultaneously disdainful of offers of sympathy (preferring to act as if there was nothing to warrant it), and resentful of what she perceived as the huge difference between herself and anyone who did not have cancer. "You're whole and I'm not, and I resent you," is how she described her attitude, even while breaking all records to demonstrate how whole she was.

"It wasn't that I thought so much about dying as that I was afraid of what people would think of me—that I had brought it on myself," she said early in 1981. A month or so earlier, she had run into an old friend who didn't know that she had had cancer, and Johanne found herself not mentioning it. "An opening never came up," she said. But that consciously disingenuous attitude alternated with an occasionally ferocious aggressiveness about being sick. "Two months ago," she told me when we first met, in March 1981, "you would have met with a lot of anger and suspicion. I would have asked you whether you were in treatment or in remission." No one who ventured to say "I understand" was to be believed, though what form of comfort she would have accepted, Johanne could not say. For a time she felt obsessed by cancer, and totally cut off from those who had not experienced it. "I used to watch anything about it on TV," she said. "If the person was dying, all the better."

But the strain of going it so much alone was awful, and at the start of 1981 she joined a small group of cancer patients who met weekly to talk. "I didn't know, to be honest, what I wanted. I think I wanted to talk about cancer—and guilt. I felt I had brought this on."

The group she joined turned out to be less interested in emotional therapy than she had hoped, but it provided more support than she had, until then, let herself look for, and it helped. Discussions often centered on nutrition and other self-help issues, including the investigation of alternative treatments and the dangers of conventional cancer medication, all of which fed Johanne's growing conviction that her disease and her cure were somehow her responsibility.

Her involvement with the group came at a time when she was feeling particularly vulnerable. Since her operation, she had felt a special closeness to her cousin Evelyn, who was about the same age and had been diagnosed with ovarian cancer a year earlier. The two women had talked often about how they were going to lick it, and Johanne remembers being inspired and heartened by Evelyn's endurance. "They were constantly opening her up," Johanne said of her cousin, whose disease eventually spread into her liver, lungs and chest cavity, "but she pretended it wasn't so." And Evelyn looked as if she was going to beat it, Johanne said. "I remember when I came home from the hospital so skinny, and Evelyn was all fat and healthy-looking after a year of it—" the contrast was all in Evelyn's favor, Johanne thought.

But while Johanne was undergoing her first months of treatment, Evelyn's disease was spreading. Its effects were devastating. She had a colostomy—"a bag," Johanne says, speaking of its results, "and that was so hard. She had a relationship with a man and it went bad. It was hard on him. And she gave up."

In the fall of 1980, Evelyn returned to the Bahamas, where both she and Johanne had been born, and before leaving, told Johanne she wouldn't be seeing her again. She stopped her treatments and died the following January. Johanne wasn't told until a few days after it happened, coincidentally the day of their grandmother's funeral. There had been a lot of deaths in the family, several from cancer, and everyone was afraid of the effect on Johanne. Finally, when the grandmother had been buried, Johanne's mother spoke to her. "'Josie, I have something to tell you,'" Johanne recalls her mother beginning.

"I was dancing through the apartment like a crazy person," Johanne says. "All I can remember is saying, 'I'm next, I'm next.' But everyone said to me, 'You're a fighter, you're different. Evelyn gave up.' So then every day, I would look in the mirror and say, 'I'm not going to die.'" But for the first time in months, she thought it more than likely.

"I started believing that I had cancer everywhere." Instead of diminishing month by month, as she had been telling herself, it was now sprouting everywhere in her imagination. It suddenly seemed pointless to continue the health regimen that she had been pursuing as her contribution to her recovery. What good were all the vitamins, the vegetables, the lean meats? "I started doing destructive things," Johanne says, "smoking, eating junk food." The comparison her family made between her and Evelyn was not lost on her, however. She was "acting out" but she was far from suicidal.

Still, with Evelyn's death the idea that treatment might prove futile had taken root. Johanne had always been worried about possible damage to her heart and kidneys, organs that were specially vulnerable to the drugs she was getting, but by early 1981 she was also suffering from more immediate side effects, and these combined with her new fears to begin to turn her against the continuation of treatment. She was chronically insomniac, but that, she was convinced, was a condition that would end with the treatment; more frighteningly, she had developed a bad case of drug-caused neuropathy, or nerve damage. It was most severe in her feet and ankles, but had also begun to edge up her legs and to be felt in her hands and wrists—a tingling sensation alternating with numbness, as if her extremities were continually going to sleep and then waking. It drove her wild at times, woke her in the night, broke her concentration when she tried to study. And although the neurologist she consulted at Memorial said there was a chance that it would go away when chemotherapy ended, on the basis of his experience with other patients, Hakes disagreed.

The outbreak of neuropathy was one reason why Johanne got little argument from Hakes when she said she didn't want to take her final treatments. Although there are standard doses, and protocols to follow, when properly given, chemotherapy is not given without reference to its demonstrable effect on a patient. Treatment is commonly modified, doses are halved or skipped altogether. In Johanne's case, all the signs seemed to indicate that she would be better off without the last two treatments. Her physical examinations showed no palpable mass; she looked well; her tolerance for chemo seemed to have been exhausted psychologically and emotionally; to administer any more might do more harm than good.

Where she and Hakes did not agree was on the question of a second surgery, to confirm her apparent remission. The "second look" is standard in Memorial's treatment of ovarian cancers; just as Johanne's diagnosis had been delayed and nearly missed because of the difficulties of detecting and testing for a hidden tumor, so it was impossible to determine by external checks alone whether she was completely clean now. The routine at Memorial was to do a confirming exploratory after the program of chemotherapy was concluded; if anything was found, it would be removed, and a second round of chemo initiated.

Johanne had known for months that this was coming and had decided against it. "They'll put up a fight," she said of Hakes and his colleagues, "but, I've made up my mind."

In fact, her mind continually wavered on the question. Some moments she was confident of her decision, at other times she was desperately anxious. She took a positive reading of whatever she could to bolster her decision and fought hard against contrary evidence. In one of her last sessions with her cancer group, in March, she performed an exercise called "traveling" that other members of the group had done previously. The idea was for a patient to lead a fantasy voyage through some part of his body, exploring his disease and his feelings about it. When it came Johanne's turn, she chose her rectum, the site of the mass that her chemotherapy was supposed to have eradicated. "We went inside, and no one could see," she said. "So I thought nothing had happened. Later on I thought, Oh, yes, it did. We got out—there was no obstruction."

In early April, before talking to Hakes about the second surgery, Johanne broke out in a bad face rash. "I look like a fish," she said. "My neighbor looked at me and did a double take. 'What's happened to your face?' I said I got washed ashore." She got an appointment with a dermatologist at Memorial the next day, and while waiting to see him, kept covering her face with her beautiful, long fingers, her dark-painted nails fluttering up and down as she laughed and made painful jokes about the puffy, blistery welts all over her face. "I've tried egg whites, Vitamin E, aloe—I doubled up on my zinc." She rolled her eyes. What chance did her remedies have against the damage being done by chemo?

She was afraid that it might be herpes, an affliction common to cancer patients because of their lowered resistance, but the dermatologist said it was a localized reaction to chemotherapy. By the following week, it had cleared up, and Hakes had agreed to discontinue her current treatment. They had still not discussed the second look, and so Johanne fixed on this interim landmark instead. She made a big, exaggerated sigh of relief, saying, "That's just how I feel," then added, "but I'll have to get over the shock," meaning the shock of being, as she took it, cured.

A week later, the reality was not sitting comfortably. Being off treatment was like performing without a net. She felt terribly exposed, and alone. She had just talked to Hakes and been startled by his vehemence about the second surgery. "He really surprised me," she said in a dazed voice. "His voice was sharp, he was very blunt. I'd never heard him like that before. He told me I might be putting myself in danger. There might be something there. I had thought of it the other way around," Johanne said. "The danger of opening me up, the painkillers. I asked him, 'What if you open me up and find something and let air in?' He said, 'We'd close you up and start you on estrogen therapy.' I asked him about the chances of its recurring, and he said I'm in the high percentile. 'And you could open me up and not find anything, and a year from now it would be back?'" she asked. That, too, was possible.

She had thought she had made up her mind months before, in part because she hadn't let in all the things she was now hearing. "It takes me back to a year ago," she said. "I'm running the tapes in my head."

Still, something pushed her to hold out, scared as she was. "It *is* my body," she repeated, to Hakes, to herself, to everyone with whom she spoke. "It is my decision. And a hundred years from now it will still be my decision."

On April 27, 1981, Johanne kept a late-afternoon appointment with Hakes to discuss her future treatment. By now they had been through it all several times. Hakes had been as frank as he could be about his fears for her, and she had been as clear as she could be about her refusal. Their meeting now had a quality of reconciliation; each came prepared to work out an agreement on Johanne's future care.

"You look very good," Hakes said when Johanne appeared in the examining room, and she smiled at him. She did look good, and she had a playful, teasing eye for him today, which she held in check as he reviewed her treatment so far. "We've given you the twelve months we usually give," he began, only slightly inaccurately. "There are no large tumors present, but there could be microscopic tumors that I have no way of detecting." Johanne nodded, lips pressed together, expectant, though this was a replay of their earlier conversations. "That's why we recommend the second surgery," he continued, explaining the procedure briefly. "The next question that people ask, is, 'Is it absolutely necessary?' The answer is no."

Johanne broke in, speaking in a musical voice. "If the tumor is gone, it's gone, if it's not, what good is it going to do me? I'm going to die anyway." Alert to pressing his case, Hakes replied, "If we find something, we can treat the pelvis with radiation, or if it's in the abdominal cavity, we can use oral medication."

Johanne shook her head. "No, no," she said with a smile. "I've decided I'll be one of those rogue patients."

Hakes's straight face broke slightly. "I have several of those."

From there the discussion moved on to the question of the medication Hakes wanted her to take in lieu of the second look. Nowhere as harsh as her previous year's chemotherapy, it would include two drugs in pill form, Leukeran, which Hakes said could depress her blood count, and Tamoxifen, an antiestrogen that frequently causes hot flashes. Hearing this, Johanne, who was already having hot flashes severe enough to soak her clothing through in the course of a long subway ride, said, "Just what I need."

Before leaving, she mentioned to Hakes that she wanted to fast for a day or two, now that her main treatment was over. "I want to get some of the poison out of me," she said. "Is a juice fast okay for a couple of days?" Hakes nodded, smiling, interested. "After I'm done with school, I'm going to set up shop next door to you," she teased. "You know, the other side of the fence." She winked and added, "I'll win you over."

Hakes laughed. "I'm a hard case," he said dryly, and told Johanne that he would see her in six weeks.

The euphoria that Johanne felt on leaving Hakes that day did not survive long past the two-day fast, which she undertook a week or so later. The fast, she reported, "really was beautiful," but the reality—and the possible consequences—of her decision not to let the doctors have a second look was torturing her. She had thought that by saying no she was defining a clear end to her treatment, and therefore to the cancer itself, but she discovered that she had done just the opposite. It should all have been behind her by now, but here she was, still taking medication, having passed up the closest thing to a certain chance to find out that her cancer was gone.

And she hated the way the pills were making her feel. "The flushing is enough to drive you mad," she said in early June. "From nowhere, I'm burning up. It's awful, it's embarrassing. I look like I just stepped out of a pool." Her solution was to take two pills a day (and sometimes one) instead of the five that Hakes had prescribed, but this carried its own insidious penalty. "Am I doing myself harm?" she would ask over and over, and when she began to feel aches and pains in her breasts, her rectum, her groin, she imagined that it had come back, and that this time it was really her fault. "I take one step forward, and then I hesitate," she said. "It tears at me, the idea of death. Now more than ever before. As long as I have breath in my body, I will feel like this," she said.

At her next appointment with Hakes, in mid-June, Johanne raised the question of the second look and confessed that she hadn't been taking the pills regularly. Hakes noticed her extreme nervousness and asked what she had been doing for the summer. "Nothing," she answered, and he said he didn't think that was a good idea. "You're used to being busy," he said. She nodded and said, "Maybe I'm having a delayed reaction."

She asked him to describe the surgery again, as well as an intermediate procedure called a laparoscopy, and said she had been thinking a lot about it. "Maybe if I let you go ahead, I'd feel more at ease." Hakes suggested that she not rush it, but think about it for another month. And in the meantime, take the pills every day.

On leaving, Johanne seemed unrelieved, despite Hakes's solicitude. She had told him she thought she would like to join a therapy group of cancer patients and asked for a referral to one of the social workers. Hakes had given her the name of Sharon Cooper, an outpatient social worker who also conducts individual therapy. Johanne headed for her office, intending to get information about a group and wound up staying for a private session that she badly needed.

She told Cooper about her previous group, which had ended just when she most needed support. "Right now," she said, sounding slightly ashamed, "I'm really having a hard time. I came through surgery and everything really good—everybody said I did—but it's difficult talking about how I feel to people who are not in the same boat."

She started to cry suddenly and, startled, lifted her hand to catch the tears as they ran down her cheeks. She described her conflict between refusing the surgery and having to continue to take the pills she hated. She said all this very fast, and then looked up and said, "I feel like a moron right now, but I guess it's just because I've had a knot in my throat for weeks."

Cooper asked her what she was most afraid of at the moment.

"Recurrence," Johanne said without hesitation. "For example," she added, "I need a job, but I'm afraid to look for work. I'm really not free of it." Cooper asked her whether she had ever talked to a therapist about this before, and Johanne shakes her head, No. "I always thought I could do it on my own. And if I didn't talk about it, I didn't have it. If I didn't talk about cancer, my mom, my brothers, my sister, wouldn't have to be depressed." Crying hard now, she says, "Sometimes I think it's my fault, if that makes sense." She described the strain she had been under the year and a half prior to her diagnosis, when the store that her mother and brother owned was having trouble. "We stayed up late, worked hard, but the business failed anyway. I didn't eat properly, didn't sleep right. So now my biggest fear is that I'll keep worrying and worrying, and it will come back."

Cooper says gently, "You're getting into a very controversial area," and later on, "You've got a real dilemma—if you take the medication, it means you're still sick, and if you don't, you worry." Johanne nods. "I get the feeling," Cooper says, "that you're disappointed not to be able to do it yourself."

"It's the way I was brought up," Johanne says. "I thought I had to do it myself."

When Cooper asks her whether she has been seeing men lately, Johanne shakes her head again, No. "I haven't had time," she says at first, then adds, "Since my illness, I've shied away. I'm not like other people. I'm useless."

Her account of herself all has to do with accounting to others, with her worth in their eyes, of her need to be perfect to be loved. It is not how she feels every moment, but it is there, deeply layered in her psyche, and her illness has made it swell. She cannot let down for a minute, or everyone around her will collapse. She cannot let down for a minute, or *she* might collapse. Before leaving Cooper's office, she attempts to explain how powerfully she has felt that others were counting on her to pull through. "When I got sick," she says, "my mother said to me, 'You're my strength.' And my brothers and sister," she adds, looking stunned even as she says it, "they said to me, 'If something happened to you, what would become of us?'"

In the months to follow, Johanne would turn the several themes from this conversation over and over in her mind, along with the problem of what to do about treatment. She was surprised by the image of herself as someone so resolutely self-sufficient, but she conceded that it was correct, motivated by fear more than anything else. "I've been running scared," she said. "I was afraid to sit down for fear I'd never get up. Sometimes I felt as though I wasn't doing anything, so I just kept doing the little things. I didn't want to burden people with my problem. I was afraid they'd think, Oh, God, it happened to her, it could happen to me. But I should have known there would come a time when I would not be able to do it alone. Now I see that in order to get on with my life, I *have* to talk about it."

She saw Sharon Cooper a few more times, found part-time

work as an office temporary for the summer, and began to climb out of her depression. But the question of her physical health remained unresolved. She was not taking her medication except in the days immediately preceding her blood work. Like a guilty child who fooled no one, she would swallow a few pills a day or two before, hoping it would show up in her blood. She was less distraught by her defiance than before, but she was still worried. "The days I don't take the medication, I think, Are you canceling out another day?' But what the hell. Even after a second look, I'd still think, Did they miss it? I believe there will always be that doubt there." She talked of finding another approach, sometimes nonmedical, sometimes just an alternative to Memorial, but she never followed through.

In September, Johanne started school again, switching to Hunter College in Manhattan, just a few blocks west of Memorial and tougher academically than Bronx Community. She kept on with temporary work when she could get it and spent many hours a week filling in for one of the staff at the drug-abuse clinic at Lincoln in the Bronx. By October she was looking ragged from squeezing so many things in. "I can do so much more when I don't take the pills," she said, as if trying to convince herself. "But my mother says I'm walking on ice."

In late November, Hakes felt what he thought was a small mass in Johanne's rectum during her checkup. He called in another doctor, a surgeon, to see whether he could feel it too, and the second doctor confirmed his finding. Johanne's reaction was subdued, as if she had nothing left to respond with, and as if it was what she had expected all along. "The last few visits, I've really been listening to their voices. Hakes never tried to pretend with me. He always laid it out." Her subconscious was less sanguine. "I'm having nightmares about it," she confessed. "I'm running and there's this huge thing sticking out of my stomach. It's a human being, an old man." She did not define her stowaway further.

Through the month of December, Johanne concentrated on staying calm, or at least keeping the news at bay. She put off contacting the surgeon Hakes wanted her to see, gathered some information about the proposed surgery, but never put it all together, as if it might somehow go away if she didn't look at it too closely. She spoke to Michael, who was very angry, and decided this meant she was going to die. After her previous recovery, like his mother he had believed that it was over. "I didn't promise him I wasn't going to die," Johanne said in mid-December. "'But you got sick *again*,' he said, and I told him, 'I didn't get sick again, it's a continuation.'"

212

Hakes and the surgeon wanted her to go in for surgery right away, but Johanne said No, it might be her last Christmas. And still she acted as if there was no hurry. The month stretched out, and the year, and she danced all New Year's Eve and finally went in to see Hakes on January 6, after a frantic phone call from his office. She had somehow succeeded in burying all that she had known for a month, so that when Hakes said, as he had said before, on examining her, that there was definitely something there, she actually asked, "What is it?"

"Well, in a word," Hakes said, "it's the cancer." And Johanne said, her voice flat and low, "Oh, God, this can't be happening to me."

They talked about what they had talked about before—about the surgery, and the fact that Johanne had wanted to wait until after Christmas. It was a peculiar replay of a scene that one would think needed only a single playing, but Johanne was not the first cancer patient to require a repeat staging of bad news for it to become real.

When Hakes left the room to permit Johanne to get dressed, she emerged from behind the drawn curtain, wearing a white cotton examining gown and trailing a sheet that she had wrapped around her waist. She moved very slowly, and muttered to herself, "All right Johanne, that's enough. Pull yourself together. Put the mask back on."

The surgery was scheduled for two weeks later, the twentieth. Ahead of time, she was busy trying to strike deals about how the operation would be done—could she just have a local, she wanted to know, and would they promise not to do a colostomy if one was needed without giving her a chance to think about it? By the time of surgery, she had given up all efforts to negotiate and was simply relieved to wake and find that her rectum was still intact, that they had found a small mass and removed it, and that they had seen a spot near, but not on, the liver, which they could not remove. She had come very close a second time.

A week later, she hears from Hakes that her new chemotherapy plan calls for alternating doses of cis-platinum and another, similar drug of lower toxicity. The treatments will be in hospital, like her first series, once a month, for an indefinite period. In the tenth-floor lounge, her arms wrapped around her still-sore belly, Johanne wears a print bandanna on her head, as if her hair had already fallen out again. Everything is starting over, only this time she knows before it starts how hard it's going to be.

Four months after Howard Mindus discovered the lump on his neck that would lead to a diagnosis of Hodgkin's Disease, *The*

New York Times ran a small article about a study done by the Harvard School of Public Health that resulted in a profile of children at greatest risk of growing up to have Hodgkin's—"those who belonged to small families," the report, published in the *New England Journal of Medicine,* read, who "lived in single-family homes, had relatively few neighborhood playmates, and had relatively well-educated parents." Jewish children were twice as likely as Roman Catholics to contract the disease, those from sheltered or affluent environments more likely to get it than the less privileged, older or single children than those of late birth order in large families.

The only child of educated German-Jewish immigrants, Howard recognized himself at once. "Except for the fact that I did not come from a background of wealth," he remarked, "I fit their description exactly."

Being "typed" thus did not strike him as distasteful in any way, or demeaning, nor did it cause him to reflect overlong on the meaning—or the absurdity—of life. Indeed, it seemed quite simply of a piece with his already strong feeling that his cancer was close to inevitable, given his father's lymphoma and his grandfather's leukemia. If anything, he was grateful that circumstances—whether environmental, demographic, or pure chance—had visited him with nothing worse than what he calls "the cancer of choice."

Given the combination of attitudes with which Howard greeted his illness, it would not be imprecise to call him a "hopeful fatalist," except that only the fatalistic half of the characterization is instinctive with him. The hopeful part was very much a product of will, a reflection of Howard's determination not to let this thing overwhelm him. Howard's wife, Myriam, has an even better line on her husband. She calls him—lovingly, but perceptively—the "great minimizer," referring not to any lightness of heart but to his deliberate and unceasing efforts to maintain control and foster the impression that his cancer was never anything to get excited about.

"My wife does the worrying for both of us," he said one day, with tongue in cheek, adopting an uncharacteristically sexist frame of reference to convey his equanimity. And at the conscious level, the level at which Howard operates most comfortably, it did appear to be true. Having decided that the best possible reading of his chances was the one most likely to prevail, he spoke of his disease as being one that was not "life threatening" at all, but more a condition of inconvenience, serious but manageable, requiring an investment of six to seven months, by Howard's advance calculations, after which it would be over. Many of the three-way contracts that Howard negotiates in his job as a contract lawyer take nearly that long to conclude; six or seven months of intermittent discomfort did not seem like such a bad deal, considering what it would buy him.

For about the first six months of 1981 Howard appeared for work at his law firm looking essentially the same as he had looked for the previous seven and a half years—loose-fitting conservative suit over a white shirt and forgettable tie; comfortable shoes; knuckles clasped around briefcase handle. Howard's is a big office, and he was never certain of how many people there knew of his illness. Beginning in late February or early March, those who knew might have glanced at the back of Howard's head from time to time and thought, Oh, right. Those who did not know would have been curious about the swath of bare scalp, a couple of inches wide, that cut across the base of his skull from ear to ear like a strip of parched field grass. If one observed him closely for a time, one would notice too that in the late afternoon certain spots at the edges of his jaw did not display the same brown stippling of beard growth as the rest of his face. These were souvenirs of radiation, the middle third of Howard's three-part treatment and the only one to leave visible marks. The radiation began in late February 1981, in the interval between two three-month rounds of chemotherapy. During each of the chemo phases, Howard received treatment twice a month, on successive Wednesdays. His appointments with Koziner were usually for one o'clock, and with any luck, he and Myriam, who accompanied him most days, would be out of the clinic by five. The vomiting would not begin for several hours yet, and it was, in fact, something of a game with him, and unquestionably a matter of pride, to see first how long he could hold it off, then how quickly he could recover from it. "There's a certain *machismo* to this," he would say in the afternoon of his last treatment, when the *machismo* had been all but used up.

Lunch would be the last meal of the day. At home, there was quiet and a pail beside the bed. Howard liked to be alone for the worst of it, and so on Wednesday nights Myriam would sleep in the living room, within calling distance. They never knew ahead of time how bad it would be. A few times, Howard was able to make it to work by Thursday afternoon; a few times not until Friday afternoon. The people who needed to know where he was knew; those he believed did not need to know were told only that he was not in the office, the presumption being that he was elsewhere on business.

The four-day-a-week radiation treatments he managed even more circumspectly. His appointments were generally for eight or eight-thirty in the morning, which allowed him to make it to the office by ten or so. Indeed, if it were not for the strip of rapidly thinning hair above his shirt collar, Howard's regular visits to Memorial would probably have gone totally unremarked. As it was, no one at work ever spoke to him about treatment, nor were there complaints about diminished effectiveness. Possibly no one but Howard had anything to complain of. "Day to day, I was not cognizant of accumulating weakness," Howard recalled of the period of radiation, "but I had a general idea that my capacity to work was being reduced. You feel worse immediately after chemotherapy than you do after radiation. But in terms of general fatigue, radiation is much worse."

Radiation is tidier than chemotherapy, less wrenching, less violent, and much sneakier. The machines hum and blink and click, but there is no sensation, no prickly skin, no blistering, no scars. In the early days of radiation, the cobalt machines left thick red burn marks on patients, as if someone with a fat thumb had taken to finger painting on flesh, and the potential dangers of radiation were nearly equal to the disease being treated.

There are still side effects, but because of improved technology, they are generally less dangerous, and also more subtle: despite shielding, Howard developed a lump in his throat from the treatments aimed at the lymph nodes in his neck, making it difficult for him to swallow. Some of the salivary glands were knocked out, apparently permanently; he takes water with his meals now, and because his reduced salivation makes him more vulnerable to tooth decay he has been getting special fluoride treatments. Months after radiation had ended, he started to feel an irritating sensitivity in his arms, which had never been radiated. Howard raised the subject first with Koziner, then with Burton Lee, the head of the lymphoma group, who saw him several times in Koziner's absence. Koziner was noncommittal, but Lee assured him that what he was experiencing is a common—and temporary—reaction to radiation of the neck area, which often affects the roots of the spinal cord, creating nerve activity in the arms.

Though he never let himself become seriously alarmed by the peculiar sensation, Howard was relieved to learn that it was a side effect of treatment rather than a signal that something more serious was wrong. Because you never know—even the most stoic of patients is hard put to stifle the suspicions that cancer sets off. One of the costs of cancer is the loss of that false security that shields us all for a time from the knowledge that we won't last forever. Not knowing the means, or not having a particular means nailed to your door, helps to prolong the illusion of immortality. Even with as nice a prognosis as Howard's, cancer erases that illusion in a swipe.

Still, Howard held to his conviction that Hodgkin's would not get him, and he held to it through several more legitimate alarms. In April Koziner found another swollen lymph node, this time under Howard's right arm. At about the same time, an interim X ray showed a shadow in his chest cavity, the site of one of his original two tumors. In the first instance, Koziner felt fairly confident that the node would reduce by the end of treatment, and he decided to postpone a biopsy until the complete restaging that would take place then anyway. In the second, Howard heard a variety of opinions, first from Lee, who happened to see the results first, then from Koziner. Lee's version was that the shadow could be nothing, scar tissue, or active Hodgkin's, all unassailably correct but not much help to Howard. Koziner was marginally more reassuring. Though he stressed that "we don't talk about complete disappearance at this stage," a marked decrease in the size of the tumor from when last checked in January suggested that it was on its way out. Slightly complicating the reading of the X ray was the possibility that the mediastinum, or chest cavity, might have changed shape as a result of radiation, a benign event that unfortunately fogged the picture. In the end, resolution of this question, like that of the lymph node, would have to wait until the summer workup.

There were other, smaller alarms. "I notice he's gotten more brown spots," Myriam said to Koziner one afternoon during Howard's examination. "That's a chronic thing," Koziner replied, without further elaboration. Consulting the list that they had gotten into the habit of bringing with them, Myriam then reported that Howard had had a slight fever, 99.5 degrees, and that he had not been sleeping well. Koziner's response is a smile and a nod. The Minduses have discovered that both Koziner and Lee are expert at "deflecting inquiries," but so far neither has felt badly served. Because things seem to be going well, they are able to absorb personal eccentricities along with the delays in clinic and the punishment of treatment. "Koziner does a lot of shrugging that's hard to interrupt," Howard said one day, more amused than upset as he described Koziner's style. "Sometimes you can't tell whether the shrug means that something *is* significant or isn't,"

Every clinic has its peculiar atmosphere. At some, the prevailing mood is forlorn, because the waiting patients are so obviously doing poorly despite treatment. The Wednesday afternoon lymphoma crowd is smaller than most, however, and many of the patients seem to share Howard's essentially confident attitude. Whatever a cancer patient ought to look like, Howard does not. He looks rather like someone on his way to a business meeting, and he has the quick leap of a man used to tightly scheduled days. His briefcase seems to grow naturally out of his right arm, and he reaches for it whenever he moves from one part of the clinic to another, as if documents necessary to his health were mixed in among his legal papers. For all of Howard's talk of Myriam being the family worrier, he is the one with the more skittery temperament of the two, she the one who centers the discussions and resolves indecision. She is also firm about what Howard needs, in spite of his claims, and makes a point of meeting him at the hospital when he goes for chemotherapy. "I don't think he should have to come alone," she says. "He says he doesn't mind, but I don't believe him."

Howard's insistence that his cancer is not a big deal prompts wry objections from Myriam, who believes that it is something of a big deal. Their differences on this question are mutually respectful, but deep. Myriam is the one who sought out the Center for the Medical Consumer to research Hodgkin's, not Howard. Howard started but never finished *Getting Well Again*, one of the popular psychological texts on cancer in good repute at Memorial; Myriam read the whole book. Myriam makes note of the conflicting survival statistics on Hodgkin's—some sources give 66 percent, some 75 percent, some 80—whereas Howard speaks of his "extremely favorable" or "nearly certain" chances of survival and quotes Koziner's estimate of "better than 90 percent." And invariably their different attitudes toward his illness have drawn different responses from friends.

From the beginning, Howard says, he has had "more attention from friends of Myriam's than from people at work," a certain result of his decision to make little of his situation and to keep it as separate as possible from his professional life. Indeed, Howard has only one story to tell about his disease and the office, and it dates to the first days after his diagnosis. "I had told the people who had to know, and the story spread like wildfire—although," he interrupts himself to say, "I believe there are still people in the office who are unaware of it." "Still?" Myriam asks. "Well," Howard responds, "there are eighty to a hundred people in the office." He meets Myriam's skeptical look and continues. "At any rate," he says, "the story spread, and shortly afterward there was a meeting of some of the partners in one of our other offices. I guess some of them were asking about it and someone said— there were twenty or thirty partners there— 'How did he discover it?' And the New York partner said, 'Apparently, he just reached up one day and found a bump on his throat. There wasn't any pain or anything.' And he said later that he could feel every hand in the room straining against the urge to reach for his neck."

It is of course possible that lawyers as a group are, like Howard himself, more reticent than most to speak of personal matters in the office, and yet it seemed odd that when Howard was in the hospital for his staging in October 1980, only a couple of people from the office called. "Everyone was perfectly decent in that they made allowances for the work load, but I was essentially ignored while I was in the hospital. But then people don't ask about the treatment either, not even, 'How are you doing?'"

"A lot of people ask me," Myriam says, "because they're afraid to ask Howard."

Howard looks at his wife in slight amusement. "Am I fear-inspiring?" he jokes. Myriam shrugs. "They don't want the hassle of confronting you if there's bad news," she says bluntly, touching on a theme that Howard consistently resists. He quickly suggests an alternate explanation. "A lot of it has to do with the fact that people don't want to intrude on what may be considered a very private matter." Myriam nods, but adds, "I also think it may be a risking of your own mortality to discuss it—to encroach upon what many people consider to be a sentence of death."

Whereas Myriam recognizes people's reluctance for what it likely is—a mixture of anxiety about a difficult topic and reaction to Howard's extreme circumspection—he persists in a mild bewilderment, unable to see beyond his own view of what has happened to him. "Basically," he says, "it has not changed the direction of my life," although he concedes that that is entirely because of his favorable prognosis; if he were to be told that he had a couple of years to live, he thinks he might well change his life radically. And though he spurns self-help volumes, he picks a copy of Tolstoi's *The Death of Ivan Ilych* off his bookshelf during this period and reads it—after several years of meaning to.

Having heard Myriam out on the subject this evening, however, he admits that he does have some concerns about the reactions of others. "I think my biggest problem has been with being unable to meet the immediate professional demands of my job, which I take very seriously." "*Very* seriously," Myriam teases, and Howard laughs. "Very seriously," he repeats. "Unfortunately, perhaps more than I should. Although I realize that, in an overall sense, what I do is not that important, nevertheless there are people who are looking to you to do the job, and I take that seriously. So I feel a little bit of a problem when I'm in the middle of a transaction such as the one I'm in now, where there are time pressures to get it done, and the people who were in the office today—well, I didn't tell them why I was going to be out. All I've told them is that I would be out of the office tomorrow afternoon and Thursday morning, and that I expect to be in the office Thursday afternoon. Which is an iffy proposition."

"Shouldn't you say something, so that people don't just think it's your whim?" Myriam asks.

"Nobody thinks it's my whim," Howard says. "They probably think it's another meeting or some professional obligation. But somehow I suppose I would not feel as bad if it *were*. I have told myself time and again that my A-number-one priority is to get well again. And in order to do that I obviously have to go for the treatments and handle that as a high-priority matter. But although in this case I've been able to persuade myself otherwise, somehow I view my responsibility to others—and that's probably wrong—as having a higher priority than my responsibility to myself."

Though he has outlined circumstances that fairly well preclude his colleagues' involvement in his illness, Howard still seems unaware that he has arranged things thus. The strength of his resistance to friendly solicitude, though he is troubled by its absence, becomes apparent to him only when the conversation shifts to the subject of sympathy. "I'm not interested in getting a lot of sympathy," he says, attempting to explain the difference, as he sees it, between a civil interest in his welfare and the kind of attention that would make him cringe. "I suppose objects of sympathy are objects of contempt in my mind. I'm not interested in encouraging that."

"I don't think it's inappropriate to give sympathy to someone who's being poisoned," Myriam says flatly.

"It's a matter of degree," Howard says. "I'd like a sense of some interest in how I'm doing, a sense of solidarity if you will, that somebody out there is rooting for me to pull through. But I don't feel the need for sympathy particularly. I don't need anybody to feel sorry for me, at any rate. If I were worse off, I could understand, but—nevertheless, I have been surprised by the fact that in the hospital and since then there really have not been too many inquiries. Possibly," he reflects, "the way I handled early inquiries was such as to discourage people."

"I think Howard is a minimizer about this particular illness,"

Myriam says. "In a way, that's a good way to deal with it, but it's off-putting when people inquire how he's doing. People say, 'How're you doing?'" she says, and she imitates Howard shrugging "Okay." "He's essentially changing the topic."

Howard laughs. "I'm a little bit more elaborate than *that*."

Myriam shakes her head. "Very often you are no more elaborate than that," she says. "Occasionally, when someone is very close, you'll provide another sentence indicating that the last treatment was really awful and you're looking forward to the end."

Howard shifts in his chair at the pinching accuracy of Myriam's summary. "There are some people I don't want to talk to about it," he says

"You are quite short with frequency, Howard," Myriam says. "And people are discouraged from asking again. I'm not saying it's inappropriate. But you are quite curt."

Howard considers what Myriam has said and admits that she is probably right. "Part of it is that I feel as though there is a professional side to my life and a personal side to my life, and unless I see somebody as a friend, or likely to become a friend, I don't know, I just don't—and particularly if I have the sense that somebody is going to feel *sorry* for me."

"I think Howard's attitude touches on something we all feel in some fashion when we're sick," Myriam says repeating an observation she has made before, with reference to her own illness and to her son's. "Which is that your power is diminished. It *is*."

So important was it to Howard that he hold himself unchanged, undiminished, that even sympathy, the most decent of emotions, had to be avoided, lest it curdle into pity, and make public proof of losses worse than he felt or could stand to feel. To keep pity at arm's length, he had to keep much of the world at a distance, too, and he was beginning to feel the pain of that bargain.

As is often the case, his body knew better than his waking brain how much he deserved sympathy, and moments before his penultimate treatment it rebelled in his behalf. Reporting on it afterward, Howard had a boyish, sheepish look. "It was the first time I had to use a doggie bag in the chemo room," he said. "I threw up *before* I got the medication. It's all psychological," he added, with a dismissing shrug. "But I'm beginning to have a reaction to this place."

The night before his final treatment, nine months almost to the day since he had first felt the lump in his neck, Howard couldn't sleep at all, his apprehension split about evenly between anxiety over getting another treatment and concern that it might be postponed because of his counts. But his checkup with Koziner went well, and his counts were high enough for him to get a half dose, all he had been able to tolerate since the third cycle. They discuss the posttreatment workup scheduled for July, which, if all goes as expected will result in at least a temporary bill of clean health. Howard is edgier than usual during Koziner's exam, and before it is over he asks Myriam if she will get him a vomit bag from the chemo room, just in case. To Koziner, he says, somewhat apologetically, "The psychological reaction seems to be getting worse." Koziner nods. "That's very common," he says quietly.

In the waiting room, Howard paces, growing paler and paler in anticipation of the injection to come. "Oh, I shouldn't have had lunch," he groans, and makes a face at the recollection. "I had an Amy-burger," he says, referring to a local fast-food sandwich of singular taste—mashed chick peas deep fried and served like a hamburger. Howard sinks into a chair and says, "I'm feeling the deep-fried part right now." He retreats to the men's room several times, checks once with the nurses in chemo to see if they are ready for him, then asks Myriam to check a second time. After some twenty or thirty minutes, his name is called. He leaps up with his still-clean doggie bag—double strength on the basis of experience—and starts for the back of the clinic reluctantly, like a diver who has no choice but to head for the end of the high board. When he returns, fifteen minutes later, he is still carrying an empty bag, but announces that he has already been through two. There is an embarrassed look on his sweet face. He looks about ten years old, and in need of all the mothering—and sympathy—Myriam can give him.

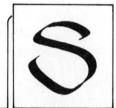omeone forgot to tell Sean O'Brien that his mother had been transferred down the hall from Room 426 over the weekend, and when he arrived at the hospital around four-thirty Monday afternoon and found her old bed empty, he felt a sudden terror that it was all over.

A few minutes later, directed by one of the nurses, he bounds into his mother's new room, so buoyant with relief that he does not at first register her changed attitude. "I was a little scared, Ma," he jokes, expecting her to pick up on it, but her only response is a sort of mumble.

It is barely an hour since Berman left, and when her eyes fall on Sean, it is as if she cannot place him in this new context. Recovered from his fright at not finding her where he expected to, Sean has reverted to the role of merry visitor, but it no longer works for her the way it did the Friday before.

She is beyond merriment now, yanked abruptly past it this very afternoon, and she does not know any longer how to respond to his offerings. When Berman was here, she was fully coherent, but in the last hour, she has begun to retreat into a stupor of confusion, or despair.

Exhausted from a few moments' conversation, she sinks back on the bed again, looking broken and uncomfortable, and yet somehow unaware of it. Her shoulders are lodged below the pillows, while her head is propped at an awkward angle above. Sean tries to ease her into a more comfortable position, but she is indifferent to his efforts and falls briefly asleep before he succeeds in resettling her. He sits beside her, crooning to her sweetly, and when Ray arrives, just after five o'clock, her eyes are still shut. Ray watches for a while, waiting to see whether she will wake, then steps outside to talk.

He speaks in a low voice, as weary as it is discreet, saying that he has just come from Golbey. "And basically," O'Brien says, pushing his gold-rimmed spectacles up the bridge of his nose, "Golbey says it's 'irretrievable.'" His eyes widen and his face contorts briefly as he pronounces the word, so remote, almost squeamish, and yet just the sort of clarifying word they have been anticipating.

Earlier in the day, Golbey had met with several other doctors to discuss whether anything more could be done. The pathologist's report Berman had mentioned to Mrs. O'Brien was discussed, as were the most recent X rays. O'Brien says Golbey told him that the cancer is moving so fast now that looking at a sequence of X-ray stills is like looking at a movie film. The cancer is taking over, squeezing out healthy cells in her bones at a terrific rate. They are keeping her going with transfusions, but there is a limit to the usefulness of both blood and platelet support, as well as a limit to their economy.

Because platelets—the shortest lived blood components—cannot be matched for compatibility the way whole blood can, sooner or later she will react badly to a transfusion. And, despite matching and other precautions, neither whole-blood nor packed-cell transfusion is risk-free; there is always a chance of infection when a patient is being given someone else's blood, and the odds that something will go wrong rise with every pint.

In fact, the expectation that "something will go wrong"—that the *coup de grâce* Golbey spoke of earlier will materialize in one form or another, and soon—is everyone's best hope. If it does not, and if her condition "stabilizes," then she could last anywhere from a week to a few months, and the problem of her care would revert to her husband.

Ray O'Brien understands this. He and Golbey have talked about the possibility. "The question is," he says, "if they get her well enough to leave here, how do we take care of her?" Golbey has advised him not to let his two younger daughters take care of her. "It's fine for you or me," O'Brien quotes Golbey as saying, "but they don't need it." O'Brien glances toward his wife's room. "Well," he says, "I'm not putting her in a nursing home, so it becomes a question of a private nurse."

There is also the possibility of Susie's caring for her mother. She has told her father that she thinks her mother should be brought home to die and that she is prepared to take a leave from work to care for her. Her father, astonished and impressed, and also a little frightened, is uncertain whether to accept her offer. It is clear that he hopes he won't have to, but nothing is certain at present.

O'Brien reenters his wife's room. She is awake now, and he bends low over the bed and gives her a big kiss on her bloody lips. He says to her gently, "You're bleeding again, Te." She looks up at him and tries to explain. "Last night," she says, "last night I had a hemorrhage." From where, he asks. From what place? She calms down, seems to think of something disappointing, and touching her fingers to her lips, says quietly, "My mouth."

Since she changed rooms, she has acquired a new oxygen rig, this one a clear plastic mask that fits over her nose and mouth like a World War II pilot's mask. She fiddles with it, doffing it like a cap to talk, replacing it when she wants air. She removes her glasses from time to time, and bumps them crooked when she tries to arrange the mask on her face. She is alternately still and twitchy, engaged with her visitors or distracted. The notes on her chart during the week chronicle the attempts made to ease her pain and reduce her confusion, but the two goals are in stubborn conflict. Golbey's last note for Monday reads: "Our primary concern is to keep the patient as comfortable as possible." Platelets are ordered "for bleeding only," and on Tuesday the order is modified to "for significant bleeding."

On Tuesday, as it happens, Mrs. O'Brien's lips are clean for the first time in several days. In the late afternoon, she sits on the edge of her bed, staring out at the nurses' station across the hall. Kak sits beside her, having no luck keeping her attention. Te is fiercely intent today, impossible to distract. She stares at visitors hard, then looks away without speaking, returning her eyes over and over to the nurses' station, as if on the lookout for some particular person. She is very angry but calm. At one point she announces in a voice with little inflection, "This was the worst day of my life," but she will not elaborate. She seems to be communicating with the world from a great distance, and the look on her face is that of a prisoner plotting escape.

Only when Ray arrives does she return to the present. She is lying back on the bed, worn out from her watch, when she turns her head, sees him, and breaks. She lifts both arms to him and starts to cry. "I want to go home," she sobs as Ray leans down to embrace her. "I want to go home." Rays stays with her while everyone else leaves the room, and soon she is dry-eyed again, more alert than she has been all day.

Her remarks have a kind of loony appropriateness to them. She points casually to Ray at one point and, with a straight face that stifles challenge, says to the nurse who has stopped in to check on her, "He wasn't here last night for the hanging of the Cross." A moment later, when the nurse has gone, she says she wants a painkiller. Sean asks her if she is in pain right now, and when she says yes, he buzzes the nurse.

When the nurse returns, and says it is too early for her painkiller but "How about a Valium," Mrs. O'Brien says, "Sure," in a bright tone. When the nurse has gone, she spins around and announces, "And then I'll have a chaser of scotch and a beer."

Tom Fahey, the internist who has treated both O'Briens, stops by, and several conversations overlap. Mrs. O'Brien is at short liberty, attached to an I.V. pole, but mobile within a five- or six-foot range of the bed, and she paces the length of the room talking to different people in turn, rarely waiting for a reply. When Sean fails to get her attention after several tries, and raises his voice, she turns to him and says, "Don't interrupt!" He laughs and says, "You're pretty grouchy today," at which she turns and says, with an ironic smile, "I wonder why?"

She sulks then, until Ray says to her, "Don't you love me anymore? After twenty-nine years, you better make up your mind. I may be the only husband you get." She gives him a sharp look. A bit later, she starts to play with the I.V. tube that hangs from overhead. She makes scissorlike movements with her fingers, saying, in impatient bursts followed by periods of silence, which no one breaks, "I need to cut this. . . . I need a scissor. . . . Would you cut this, *please?*" she says finally, annoyed that no one else sees the need.

When Dr. Berman arrives, Mr. O'Brien steps outside with him, followed by Chris and Sean. There is no new information of substance, but Berman explains that, despite the fact that her gums are not bleeding today, her platelet count is very low, and that, along with the painkiller, may be contributing to her mental confusion. "There could be bleeding in the brain," he says. "And eventually platelets become useless in her case. Unfortunately," Berman adds, "we have people who are literally bleeding to death for whom they will work." The implication is that it's time to stop. When Berman has gone, Chris and Sean look at their father. He purses his lips, blows out, and says dully, "Hot dog."

The boys ask what will happen now, and he says they will keep on making her comfortable.

His sons stare, and O'Brien goes on. "What could happen," he says, backing up to the doorjamb in the hall and aligning himself with it unconsciously, "is your mother could die of a stroke." The boys do not flinch. "That's how Johnny Sheridan went," he tells them, speaking of a family friend and needing to make it a plausible event for them. He wags his head from side to side and says, "Listen. That's not a bad way to go. You don't feel anything. It's better than—" He jerks his head toward his wife's room and does not finish.

Back inside, O'Brien is loving and playful with his wife, getting a reaction only some of the time. He turns to his sons and asks them whether they can make it home early tomorrow, because it is Carol's eighteenth birthday, and he wants to give her a party. "It *is* her birthday," he says, though no one has objected. "If we don't do something, she'll think we don't care about her," he says, instinctively appropriating his wife's usual role. He asks Chris and Sean whether they have spoken to Raymond or Susie, because he would like to get them to come out too, if they can, and Chris says they were both in to see their mother last night. O'Brien shakes his head. "See, your mother was saying she hadn't seen Ray for three months." It is getting harder and harder to know what counts, what registers, and whether any of their efforts are making a difference.

Golbey's chart for June 9 is brief: "Situation as above [referring to the previous day's entry]. Confusion increasing." He might have remarked as well on her still powerful resistance. Later that night, when the floor is quiet, Mrs. O'Brien gets herself out of bed, leaves her room, and makes a run for the elevator and freedom, trailing I.V. stand, bottle, tubes, needle, and tape past the nurses' station, heedless of the wild bouncing of her paraphernalia until the bottle breaks and cuts her hand. "I really gave them a fright," she reports the next day, speaking of the nurses who corralled her and returned her to her room. She holds up her right hand to show a thickly bandaged thumb, but, despite her excitement, the chart indicates that the cut was slight, the bleeding minor.

"I tried to leave, yes," she says. She sits in the big aqua easy chair next to the bed, wearing a fresh summer nightgown and a quilted bed jacket, small but strong, steely rather than frail, and eerily rational. "Yes, I wanted to get out in the worst way," she says. "I thought the most unimaginable thoughts a human being can think, and then I screamed. I thought, I'm going down fighting. They're not going to have me."

She looks very proud as she pronounces these words, but the result of her escape attempt is unhappy. Her chart for June 10 indicates "companion," meaning that the staff believes it can no longer control her, keep her safe, without help. From now on, unless someone is with her, as Kak has been all day, she will have to stay in her bed, with the railing up. If she refuses to stay put there, she will be confined in a "posey," a light mesh wrap-around vest, white with green piping, that can be tied to the bed. The posey looks like a very genteel loose-fitting straitjacket, which is exactly what it is. So that she will not have to be confined, the O'Briens have hired a companion for the night, who will arrive at eight o'clock.

Of these details, Mrs. O'Brien seems oblivious. But she has not relaxed her suspicion. If anything, her paranoia has increased. "Something's up," she says nervously to Kak, her eyes darting around the room and to the door to the hall. She says she thinks she's going to be sick, bends over the bedpan Kak hands her in her lap, then changes her mind and tries to look under the bed. "What's there?" she asks. "Nothing, Te," Kak tells her.

A few minutes later, she is back in bed, and starts to panic. "Where's Ray?" she asks suddenly, with a wild look. "Something's up, I know it." She is crying now. "Where's Ray? He didn't leave me, I know it. Something's up." She does not remember that it is Carol's birthday, that Ray has been and gone already today, trying to take her place at home. All portents are bad for her, and she trusts no one. Including God. "Huh," she says with a shudder and a look of disgust. "Did I tell God what I thought of *Him*. I told Him I didn't know if I wanted to be with Him or not. If this is the way He's going to act." She is down to herself.

In the late afternoon, when the painkiller starts to wear off, she sits up and buzzes the nurses' station. When no one comes immediately, she starts to fret. Kak tries to soothe her, but she won't allow it. In a short while, a nurse comes, and says it is too soon for her painkiller, but she can have her Tylenol early. She gives her two pills, and returns a half hour later with the more powerful medication. She holds three pills in her hand and asks Mrs. O'Brien whether she thinks she'll be able to swallow them. Mrs. O'Brien stares at the hand outstretched before her and declines to remove the pills. She looks up at the nurse and asks, "What are they?" The nurse and Kak assure her that the pills are the medication she's been asking for.

"I want to know what's going on," she says.

"Okay," the nurse says.

Kak says, "It's six o'clock. At six o'clock, you're supposed to get your pain medication. Remember, you were asking for it a while ago."

"What kind?" Mrs. O'Brien asks.

"Dilaudid and Zomax," the nurse tells her.

"Look at the pills, Te," Kak says.

Mrs. O'Brien says there are too few, and the nurse explains that she usually gets them together with the Tylenol, but that she's had the Tylenol already.

"Te," Kak says, "I wouldn't tell you to take anything you weren't supposed to. I swear to God."

"Look at my Irish face," the nurse says. "How could you not trust this face?"

"I swear on Mom's body," Kak says. "It's just to ease the pain."

"Yeah?" Mrs. O'Brien's voice is thick and hoarse. She is truly frightened. "To ease the pain to Hell?"

"No, no way, honey," Kak says. "It's just for now, I swear."

Her sister looks at her disbelievingly. "Yeah, she takes the pills, and in a half hour Satan takes her!"

Kak despairs. There is nothing more she can do. But suddenly Te's look of wariness vanishes, and she swallows the pills, one at a time, her eyes falling on Kak after each.

Within the hour, there is a second crisis. Kak has arranged to meet Mickey, her husband, on a corner at seven. He is driving in from Long Island and they are to have dinner. Knowing the new rule, and worried about her sister's frame of mind, she lets the nurse know that she has to leave before eight. The nurse nods and says quietly to Mrs. O'Brien, "You won't mind getting back into bed for an hour or so, will you?" Mrs. O'Brien catches on. "Okay, you stay, then" she says to the nurse, who replies, "I would, Mrs. O'Brien, but I have ten other patients."

Mrs. O'Brien turns to Kak and says she has to stay.

"But I have to meet Mickey," she says.

"You can't go."

"But I have to, Te," Kak says.

"No," Te says firmly.

Kak looks helplessly at the nurse. "Mrs. O'Brien," the nurse says, "she has to go. It'll just be for a little while."

Mrs. O'Brien is sitting in the big chair next to the bed, facing her sister, who is balanced on the edge of the bed. The nurse hovers at Mrs. O'Brien's side. Staring at Kak, Mrs. O'Brien says to the nurse, "She'll stay." She pauses. "She's my sister." She never takes her eyes off Kak as she says, "He's not heavy. He's my brother."

Kak sighs and repeats the line. "He's not heavy, he's my brother." She's caught. She says to the nurse, "If I can just go tell Mickey I'll be late." The nurse is torn; she can't stay. I offer to wait with Mrs. O'Brien until Kak comes back. "Will you?" Mrs. O'Brien says, suddenly coherent, turning to me. "Thanks." She releases Kak, whose place on the bed I take.

She seems distracted again; the effort of will she has just made could not have lasted much longer. A line of blood has appeared on her lip, perhaps for the tenth time today. Her face is drawn and tiny, her body hollow and limp. She looks far away. I touch her hand, which lies palm down in her lap. "Are you all right?" I ask. She looks up, focuses her eyes and is lucid once again. She leans forward and touches my hand. "Thank you," she says. "Thank you very much." She settles her bright gray eyes on mine and repeats, "Very much."

Her sudden, unpredicted returns to clarity—to her real self— are almost as startling as the confusion they interrupt. What she says or does in these moments are like stage directions, or negotiations under truce, and they remind one of the terrific force of character that remains in this small, battered body. She cannot be written off yet. She is still there, just as her blank-faced mother is still there downtown, commanding regular visits from children she never acknowledges. It is not hard to imagine Terry O'Brien holding her family that way, and it suddenly seems plain how she came to the sense that she deserved a biographer. She does.

She is quiet for a while, then politely asks me if I will get her suitcase from the closet. "What for?" I ask. "I just want it," she says. I tell her she doesn't need it, backing away from the request. It frightens me, because I would so like her to escape, and I dread participating in something that will get her hopes up. I say she isn't well enough to go anywhere, and she says, "I know. But do it anyway, will you please?"

I can't think of any way to resist, and like Kak earlier, I give in. "Okay," I say, "but then"—my response more absurd than her request—"I'll put it right back in the closet."

The suitcase is the same, stiff gray-green zipper case that she has been bringing to the hospital all spring. I balance it on my lap and start to fill it with things from her night chest. First a yellow Fair Isle sweater, then a gray shetland. There are nightgowns and bed jackets—both Ray and Kak have been supplying fresh ones daily—a girdle, a bra. I lift out the Ken Follett book that has accompanied her unread for weeks and ask if she wants it. "No," she says. "Leave it here."

The drawers are quickly emptied. There is little in them, and she doesn't want it all, anyway. As I finish, Kak returns and nods at the suitcase, understanding. She has taken part in a similar ritual earlier. When I zip the case and return it to the narrow closet near the door to the hall, Mrs. O'Brien nods her approval. For the moment, she is appeased.

Susie O'Brien came in to see her mother several nights that week, usually toward the end of visiting hours. What she found most nights was "a typical senile person," not unlike those she had seen while working in hospitals. Although aware of the probable medical causes of her mother's senility and paranoia, Susie felt they were probably aggravated by being in the hospital. "It wasn't like she was always begging to go home," Susie recalled later, "but being upset like that is not uncommon in elderly people in the hospital. It's not a familiar environment, there's nobody around that you know except when people come to visit. In the last months, my mother always wanted to come to the hospital when she felt sick, but then she always wanted to go home again."

This time, it was clear to her that there would be no going home, at least not in the sense of a real recovery. Going home had always meant not dying—each release from the hospital worked to confirm her private certainty that she would make it. And though it was against all logic, Susie remembers that her mother somehow thought that, having "beaten" lung cancer once, she could beat it again. Her desire to escape from the hospital was perfectly sensible seen in that light—a departure would mean survival for another while, at least.

Susie's idea was that her mother should be brought home specifically to die. Even as she raised it with her father, she knew that it was an impossible choice from everyone's point of view but her own. "I think if I were not a doctor, if I didn't see people dying all the time, and someone said to me, 'Let's bring her home to die,' I'd be terrified. If I were not a doctor, I'd probably think, That's crazy, dying people belong in the hospital. Now I feel just the opposite."

Ray O'Brien was concerned about several things—his younger daughters foremost, the management of emergencies next in importance. "He'd say, 'What are we going to do if *this* happens?'" Susie recalled later on. "I said, 'Nothing.' He said, 'What if she started to hemorrhage?' I said, 'So?'

"I couldn't see her needing anything more than oxygen, for comfort, and pain medication. He was worried, but he said he'd think about it," Susie said. "But then she went downhill so fast it never happened."

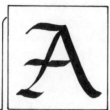t his most outrageous, Sal Giovia remained essentially impossible to dislike. He provoked exasperation in almost everyone who knew him—exasperation and the impulse to shake him hard and get him to grow up fast so he would start to take care of himself. But he also provoked delight and amusement with his bravado, his angry edge and his blunt, sometimes rude assessments of people and situations. He was funny oftener than he was not, and even at his most wrathful. He was cocky when he had no reason to be, and when he occasionally gave way to the frightened boy inside to ask questions of such innocence that it was painful to hear them, the difference between how he must really have felt and how he pretended to feel seemed immeasurable, and devastating.

From the beginning, his parents knew that he was unmanageable, and so did Dr. Gee. "He's not a child," his mother said one morning while they waited with the Polacks in clinic. "I let him go out, have a good time. You gotta let them live. You really do. Because they're so scared."

Sal would never admit it. All his fear was converted to fury and bluster. He bebopped through the clinic as if it were his private club, harassing the blood room for his counts, nailing Dr. Gee or Kathy Dietz in the corridor, demanding attention. He was competitive with Jimmy over their respective reactions to chemo and their quickness to recover, boastful of his ability to "beat leukemia" with or without medication. He was also inordinately perceptive about what went on around him. "This is the outlook I've got on the fellows," he said one day. He was in an especially good mood, about to start the last of his inpatient treatments in late March 1981. He had been out very late the night before, wandering Times Square with three of his friends after checking into the hospital earlier in the evening, and he was feeling worldly and full of himself. Referring to the fellows, of whom he had seen four since becoming Dr. Gee's patient in late December, he said, "Most of 'em are afraid to get too close, 'cause, God forbid, something could happen." He raised his eyebrows, the only hair on his head, and smiled meaningfully. "Small and Gabrilove aren't like that," he said, naming Dr. Catherine Small and Dr. Janice Gabrilove, two women who had been Gee's fellows in succession during Sal's first two months of treatment. "They come around. They're glad to see you."

Once in a while, his terror would seep out, though he usually announced it parenthetically, or as a joke. One day he emerged from a checkup to tell Jimmy, who was waiting his turn, that "Kathy [Dietz] says not to worry about the dreams. They'll disappear when we get to maintenance." He has never mentioned having bad dreams, and when asked about them later, lists them rapidly, as if hoping they will not be counted as significant. There are three, recurring since the night he was admitted to Memorial. "I dream about a big cell eating me up," he says first. "I dream about dying in my sleep, and also that everybody was bald." A short laugh closes the subject.

Even with bald heads, a lot of young leukemics manage to look rosily well through much of their illness. Karyn Angell did certainly, though Jimmy Polack did not in the early months. Sal, tightly built and tightly wound, his lean face so much older than his years, rarely looked ravaged, though he sometimes looked improbably pale for someone so full of energy. It was easy to believe, for that reason too, that he was as tough as he acted, so it was shocking one day to see him at the clinic after a ten-day siege of nausea that had left him haggard and limp. His motor seemed driven by rage alone, and the look on his mother's face as they raced from the elevator to the bathroom on arriving suggested that the two-hour drive from Smithtown had been hell for them both.

The last cycle of treatment had been the worst so far, and Sal's reaction was so violent that his desperate father had left the hospital one afternoon in search of marijuana, a drug with which none of the Giovias was familiar. It didn't help, and the residue of the treatment was as bad as its initial punishment. When Sal left the hospital at the end of five days he was still retching, and his throat was pocked with ulcers from the chemotherapy. The first condition aggravated the second so severely that he could not even swallow water, and his parents' chief concern, besides his weight loss of twenty pounds in ten days, was dehydration.

Waiting to see Dr. Gee, Rose Ann Giovia calls her husband at home to tell him that they have arrived. "I'm going to tell Dr. Gee, 'Don't believe anything he tells you. He's lying. Put him in.'" She thinks she has brought in her son half dead and that salvation will come only with his hospitalization. But Sal, however miserable, has sworn that he will not go back in, and they have fought this battle all the way in in the car. Now they sit wedged together in a chunky loveseat in the southeast corner of the waiting room, knee to knee with Jimmy and Valerie Polack. Rose Ann strokes his leg from time to time, but Sal wrenches his thigh away as often as he submits, flinging his body first against the arm of the couch, then against his mother, then tossing his head back against the wall. He looks awful, close to what one imagines a leukemic would look like if he was never going to get well again. He holds a gauze pad to his parched lips; there is no trace of animation anywhere in his face. His faded skin is drawn tight around his mouth, and he stares balefully out at the room with flat, dulled eyes. His throat is so sore and scarred that he can barely speak, capable only of hoarse, croaking muttering whenever anyone says something he doesn't like. He spots a fat woman eating candy from a bag and snarls, "I hope she chokes."

His friend Jimmy sits diagonally across from him, palms resting on thighs, also pale, but not suffering the way Sal is. He says he is surprised at how low his counts have fallen, because he doesn't feel as weak as they would indicate. In fact he feels pretty good, but he is careful not to say so out loud after Sal arrives. The last treatment hit him hard, too. "Never in my life have I felt so shitty for so long," he says, "After a marathon, you feel pretty awful," he says. "Sometimes I throw up. But you know you're going to feel better soon." He smiles ironically. "If you're an old man it doesn't matter," he says. "They're ready to knock on heaven's door anyway. But to feel this as a *young* person?"

From his slumped position, Sal spits out in a raspy voice, pointing a finger at his throat for emphasis, "When I'm better, I want to talk to you about this whole Methotrexate period." He shifts jerkily in his seat. "I've never felt worse. Emotionally, physically, every way."

Each in his own fashion remains incredulous. How did they wind up here? Or as Jimmy is fond of saying, "Nobody deserves this kind of abuse."

It is not hard to imagine that Rose Ann Giovia would prefer to leave her son here rather than take him home, but Dr. Gee checks him out and says that, despite appearances, he is not in danger. His counts have not fallen that low—Sal's interpretation is that the chemo didn't work, and that "maybe they'll have to give me more Methotrexate"—and he would have to lose another ten pounds before it became a problem. Gee says to bring him in again on Thursday, three days hence. In the meantime, try to get him to drink liquids, but don't worry. As Rose Ann departs with her triumphant invalid limping behind, one wishes that she could have the bed rest he spurns, so frazzled and worn-out does she look.

On Thursday, Sal senior brings Sal in and the younger man looks reborn; he is upright, tingly with energy and eagerness to be done with the clinic, still edgy but aware of it and self-mocking. His white count is good but his platelets are low, and Dr. Gee has said that if he wants to stay out of the hospital he had better get an infusion of platelets as an outpatient today. At twelve-thirty he and his father are still waiting for the six-unit order (5,000 platelets to each unit) to be ready, and Sal is pressing one of the nurses to call downstairs for the second or third time. "Morons," he says with a grin, then adds, "Write that down."

When the platelets are ready, father and son take the back stairs to the third floor, to the outpatient transfusion room at the back of the surgery clinic. With only one nurse on duty, there is another short delay. Sal senior notices that Sal's chart has been placed on one of the beds and he flips through it with interest. On the emergency admitting form used in Bedholding there are multiple-choice listings for a patient's physical and emotional condition, and finding one of Sal's sheets, he starts to read off mood descriptors. "Irritable, confused," he begins slowly and Sal laughs and says, "*Irritable*, that's it. Write that down." They clown together over the chart until the nurse, a stiff, correct woman, returns and says they are not supposed to read it. Sal senior raises his eyebrows and says with mild irony, "Oh, we thought since it was about him . . ."

They have been up since six-thirty this morning, arriving at the hospital at ten-fifteen. Sal senior has a business appointment in the city and is worried about the time, but both he and Sal are in fairly good moods. They have been through the worst the last couple of weeks and are like survivors of a storm, grateful to be alive. "Yesterday we almost broke," Sal senior says. "Rose Ann was really on the edge. We sat down, Sal, his brother, my wife and I, and we said, 'We know it's not your fault that you feel this way, but you've got to help us help you.'" Sal listens to his father attentively, then tries to explain. "I don't know what happens to me on medication—I get emotional. I get upset easily." He grins at his father. "Yesterday I couldn't find my girlfriend. I was calling everywhere. He saw me. I was crazy." He looks ready to be forgiven.

But the physical battering continues. The next drug scheduled is one called L-Asparaginase, which he is supposed to get as an outpatient three times a week, two weeks running. But his reaction to the drug is so bad that Dr. Gee takes him off it almost immediately. "I was getting nauseous just thinking about coming here for the L-Asparaginase," Sal said in mid-April. "When Dr. Gee called up and said, 'How you feeling? No more,' I wanted to run over here and kiss him."

His girlfriend, Ginny,* has come with him today, a sweet-faced redhead two years younger than Sal. She has known Sal for a year or so but has been his girlfriend only since a few weeks after his diagnosis. Sal's former girlfriend, Ginny says, "broke up with him the same night he shaved his hair off [when it was starting to come out from chemo]. So what are you supposed to think?" she asks.

Ginny puts Sal in delicious spirits, and he talks about his counts, predicting how high they will be, then predicting that "By the time I'm in maintenance, I'm gonna have a Rolls. I've already got a driver," he says, referring grandly to the man who drives his father to and from engagements in the Catskills when the senior Giovia is exhausted. "I know I'm gonna get it," Sal says to a dubious look. He laughs. "My father says, 'You have a way of getting what you want.'"

He plays with Ginny's ear until she tells him he's driving her crazy, announces that he's already bought the bid for his senior prom and, with barely a missed beat, turns and asks, "If I slipped out of remission, would I know?" Before anyone can answer, he says, "Yeah, my gums would probably start bleeding again." He shrugs and tugs at Ginny again, who squirms in her chair and sighs. "But even if I did," he says, "the treatment would probably be better by then."

Jimmy is getting his last consolidation dose today, and his grandfather has come with him. They visit with Sal, Mr. Polack nodding approvingly at Ginny, and Sal mentions that he and his family are going to a "healing Mass" out on Long Island the following week. He tells the Polacks what little he knows about

---

*Pseudonym

the service, and Jimmy is interested. Morris Polack's eyes narrow with skepticism. "This I have to see for myself," he says, and he cautions Sal, "It's okay as long as you keep doing what Dr. Gee says. He's a priest, too."

The healing, as Jimmy and Sal speak of it, is on a Tuesday night in April, at a big red-brick church that rises from the center of a huge suburban parking lot like a drive-in bank. The Giovias, who have not been ardent churchgoers, have become at least occasional communicants since Sal's diagnosis and also close to a young priest they call Father Frank, at whose Mass for teen-agers Sal spoke earlier in the year. They have raised the subject of the healing with him, and reassured that he does not think of it as a wacko event, they go with a willingness to believe and a need to do this thing as a family.

The Polacks come for their own reasons. Jimmy is in need of a change of scenery and some fun, as eager to be leaving the city for an evening as he is expectant of any miracle. Though he muffles his anger better than Sal, he has been much less guarded about his other emotions and has not hidden his feelings of despondency from himself or his family. His isolation in New York has grown more painful each week, and though he has explored the city some—and already knows it better than Sal, to whom Manhattan is as exotic as Bali—he longs for home and friends, even as he reiterates his reluctance to be seen by them in this condition. And, as he has done from the beginning, he thinks often of death—his own—specific and not at all far-fetched to him. He talks about how he used to take crazy chances with his life— riding motorcycles and driving souped-up cars, leaping into hidden water from high places. He talks about how hard it is to stick with "this abuse" without any guarantee that it will work. *Fifty-fifty* sticks in his throat as a meaningless statistic.

Jimmy has none of Sal's innocence, feigned or real, and none of Karyn's single-mindedness. He is thinking it through as though it may really happen, a nervy and dread-filled exercise. So the healing for him is a diversion and a possibility so bizarre as to be apppealing, and on the way to the church he sits in the back seat of the Giovias' Cadillac prepared for anything. His eyes seem glued open, the pale shadows underneath a perfect match to the buff-colored high-sitting cowboy hat on top of his head. The hat belongs to Sal's younger brother Guy, who, like the rest of the Giovias, has a habit of including Jimmy with such gestures.

Forewarned, the Giovias and Polacks arrive at the church around seven for an eight-o'clock Mass. The pews are already full a third of the way back, and there is in the air the kind of expectancy that precedes a theatrical performance. Sal, who has had his last consolidation treatment just the day before, sits near the end of the pew with Jimmy, Ginny and Guy, rubbernecking furiously and reporting on everything he sees. A terribly tall woman enters a pew a few rows back and Sal turns to Jimmy and says, "She's here to get short." A couple of his cousins are seated immediately behind him, and he whispers loudly to them that he and Jimmy won't be the first to go up. "I want to see somebody in a wheelchair walk," he says excitedly. "If that happens, it's gonna freak me out." He laughs. Stroking his shiny scalp, he adds, "It'll make my hair stand up."

Earlier, Sal had said, "How will we know if it worked? I mean the leukemia is already gone." He thought for a moment and came up with an answer. "I'm not saying this will happen, but maybe in a year, Dr. Gee will say, 'You don't need no more chemotherapy.'"

The singing starts around eight o'clock, led by a small group clustered beneath a banner of the Sacred Heart. There are guitars and tambourines and widespread rhythmic waving of hands above the crowded pews. The procession begins—a line of banners carried by young people, a phalanx of somber women dressed in blue robes and looking like deacons in some decidedly non-Roman rite, and finally three priests walking slowly abreast down the center aisle in full regalia. The one in the center is the starring attraction, the healer from out of town, rumored to be a Father D'Orio trainee, a middle-aged priest with a professionally composed face beaming piety.

As the three priests reach the sanctuary, a great babble rises from the congregation, signifying speaking in tongues. The head priest joins in and raises his hands in the style of the charismatics before him. The Mass begins. After the Gospel is read, two speakers address the congregation. The first is one of the women in robes, whose language can be interpreted as either symbolic or actual and whose intent is hard to make out. She speaks with expert ambiguity of spiritual and physical health, spiritual and physical healing, yet seems unmistakably explicit when she addresses "someone here tonight with cancer of the breast" and assures the unidentified woman—there could be thirty in the congregation—"You don't have to worry. Because it's already taken care of."

The main priest speaks next and he is more careful; honing close to a traditional line on the meaning of salvation, he alludes to the conflict between God and Satan, speaks of evil and suffering, then takes some heavy swipes at science, which he can safely presume has failed many in his audience. "Maybe what we have to try is holistic medicine, biofeedback, acupuncture," he says from the pulpit. "As Jesus said, Go back, tell them what you have seen." As if choosing his words with an eye to possible lawsuits he says, "Jesus touches the cancer that grows on men's souls, because He wants you to be whole."

The healing itself does not begin until almost ten o'clock, when the head priest, his two concelebrants, and a half dozen lay assistants leave the altar and form teams of three just inside the altar rail. Though no instructions are given, everyone in the congregation seems to know what to do by instinct, and lines of those who wish to be healed quickly form in the aisles. This is not an assembly of the lame and halt; everyone is upright and self-propelled, making one wonder what hidden wounds or sorrows have brought them all here, and in fact their bald heads make Jimmy and Sal two of the most conspiciously ailing members of the congregation.

Characteristically, Sal has decided that he will settle for neither of the auxiliary healers and will present himself to the main priest only. Fortunately, popular sentiment is less exclusive, and the center line is no longer than the others. Still, the traffic seems unceasing; lines of supplicants run all the way to the back of the church for over an hour, while at the front a nearly identical scene is repeated in triplicate every few minutes. The person seeking to be healed approaches the healer, who is flanked by two assistants. The supplicant is drawn close, sometimes in a three-person embrace, states his problem, is prayed with, and anointed on the forehead. The result is almost without exception a swoon, and the chief duties of the assistants are suddenly clear: to catch the falling bodies.

The Giovias and Jimmy approach the main healer shortly before eleven o'clock. Later, Rose Ann and Sal senior will confess that they were reluctant and skeptical, particularly of the swooning, but Jimmy and Sal are caught up in the event and prepared for something to happen. The Giovias step forward as a family, while Jimmy waits behind them. Sal tells the priest that he has leukemia, is clutched to the clerical bosom, is blessed, and keels over. His brother Guy declares himself, receives the same treatment, and follows Sal to the floor. Rose Ann and Sal senior come closer, trembling. The priest says something Rose Ann can't remember afterward and shocks Sal senior with a message about guilt. They too are held close and blessed, and each in turn executes a dive.

When Sal senior is on his feet again, he turns and presents

Jimmy to the priest. Jimmy remembers telling the priest that he is Jewish, and that he has leukemia. The priest embraces him and anoints his forehead, and Jimmy drops. His grandfather squints hard from the first pew, where we have moved to get a better view. He is trying to figure out the trick as he perceives it. His eyes search the priest and his attendants for some stunning instrument (a cattle prod, perhaps?) and scan the air overhead for wires. Earlier he had grunted his admiration for the way the crowd had been slowly stirred to credence by first the music, then the sermons; now he says "These people are very clever. I wish I knew how they did it."

The Giovias and Jimmy stumble in turn from the sanctuary in various states of recuperation from the experience. Rose Ann and Sal senior seem stupefied, their sons greatly excited, slapping each other and whispering to their cousins. Jimmy looks as if he has been hit by a two-by-four, his eyes both bugged out and glazed over. He walks as if in a trance, and his grandfather, seeing him emerge from the crowd around the altar, says, "I think they've all been hypnotized." Jimmy stops in front of us and stands staring toward the back of the church without speaking. He does not respond at first when his grandfather addresses him and requires a touch on the arm to bring him to attention. He says he feels fine. I ask if he passed out as he went down, and he says "No. I just keeled back." Then he tries for a fuller description. "It was like a cliff slowly crumbling underneath," he says, an image that he will repeat to general agreement later on, when the healed start to compare experiences. Though he cannot articulate further what the moment represents to him, he says over and over, "It was a-mazing."

Afterward, over dinner at Lennie's Clam Bar, there is little theological reflection, only a general glee and sense of togetherness. No one is eager to define what has taken place, nor to pin cures for Sal and Jimmy on the service. Yet it has given them all a lift, a sense that they have finally done something for themselves, made some positive move that does not include pain and confinement. And that is a lot.

Coming at the end of Jimmy's and Sal's consolidation, the healing service is also a useful punctuation, helping to bolster their belief that the hardest part of treatment is now behind them. Because maintenance, barring catastrophe, does not require hospitalization, it stretches before them like a long holiday: there will be pills to be taken and periodic injections of many of the same drugs that have knocked them flat before, but the schedule is much looser, the doses lower, the intervals longer. With maintenance comes relative freedom once more and, best of all, hair.

Sal would have liked it to come sooner, in time for Jerry Cooney's May 11 fight against Ken Norton at Madison Square Garden. Cooney and the Giovias have a mutual friend, and when Cooney learns of Sal's illness, he dedicates the fight to him. Sal is thrilled. Sylvester Stallone's *Rocky* has been one of Sal's idols for years; now this real-life Rocky turns up, in the Giovias' backyard, with a taste for sentiment and symbolism that Sal himself could not improve on. A couple of Long Island boys destined to be superstars—What better combination could he have dreamed up?

The fight is on a Monday night, a week after Sal is scheduled to get a treatment of Vincristine. With Dr. Gee going to the fight as well, Sal has no trouble getting a week's postponement, allowing him to appear in the center of the ring before the fight with his counts and energy high. "Did you see me," he asks the next day, "that little bald head shining in the lights?" In fact, his brief moment did not show up on cable television; it was like the fight itself—you had to be there to appreciate it. Cooney and Norton held the floor exactly fifty-four seconds before Cooney nailed his opponent with a *thunk*. It was not the kind of fight that most fans consider worth the price of admission, but Sal takes the speed of victory as a sign. It's just like the leukemia—a few well-placed blows and it's gone.

The euphoria holds another couple of months. Sal prevails upon Dr. Gee to switch the two arms of his first cycle of maintenance to avoid having to get Adriamycin before his prom and graduation, thus husbanding his new growth of hair. By the end of June he has a beautiful close cap of fine brown hair—not quite combable, but no longer see-through. He brushes it straight back from his forehead and pats it frequently, as if to reassure himself that it is really there.

School has never been a big part of Sal's life, but his graduation from high school, like any other landmark, has taken on unexpected significance because of his illness. The Giovias decide to celebrate it big, renting a hall and inviting all Sal's friends and theirs. It is called a graduation party, but it is Sal's survival that they are celebrating. Dr. Gee is invited and shows up with his wife and four children. Kathy Dietz comes, and Dr. Small and her husband. Jimmy has flown in from Seattle, combining this occasion with a checkup with Dr. Gee after a month and a half away.

Rose Ann and Sal senior greet guests at the door, pinning flowers on the women and handing out small printed cards that say, "Thank you for coming and sharing in the celebration of my Graduation." The main attraction sits in a small bar off the entry to the hall, hiding out until all his guests are here and it is time to make his entrance. He is as nervous as if he were about to make his debut as a comic, but he looks beautiful, and he is reasonably sure of that fact. He wears a creamy-white shirt and black tie, white beltless trousers that button at the waist and white patent-leather shoes that taper toward the toe. Hanging on the back of his chair is a soft-brown sports jacket, and around his neck, easily picked out against the black tie, is a gold pendant from Ginny.

Sal greets Jimmy happily, eyes Jimmy's scalp, and observes gratefully that he has not been outdone. Jimmy's hair has come in glossy and black, with an unruly corkscrew of a topknot hovering over his brow. Too precious to cut back, it sticks up in defiance of cream or comb, and Sal teases him about the proper maintenance of postchemo hair.

It is another half hour or so before the big hall is full. The doors close, and the band, a good one, plays a flourish to gain the guests' attention. There is a pause—the timing of this moment has been impromptu, with several last-minute changes of heart—and then the band picks up again, with the opening theme from *Rocky*. To its left, double doors burst open and the four Giovias, arms linked, stride through. They are all as smartly decked out as Sal—Guy and his mother in white, Sal senior in powder blue—and they are all of a height, and all four wear the same joyous look. They bound to the center of the dance floor as their guests stand and applaud, and then, as if struck simultaneously by the same thought, their look changes to astonishment, and all four burst into surprised tears.

There are speeches later in the afternoon, after everyone has eaten and danced; telegrams are read. Sal senior is the emcee, and he is both very good and very happy to be doing it for his son. His brother, also a professional entertainer, sings a song, and then Sal senior invites Sal to join him on the floor. The father has a lovely strong voice, a club voice that he knows how to use, and he starts the song slowly—it's a Sinatra song, "For Once in My Life"—and his eyes are glued to Sal's as he tries to bring him along. Sal is nervous, his body in position as if by instinct, but his voice is nowhere to be found. He joins in uncertainly, his voice carrying flat over the mike, but his eyes are fixed in faith on his father, who bobs his head to give him the beat. Sal picks it up as they sing, gaining confidence from his father with every note, enjoying himself by the time they have sung their way to the refrain. Sal senior signals the band to speed up its tempo, and the two of them swing back to face the audience, rocking on their heels and belting it out, in perfect body synch, if imperfect vocal harmony.

Father and son have the same light step, the same grace before an audience, a sense of timing that takes years to develop, and they are having such a good time together that they don't notice the effect they are having on their audience, half of which is sniffling into shredded paper napkins.

The day has been so good for them that the Giovias do not let it end when it is time to vacate the hall in the early evening, inviting all who would to come back to their house for more food, more dancing and a swim in the backyard pool. The last guests depart sometime around midnight, and Rose Ann reports later that it took several days before her face returned to normal, so over-worked was it by smiling on that day.

Like their son, the Giovias are tempted by the thought that maintenance inaugurates the "easy" part of having leukemia, the moment when life returns to normal, or almost that, and the drama and tension let up at last. In part, the party was to mark such a new beginning, and for Sal senior it did. In early July he leaves for Las Vegas to open his first show there, something he has been working toward for years. Sal could have used a comparable engagement, or at least a summer job. Without the frame of illness or school, order disappears from his life. He has no "normal" life to resume, and nothing to move on to. On hearing early in the summer that Karyn Angell has found a part-time job and is planning to return to school in September, Sal makes a disapproving face and says, "I think she's making a mistake. Suppose she gets sick and has to quit? She'll only be disappointed. The way I look at it, I already have a full-time job: getting well."

Of course, this talk of making his health his main business contradicts all Sal's prior assertions that the leukemia is gone forever, and is shortly contradicted by his behavior as well. It is hard to say what Sal is waiting for, but it seems almost as if he has remained idle in order to be available for some form of compensation due him for having gotten this illness in the first place. And when this is not forthcoming, he is bewildered, disappointed, and angry. He makes no move to take charge of his life, to push it ahead in any way, even to try to imagine the future beyond leukemia. He is stuck, and the hard thing, the dangerous thing, is that in the absence of all other serious interests, what he is stuck with is treatment, the part of his life he most resents. How much of this may be even dimly apparent to him he does not say. His tone through the summer months is breezy and willful, and he entertains one unrealistic dream after another.

Meanwhile he's doing his best to have a good time, and part of his pleasure is to let treatment slide a little. He makes no open declarations, but he grows sloppy with the schedules and skips a couple of clinic appointments, pretending forgetfulness and fatigue. Midway through the first cycle of maintenance is a month-long sequence of pills, which Sal himself is responsible for taking, followed by four weekly doses of Methotrexate as an outpatient. While he is taking the pills, his platelet count drops, and the fellow working with Gee that month tells him to stall the pills until his count is back to normal. Sal takes this authorized delay as the basis for stalling still further. "The truth is, I stopped taking the pills two weeks ago," he says in early August, "but what I'm going to tell them is that I stopped four days ago, and then ask them to stall another week." He seems surprised that this admission draws a reaction of concern, and he laughs and says, "Come on. I'm not gonna die. I know I'm never coming out of remission. Dr. Gee put me off for four weeks once. If it was really dangerous, they'd be calling up, saying, 'Where's Sal Giovia?'"

Though this attitude seems spectacularly self-deluding, its appeal—even necessity—to Sal just now becomes obvious when he starts to recall how awful he felt during the early months of treatment. "I used to joke about it," he says, "painting my head when I was bald and all, but deep down inside I hated it. If I had said what I was thinking inside I'd have been arrested. I didn't want people to think it bothered me. I didn't look good—I knew it. But the best thing is to show courage, and then—God forbid it should happen to somebody else—they'll say, 'Hey, remember how Sal handled it.'"

Confessions of weakness or error are most easily made in the past tense by all of us, and over the next year, Sal would report with comparable frankness mainly on feelings and attitudes that no longer troubled him. Repeatedly, resolution of an idea or a problem seems to free him from the need to dress up his motives or disguise his fears; every time something comes clear to him, his instinct for bluntness reasserts itself, and his appetite for reality takes stronger hold. A few weeks after making light of treatment, he reports with no embarrassment that he is back on schedule. He explains that he has heard from Morris Polack—"Who else?"—that one of Dr. Gee's older patients went off treatment, suffered a relapse, and never recovered—or, as Sal summarizes, "The jerk died." There is no reference to his earlier boasts of immunity from relapse.

In the middle of the summer Rose Ann hints of the explosion to come: "When Sal is in a good mood," she says, "he's a big help. When he wakes up with horns, he's awful." The mornings with horns grow more frequent, and in mid-September he blows. "I just went crazy," he reports late the next month in clinic. "I really did." He has come in for a treatment he particularly hates, a drug called BCNU that requires constant monitoring to prevent painful freezing or burning sensations as it goes in. "It's always been like that," he says—meaning that he has had his outbursts over the last year—"but this time it was worse." Without the slightest hesitation, he says, "I've started seeing a psychiatrist. I started last week. *My* choice. I had to," he says. "I didn't want to go insane, or have a nervous breakdown."

A couple of months ago such a choice would have represented intolerable weakness. Now that he has made it, it seems as natural as hanging out. His report on his first session is necessarily an innocent's, but also shrewd. "The doctor I'm seeing says there's a possibility I'm a very frustrated person, that I'm afraid to go out and accept the open world, and that it stems back to when I was a kid. I'm not myself, I'm trying to be my father. Also, she said she could see that I don't like myself, and I'm only out to impress." He lets that sink in. "Sounds like the truth," he adds. He strokes his arm as he lies on the cot, distracted for a moment by the sensation of the medication working its way through his veins. He looks up. "I don't care," he continues. "It's not my fault—I didn't do it intentionally. I didn't understand why I was screaming and carrying on." He shrugs. "And that's about all she said—until next week." He smiles. "There should be more." He says it was a terrific relief to talk to someone who never knew him before. "I'm always under pressure around the family. I'm home in the house too much. I'm isolated. I feel like I'm in a box."

He clutches his arm and lifts his head a few inches off the pillow. "Excuse me," he says politely to one of the nurses, who is busy with another patient. "My arm's freezing. It feels like there's ice on it." The nurse slows the flow of water that mixes with medication, but Sal winces and says, "Now it's burning-o-o-oh, badly, very badly—a-a-h—*damn!*" he says hoarsely, coming up off the cot in pain. "They make a sick person sicker," he says. "O-o-oh, stop it, you gotta stop it," he says, as the nurses fiddle with the BCNU flow. "Ah, shit," he whispers, clenching his fist and throwing his head back. When the flow has stopped, he says to the nurse, who is rubbing cortisone ointment on his arm, "Put it in really slowly, please."

I say to him, "It never gets routine, does it?" and he shakes his head. "This stinks," he says. "I mean it really does. Each time is different, because every day is different. Now I'm getting it in October, when it's a little colder, my chances of getting a fever are better. Plans have to be canceled. But if I get a fever, I take Tylenol. I don't call. I won't ever come back here [as an inpatient]. Never."

He returns to the subject of his emotions, enjoying the sudden liberty to talk of them. He talks about his line on leukemia, of how he's got it beat. "The problem is, I got to believe what I say." Maybe some of it is bravado, I suggest. "Of course it is," he says. "You know that as well as I do."

It is possible to come away from Sal with a different reaction ten times running, assured on one occasion of his essential sanity, another of an adolescent *hubris* that chills the blood. The truth is that he is sorting things out in slow stages, and in full view of those who care about him and can do nothing but hope and wait it out. Despite the discoveries of September and October, he passes the winter in a state of constant war with himself, his parents, and his treatments. He threatens to quit chemotherapy altogether, but after talking with Dr. Gee he does not. He is briefly employed, first at a Burger King near home, then as a waiter at Jerry Cooney's restaurant in Huntington, but neither much agrees with him. A few days before the first anniversary of his diagnosis, Sal reports predictably mixed feelings. "Coming to this time of year, you get the jitters, you know? Saturday it's one year. I'm going out after work and get bombed. I mean, who would have thought a year ago that I'd be alive now?" It is a rare allusion for him to the fact of leukemia's traditional result, and he follows it with a more typical remark. "People ask how I'm doing, I say fine. I say I've got leukemia, and they say, 'Oh, my mother died from that.' Thanks a lot."

By the end of the year, he has completed two sequences of maintenance and begun the cycle over again. He is going for chemo regularly now, but still reluctantly. There is frequent confusion about appointment days, and his previous sense of identification with Dr. Gee and the hospital has been dissipated by his resentment of treatment. He keeps everyone at a distance with his anger, and it is hard to know what he is thinking, or where he imagines his resistance is going to take him. He seems only to know that he needs to resist. Dr. Gee has seen it happen before. Patients have quit treatment altogether, disappeared for months or a year at a time, and any patient who is in remission and feeling good is in a state of constant temptation. If he is smart—as Sal is—he will not have missed a detail of Gee's explanation of the limits of current knowledge about leukemia and its treatment, and he will know that neither Gee nor any other doctor can promise that if he stays in treatment he will not relapse.

Most patients who relapse do so within the first six months, but there is no time limit on the possibility. To stick with treatment under these conditions of ambiguity requires, if not absolute faith, at least a suspension of doubt, a laying-aside of the impulse to take exception. A patient must relinquish the habit of deciding what is best for himself—or, rather, must decide once and live with his choice. For some, it is simply impossible. Doubts swell, fed by anger at the injustice of having been handed this piece of fortune, and by the physical beating of treatment itself. Grandiosity tempts—I *know* it's gone, Sal said often in the first year of his illness, as if to say it was to make it so. The need to deny, essential at some level, can get out of hand; the necessary mantra of the cancer patient—I'm going to survive—hardens into delusion—This thing cannot kill me.

Sal had taken refuge in all these forms of resistance, not out of obstinacy but out of urgent need. "I was always right," he would say later. "But nobody's always right." It isn't that he didn't know all along that he was bluffing to cover up his terror, only that he didn't know how else to handle it. "I wanted to believe what I was saying back then," he says. And so even his phone call the first of March 1982 strained at a lightness he could not possibly feel. "I got something for the book," he said, in an excited voice that could have foretold almost any kind of news. "Are you ready for this? You can put it in: 'And in February 1982 he had a relapse.'"

It happened almost two months to the day after his eighteenth birthday, fourteen months after he first went into remission. Before the original diagnosis, there had been months of warning, a terrible debility, bleeding and lethargy. This time there was no advance signal, only the permanent warning that having leukemia constitutes. He had gone in for a Thursday-morning appointment expecting a checkup and a dose of medication. His last bone-marrow had been clean, but Dr. Gee did not like the feel of his spleen and decided to take another bone-marrow right then. So scant was the evidence of disease at that stage that when Dr. Gee presented Sal's slides to the Hematology group later in the week there was no agreement on what had actually occurred. There were "suspicious" cells in Sal's marrow, but not in great enough number to confirm a relapse (immature cells are frequently found in the marrows of patients who remain in remission). But an enlarged spleen is in most patients an indicator of relapse, and as Gee pointed out, Sal's spleen had been normal at diagnosis. It was the combination of the spleen and "dirty" marrow that led Gee to speak to Sal and his parents of a relapse. He might have hedged on the word for a while, but he did not, and the Giovias understood the warning. Even Sal. He knew that Dr. Gee would not tell him such news lightly; in fact, it seemed almost as if he had been waiting to hear it, as if only a relapse could account for the terrible upheaval of recent months, as if only a relapse could make the treatment seem plausible and necessary again.

Sooner or later, Sal would have called Jimmy Polack in Seattle to tell him of the relapse, but, as it happened, Jimmy arrived in New York a couple of days after it was discovered, and for the first time in nine months, the two of them met in clinic as they used to. As usual, Jimmy was there first. With him on this trip were his aunt, Valerie, and his girlfriend Brenda, whom he had been seeing for about six months and had once dated in high school. As always, Jimmy had taken a blood check for Sal, and waved it in the air when Sal arrived in clinic with his friend Vinnie around eleven o'clock.

Despite the relapse, and despite the heavy dose of Adriamycin with which Dr. Gee was treating him, Sal looked perfectly healthy, only uneasy. He joked with Jimmy and they reminisced about the year before. It seemed to them both as though their acquaintance with leukemia extended much further back, and also as if the days of their worst misery had taken place in another life. A few days before, when Jimmy called Sal on arriving in New York, Sal had told him of the slip, and for a while during this first visit neither mentions it. But as they talk about treatment, exchanging accounts of the months they have not shared, Sal suddenly announces that he never took one of the drugs Jimmy mentions. "I never took the first half of maintenance," he says with a strangled laugh. "Remember how I asked Dr. Gee to switch me, so my hair wouldn't fall out for graduation? Well, I took the second half first, and then I lied and said I had taken the first, and so they gave me the second half again." His eyes flicker, and he laughs uncomfortably. "Maybe that's why I relapsed," he says.

The burden—imagined or real—of having brought on his own relapse sits heavily on him, and though he looks far older than his age, dressed as for an important engagement today in jacket and tie, a white double-breasted coat thrown over the back of his chair, he wears an expression of chagrin appropriate to a little boy. The relapse has drained him of most of his customary cockiness, but not all; when Vinnie, whose twenty-inch neck and sweet, stolid loyalty to his friend have earned him the title of Sal's "bodyguard," makes a remark about caution in some area unrelated to leukemia, Sal snaps at him. "That's the trouble with you, Vinnie," Sal says. "If you had leukemia, you'd give up."

Sal is demonstrably not ready to do that and is already building a case for himself. He reminds Jimmy of how quickly they were both brought into remission the first time and says that he is sure that his relapse will be nipped in the bud. In fact, he is right. When he emerges from his checkup with Dr. Gee, he reports that he is clean again. "See," he says to his mother when he calls her to tell her the news. "I told you there was nothing to worry about. Last time it took two weeks to bring me into remission. This time it only took one."

The truth is that the duration of a relapse is meaningless in the long run. What counts is whether Sal's remission has in fact been broken; if it has, everything is changed. All the evidence shows that once a relapse occurs with ALL, the disease takes a different course; the patient can be brought back into remission and, depending on how well he does from that moment, can expect to live for several years to come. But long-term survival, an expectation that was once unthinkable with respect to leukemia, depends on an unbroken remission, and it is no longer clear that Sal has that going for him.

He does not look at it that way, but his denial this time around is a chastened and hopeful denial, in which his determination to stick with treatment, and a surging maturity, combine to make his day-to-day attitude as realistic as it need be. "The relapse changed everything," Sal could report a few months later. Within a few weeks of his scare, he was working full time as a mattress salesman at a friend's father's store, a few miles from Smithtown. "He called and said he needed a guy with personality," is how Sal described the hiring, and remarkably, considering the sea-change that has taken place in his psyche, the old personality remains essentially intact. What is gone is the anger and the edge, and the need to pretend that having leukemia was no big deal even as he blindly sought to avenge himself for what it had cost him.

"I hated people who were well," he said one hot day in the second summer of his illness, almost six months after the scare in March. His forearm, freshly bandaged after a treatment, was the only evidence that he was not an ordinary suburban kid in the city for a day. "I hated my brother 'cause he didn't have it. I hated losing my hair. But I always covered up. I felt I had to, to show the people around me I was strong. But deep down I was bleeding. I cried every night. I couldn't handle it. When you're first admitted, you're so low. The infiltrations, the bone-marrows. I thought my backside would cave in. But I couldn't say so to them," he says, remembering his contempt for anyone who complained. "I didn't want to believe it could be so bad."

The way he looked at it back then, he says, every treatment was a reminder that he was trapped by illness. "That's all gone now. Now every shot brings me closer to the good things. People without arms and legs have to live with that misery every day," he says. "But I only have my misery until I'm finished with chemo. This time next year, it'll be over. You know how good that's gonna be?" he asks, and then, as if to drive home how equitable an arrangement it has turned out to be after all, he adds with much the same disarming smile that I remember him loosing on me at our first meeting, "When it's all over, I'll still only be nineteen."

In the early months of his illness, Jimmy Polack spoke of Seattle often and longingly, like a homesick soldier who has been shipped overseas. It was a reference in nearly every conversation, used interchangeably with the word *home*, and standing for everything that leukemia and a long winter in New York had stripped him of. Seattle meant health, friends, liberty and absence of dread, and in the beginning, it was easy for him to imagine that a return to the one would mean an automatic restoration of everything else, as if in fact two Jimmys existed, one well and one sick, and that they lived in separate places. At some point in the future, the sick Jimmy would disappear, to be replaced by the well Jimmy of before. But as the time when he would be free to leave New York approached, it became clear that no such exchange was in the offing. There was only one Jimmy to cart across the country, and suddenly he began to talk about not returning to Seattle after all, but moving to Los Angeles, or even staying in New York.

When Sal heard of this change of heart, his reaction was immediate. "I know why he doesn't want to go home," he observed. "He doesn't want to go through what I've already been through. With his friends, with people who haven't seen him bald."

As far as it went, Sal's reading of his friend was accurate. Jimmy had a real, openly confessed dread of appearing among his friends hairless, with still-puffy face and thick belly, incapable of his former feats of energy and grace. Because he felt not himself any longer, he could not imagine what place he would occupy if he returned home. What he could imagine—and in this he was his grandmother's true grandson—was that he would be to his friends an object of pity, something he knew he could not stand.

But there was more to it than that, and it had to do less with other people than with the changes worked in Jimmy during this long period of peculiar isolation. Though their circumstances were in most every other respect greatly different, he shared with Karyn Angell the experience of being torn from normal life by leukemia. Both had grown accustomed to great personal freedom at an early age and, unlike Sal, both had left home emotionally before getting sick.

In Karyn's case, the departure had been geographic as well, but for Jimmy being yanked back into the womb of the family proved even more unsettling, throwing up questions about the conduct of his life and future that had never occurred to him before. If he was oppressed by illness, he was almost equally oppressed by the constant, unanswerable attentions of his worried grandparents, who, with his aunt Valerie, comprised his shrunken daily world. Whatever pressure he had been under before, it had never seemed so all-compassing as it did now, when he felt himself to be the endangered center of all hope for his family. It began to seem to him, looking back, as if his entire life had been settled from birth, requiring nothing of him in the way of reflection, or choice, until this moment.

Now, for the first time ever, he was hit with the realization that other outcomes were actually possible. Preeminent among these was, of course, death, a consideration that Jimmy alone of his family entertained openly (though it was a huge, unspoken preoccupation in the foreground of his grandparents' imaginations). And once he had let that in, and played with it a while, nothing in his life seemed as immutable as before. He began to consider alternatives to what had always appeared foreordained. Suppose he didn't take over the business? Suppose he never went back to Seattle? Suppose he took up fixing cars instead of going back to school? Suppose, went one of his favorite fantasies, he moved far north of Seattle into the wild and became a hermit?

To his grandparents, these modestly rebellious notions were frightening indicators that Jimmy was depressed, and to some extent they were right. Certainly all these unfamiliar fantasies had an underside of despair—Jimmy could allow himself to imagine them precisely because he believed that the future laid out for him might never come about. The Polacks, meanwhile, continued to hold out that same future as the main incentive to getting well again. It was as if they had begun to speak different languages. In small ways and large, Jimmy had begun to look at the world differently from his grandparents, and while the reality he woke to in the early months of 1981 was depressing, the experience of seeing things freshly for himself was intoxicating. Soon it was apparent that whatever he decided to do, there was no going back to how he was before. Because they read it initially as a loss, his family was both mystified and alarmed by this change in Jimmy. But to Dr. Gee, there was nothing inappropriate in Jimmy's reaction. He had reason to be depressed and in fact would most likely benefit from letting it sink in for a while. "There's no spirit there," Valerie reported her father saying to Dr. Gee. "No," Gee answered calmly. "You're just missing the buoyancy of youth. He'll be all right."

And in fact, to eyes other than his grandparents', there seemed nothing terminal about Jimmy's frame of mind. Even though she too mourned his loss of innocence, Valerie saw early on that he had to break loose in some way. "If he were back in Washington," she said, "he could go out in the woods and be by himself. But here he has nowhere to go. At first, we never thought of not being with him all the time," she said, referring to the virtual vigil that she and her parents had maintained. "And he wanted us there. But now he needs to be alone. And he lets us know it."

Though he has begun to withdraw from them, it is not into the guise of a stranger but into that of a grown child. He is no longer docile, no longer the boy asking favors, but the emerging man saying what he thinks and wants. The change is most obvious in his relations with his grandfather, whose hold on him is slipping, despite the mutual tenderness that persists. Morris has been at Jimmy's side for months, arranging, insisting, comforting, with two goals in mind. The first is, of course, Jimmy's survival, for which Morris would do almost anything; the second is so closely connected, so pointless without the first as to be otherwise meaningless—Morris wants to give Jimmy the poultry business, wants to fulfill his intention of twenty years. It is an old man's desire, so strongly felt that it takes many conversations before he can begin to believe that Jimmy may mean it when he says that he isn't sure he wants to accept. He has the same kind of difficulty in conceding the changes that leukemia has wrought.

One afternoon, he brings out a pile of snapshots from the trip that he and Jimmy took to Israel and Egypt last year. (Mrs. Polack, trying to pin leukemia on some event, mused one day to Rose Ann Giovia, "Jimmy went to Egypt last summer—I wonder if that's where he got it?" Rose Ann blinked and laughed hard. "Well, Sal's never been to Egypt, and he sure got it, didn't he?") The photographs are mostly of Jimmy. He stands before a dozen dimly familiar landmarks of the Middle East, a boy not shy of the camera, used to having people look at him and smile. He is slim and dark-haired, and in several of the pictures he is bare-chested, showing a tan, muscled torso that is the product of youth and intelligent exercise. He looks four or five years younger, and nothing like the pale Jimmy who sits across from his grandfather wearing a reflective expression on his face. "Isn't he handsome?" Morris says, pointing to pose after pose. "He sure was," Jimmy laughs. "You wouldn't know he was the same guy."

Morris looks up. "You haven't changed at all," he says firmly, and Jimmy smiles and says, "Sure, Grampa."

A couple of weeks later, when Jimmy is in for a fever and at his lowest, Morris begins to grow more anxious. His every comment has a point—you must fight to survive—and he watches Jimmy like a hawk, waiting on him touchingly, careful not to push too hard, but always there. Every night he or Valerie takes Jimmy's food order. The spoiling that is going on is almost comic, and Jimmy milks it for all it's worth. When he wants to take a shower, his grandfather collects a clean pair of drawstring pants and a towel for him, and waits like a valet for him to finish. "Will he come back and work for me or not?" he asks out of Jimmy's hearing. "I'm holding on by the skin of my teeth for him," he says, "but the business needs a boss, and I'm getting tired."

Out of his grandfather's hearing, Jimmy says, "I get a little more depressed every day," but it is clear that while he is telling the truth, he knows that he is getting something valuable out of his suffering. Just what, he cannot yet say. "I don't know what I'm interested in anymore," he says. "You tell me. What am I interested in?" He pushes his I.V. pole along the corridor, doing laps for exercise, and to get away from his family. After a few laps his gait grows sloppy, and his legs seem to flap with each step. He says it's because he has done so little walking the last three weeks. Trying to avoid a fever, he confined himself mercilessly after his last treatment, a show of stoicism that suggests what a fierce physical competitor he is when he wants to be. But his family came and went as they had to, and food came into the house, and newspapers, and he got the fever anyway. Dr. Gee had warned him that there was no way to totally protect himself and had advised him to enjoy himself while he felt well enough. But Jimmy was so determined not to come back that he locked himself in and tried to beat it. That he did not is one more example to him of the futility of making plans. "If I was sure I was going to make it," he says. "then all this would be a pleasure. Or if I knew I was going to kick, I could just go out and have a great time. But not knowing . . ."

How long do people whose leukemia comes back live, he asks, knowing that the answer is variable. For the sake of argument, he

253

picks three years, roughly the length of time his total treatment will last, and he says, "In three years I could do a lot of things more enjoyable than this." He has been fascinated by the numbers related to his disease from the beginning, and quite naturally for someone so young, he cannot get over the possibility that his life could be finite. Having conceded it, he plays with it relentlessly, as if such a fate belongs only to him. When it is pointed out that his chances of living three years are probably better than his grandfather's, he is suddenly returned to a larger reality. "That's true," he says, "I hadn't thought about it that way."

One of Dr. Gee's Monday-night groups is scheduled during Jimmy's stay in the hospital for fever, but, despite the urgings of Gee and Kathy Dietz, he refuses to attend. His grandfather goes and talks several times, mainly of what a good boy Jimmy is and of how worried they all are about his depression. One of the patients at the meeting is a man about thirty-five named Tom Connolly,* who first became a patient of Dr. Gee's eight years earlier. He, too, had ALL, just like Jimmy, and was treated with the first protocol to result in long-term survival. With him is his wife, who is pregnant with their fourth child, their second since treatment. Morris takes the younger man's presence as an opportunity not to be passed up, and when the meeting is over, he solicits Kathy Dietz's aid in persuading him to speak to Jimmy. Though it is after eight o'clock, Kathy leads the way back upstairs to Jimmy's room, where Connolly, who is a big, handsome man with a powerful chest making light of a swelling middle, has to say very little to achieve the effect Morris wants. He and Jimmy talk in brief sentences about the treatment. Connolly says the initial in-hospital stay eight years ago was much longer than it is now, and Kathy Dietz, who knew him when she was a floor nurse, vouches for the fact. "I used to get mad," Connolly says mildly. "I kicked a few things around. But it was worth it." Jimmy can't seem to think of any specific question to ask, but he is clearly impressed. Connolly's great size—and his wife's current dimensions—combine with the length of his survival to make a great case.

A couple of days later, Jimmy speaks of Connolly with undisguised excitement. "He was a *big* guy," Jimmy says. "It's hard to believe he could have been so sick." Circling the floor again, Jimmy talks this time not about death but about options, and about getting out in a day or two. "This little sickness of mine

---

*Pseudonym.

gives me the opportunity to refuse a few things," he says, referring to his discussions with his grandfather about not taking over the business. A few days later, Morris Polack concedes the inevitable. He says that Jimmy is thinking of staying in New York to go to school, and adds, "It's okay with me. His grandmother and Valerie can't believe that Jimmy can get along without them. I know he can get along without me." He is worried about Jimmy's ability to care for himself, but remembers that "when I was his age, I didn't have anyone to take care of me. I'm very much concerned, but I have a lot of faith in Jimmy," he says.

By the end of the week, Jimmy's fever is gone and he is released. The following Thursday, he comes in for his last consolidation treatment, a dose of Cytoxan, which takes almost an hour and a half to administer. The next week is the healing, and in its aftermath, Jimmy is more optimistic than he has been for five months. On the twenty-seventh, he and his grandfather come to the clinic for a checkup, and Kathy Dietz tells them that Dr. Gee says he has three weeks before he needs to start maintenance. If he is planning to go home, or to California, his newest first-choice destination, he has that much time to arrange things. The message is one of liberation, and Jimmy reads it perfectly. "Outrageous," he says, smiling and laughing, and looking at Kathy in astonishment. The news that Jimmy is free to go has quite a different significance for Mr. Polack. He is trying to stifle his agitation but cannot, and the tears start, with a barely controlled heaving of the chest. With no hint of alarm in her voice, Kathy says to him, "Mr. Polack, now when did you last have your blood pressure checked?" She eases his jacket off, slips a cuff over his arm, and checks his pressure while he is still keening over this good-bad news. "I think Jimmy is mature enough to take good care of himself," Kathy says. "Don't worry so much." Because he adores Kathy, Mr. Polack is forced to hear what she says with an open mind, though he would probably like to block it out forever if it would keep Jimmy near him. While he sniffles and submits to Kathy's slow checkup, Jimmy's excitement grows. "I feel great," he tells Kathy. "Yesterday, I walked to the World Trade Center." She looks impressed; it is a distance of four or five miles, almost half the length of Manhattan, and nobody walks it. As he watches Jimmy, Morris grows resigned. He has, after all, been praying for Jimmy's spirits to lift, and they have lifted.

The next Monday, after clinic, Jimmy and his grandfather pick up a rental car for a trip to Washington, D.C., something they've been planning to do for months. Confined to the city because of Jimmy's treatment, they have seen little of the rest of the East

Coast and are eager to see more. Of greater interest to Jimmy than where they are going, however, is the fact that he will be behind the wheel of a car again, the pleasure he may have missed most of all since coming to New York. Since they are not to leave until the following day, Mr. Polack allows himself to be dropped off, giving Jimmy the car for the afternoon, to go wherever he likes. He is a bird let fly in the small sedan, an expert driver seeking to remind himself of his skill with sudden stops and cornerings that border on terrifying but are nicely completed. He heads north in Manhattan, needing little instruction to find his way to the George Washington Bridge.

Jimmy's mood, which has been climbing steadily for weeks, is euphoric today, the result of having spent most of the previous night on the phone to friends in Seattle. As he drives north along the Jersey Palisades, he seems almost dizzy over the remade connection. "I hadn't realized how much they knew how to talk to me about this," he says. "They're the people I should have been talking to all along. Some of them did cry, but mainly they knew what to say."

In the months since he left Seattle, his contact with most of his friends had been minimal and unrevealing. "Some of them had wanted to come out and visit me, but I wouldn't let them. I didn't want them around. I couldn't tell you why then, but it was my feeling from the start that I wanted to be alone and fight it alone. I didn't want a lot of people around me feeling sorry for me or pitying me. As it turned out, I got less of that from my friends than I did from my family."

He talks in a flood, saying more in a couple of hours than he has said in several weeks, spinning theories about why he got leukemia and what it has done for him, how it has changed him, and broadened his life.

"Dr. Gee told me, 'We don't know why people get leukemia,' but I know why *I* got leukemia," Jimmy says. He has read *Getting Well Again*** (and, courtesy of his grandfather, has donated several copies to Memorial's patient library) and is firmly persuaded by its argument that stress is a major cause of serious illness. "I remember approximately six months before I was diagnosed, I was starting to have problems with school, I was starting to have social pressures, and then I was moved from the docks to the office [at Acme, the family poultry company]. I didn't like that at

---

*By O. Carl Simonton, M.D., Stephanie Matthews-Simonton and James L. Creighton (Bantam, 1978).

all, but I couldn't tell my grandfather I didn't like it. The combination of that and my grandfather wanting me to learn Hebrew and take me to Israel and to all these dinners really got me in a depressive state the whole summer. On top of that, Grampa kept pounding into my head the idea that he was seventy-five and going to die. My uncle had just died. So I had to get my shit together soon. I think that's it, because, before I got sick, I was in the best physical condition I was ever in in my life. Then once I got sick, I didn't care about *anything*, and that immediately released all the stress. I had the chance to start over."

Looking back, he recognizes his own role in his privileged subjugation. "I had a fear of trying new things in some cases," he says, "or actually considering a different life. Like going to school in L.A. That was something I wanted to do, but I knew I'd never do it. Now I feel as though I can justify anything by this disease. I'm saying I can be free. I can study something else besides business, pursue my other interests, and maybe work at them. And I feel I can do those things without hurting my grandparents."

Asked if he means that getting leukemia was a subconscious choice, or an overwhelming of the body by stress, Jimmy says, "It's hard to say. I don't know. Before I got cancer, I had thought about *escaping*. I don't think I would ever intend to get cancer, even subconsciously, but maybe it was a way for my body to combat stress that I didn't know how to handle.

"Now, even if I wind up stuck in Washington, I won't mind," he says. "I feel really good. The only drawback is the hair loss." He is still bald, and it isn't clear how soon his hair will grow back, or if it does, whether it will fall out again. He still cares, but he is able to put it out of his mind for days at a time now. He looks forward to getting back in shape with weights and running. "That's nothing," he says confidently. "It will take me two months."

Crossing back over the Hudson farther north, we head south through Westchester County, which astonishes Jimmy by its lushness. He is bordering on nostalgia for New York already, which is linked forever in his mind with illness, but also with change. He tries to sum up what has happened to him so far, aware that many surprises are yet to come. "This is how I feel right now," he says, "I know I'm going to get well. I know I'm going to beat this. I'm taking stock and reevaluating my entire life, and I believe I'm going to be able to enjoy life more now. I don't like to say this, but, in a way, this disease did something good for me. In a way it almost discontinued my life. But in a way it kind of saved my life."

When Karyn Angell first began to sort out what having leukemia meant and how she was going to get through it, she seized optimistically on the idea that, so far, change has always been good for her. At seventeen, she could regard herself with some justice as having more than simply adjusted to her family's move to Paris from a farm in upstate New York: she had thrived. And though the circumstances were hardly similar now, she took hopeful comfort from her history of flexibility.

In 1981 alone, she would spend six months in the hospital, with seven separate admissions, both planned and emergency, and so many visits as an outpatient that she would lose track of their number. Her hair would grow back, a bit of it, and fall out again before she could comb it. She would grow thin several times over, and then regain most of her lost weight. She would spend weeks at a time in a hospital gown, lapse into a lethargy deep and alien, and burst forth with purpose, if less than full energy, after every discharge. Her muscles would ache from disuse, her backside from bone-marrows and botched spinals. There would be careful nurses and less careful ones, skilled interns and clumsy ones, more new faces than it was comfortable to have to be pleasant to. Eventually, even that natural response would give way on occasion to an unfamiliar and necessary sharpness when she had finally suffered too many pokes, too many abortive attempts at sinking a line into one of her worn-out veins.

But the physical part was the easiest by far, her resilience a genetic gift. She was more prone to fever than either Jimmy or Sal—and wound up in the hospital a second time after virtually every treatment—but her recovery after each of these episodes was swift, and only very rarely did she look anything but well. Between hospitalizations, she exercised—when she had the strength, she ran, and for several weeks in the late spring, she and her mother hauled themselves to a 7 A.M. aerobic-dancing class before driving to New York to attend clinic.

What was far worse was the isolation and the sense of normal life suspended. The day Reagan was inaugurated she was a patient at Memorial, and she was there the day he was shot two months later. When the Pope was attacked she was an inpatient, and when her friends were on Easter break she could not arrange to see them because she was on hold for a bed at the hospital. When things got much better they got better accompanied by complications that would have seemed absolutely unnegotiable if someone had laid them out for her ahead of time. It turned out that she was very good at negotiating, at making do, at change, just as she had judged herself to be, but that did not mean it was easy.

A month after she was released from Memorial for the first time she returned for her inaugural consolidation treatment, one of six that would be strung out until late August or early September. A yellow stream of Methotrexate flows into her left arm, a nasty mimicking of the sun that falls at a sharp angle onto her bed for several hours every day. The Methotrexate stings as it goes in, fair warning of what will come. The other drug scheduled for the week is called Ara-C and is given in a continuous drip for five days. Since both are new for Karyn, the nurse who is monitoring her chemo tells her what to expect. "The Methotrexate is what will give you the trouble," she says, "not the Ara-C." The trouble will be nausea, fever, chills, the nurse says, and Karyn answers, "Oh, great. Now I've got something to look forward to."

She has had leukemia now for three months, about the same length of time she was away at college, and it has become more real than not by now. She has passed a birthday, her eighteenth, and winter has given way to spring. She takes the passing weeks as markers of progress instead of lost time, and though she chafes at the long consolidation ahead and worries that it will drag on into the fall, she says she is glad to have drawn the long protocol after all. "I was upset at first," she says, "but now I'm not. They've only been using the new one for six months. This way I feel less like a guinea pig."

In early April, a week after Karyn finished up her Ara-C and Methotrexate, the Angells set off on a brief vacation, planning to spend a week at a friend's house in southern Vermont.

Karyn's counts were heading down, and she had been plagued with mouth sores for several days, but under the circumstances, anything like an ideal moment for a vacation was unlikely to present itself for a long time to come, and the Angells believed, with Dr. Gee, that the therapeutic value of the trip outweighed the risk that Karyn would get a fever and have to be hospitalized. In fact, as Jimmy had learned, she could as easily get a fever at home in bed as in Vermont, and in either case the result would be the same. With the feeling that it would be better to have tried than not to have tried, and equipped with the names of two hospitals, one in Rutland, the other across the Massachusetts border in Dartmouth, they set off.

They arrived on a Saturday and spent the afternoon skiing—everyone but Karyn, who could not risk an accident while her platelets were low. The next morning, she did not feel well, and Dee Angell drove her in to Dartmouth to get a blood count, the start of a nightmarish eleven-hour stay in the emergency room there. Karyn's counts, it turned out, were low enough to warrant a transfusion, but a succession of nurses and doctors on weekend duty repeatedly tried and failed to find a vein through normal means before finally performing what is called a "cut-down" in hopes of getting a line in. Two deep, lateral slashes were made on the side of Karyn's left ankle, exposing tissue nearly to the bone. The subsequent probing for a vein through this aperture seemed endless, and blind, like something one imagines taking place on a blowy mountaintop. Karyn and her mother were appalled. No procedure they had ever seen had gone so badly, and Karyn had never been put through so much pain. Finally she blew. "I never heard her talk that way before," her mother later reported, amused and admiring. "The obscenity was incredible."

The problem was not really incompetence—though to do a cut-down was probably going too far—but the fact that by this point in Karyn's treatment her veins were simply too frail and over-worked for anyone but the most experienced specialist to succeed in getting a line in. Ten days later, the bruises on the insides of Karyn's arms are still countable, each sickly yellow splotch a souvenir of a separate puncture that led nowhere. Two lines of black stitching edged in tender red track across her ankle; below them a fat round of black and blue has barely begun to fade. Karyn is once again sitting cross-legged on a bed in Memorial, at the tail end of a week's hospitalization for fever that the Dartmouth episode—she did eventually receive a transfusion, not through the cut-down but through a vein in her hand—did not prevent. When her counts dropped again after the transfusion, the Angells decided that they wanted her back in Memorial, where there would be no crisis over finding a vein, and on the fifth day of their vacation, Dave Angell drove her back to New York. For three days she ran a temperature of 105 degrees, rocking the bed with great trembling chills.

No chances were taken with her veins: a central line was installed immediately, and a week later it is still in place. A piece of pink tubing curls forward over her right ear, and, hugging her cheek, extends down toward her collarbone, where it enters her body through a small cut in the skin. The line feeds directly into one of her main arteries and is held in place by a stitch and some tape. The incision is tidy, and the rigging, now that Karyn has her color back, has an oddly decorative look, set off against her bald head and huge blue eyes like some ceremonial headdress. She and her mother make a gay pair recalling the grisly details of their Dartmouth adventure, but although they have put it in the past—

and with Karyn, this effort seems so effective that it is sometimes hard to connect her, as she tells such stories, with the person who suffered them—the moral of the story is bitter. They had wanted badly to believe that they could pull off a normal outing, but it had not worked out, and they were forced to look at how circumscribed life really would be for a while. "Next time we won't be so cocky," Dee said.

With good reason, Karyn's mood this stay is gloomy. She is disappointed over the broken vacation, and feels guilty about "ruining" it for the rest of the family. Unlike a hospitalization for treatment, which has some positive purpose, being in for a fever is like a punishment, reminding you that you are sick and vulnerable. The stoicism that she brings to the first is harder to muster for the second, and she seems slightly annoyed with herself as well for failing to be cheerful. When Kathy Dietz stops by in the afternoon before Karyn is scheduled to go home and asks whether she has been out of bed all day, Karyn shakes her head, No. "I'm always like this the last day," she says quietly. "I can't seem to get myself going. But," she adds, "I'm never like this at home."

It is true, and when a friend invites her to a dance at Wellesley after she is released, Karyn surprises herself by arranging to have her next treatment moved forward a few days so she can accept. It is the first time she has asked for special consideration of any kind, and it is hard for her, but she so wants a break from confinement that she screws up her nerve. "I think it's really important that you not feel like an invalid if at all possible," she says midway through her rescheduled treatment. The week before, she had had a taste of freedom, driving to Mount Holyoke for the first time since she left, to visit her friends, and she is struck by how incredibly her world has shrunk in a few months. It is noticeable in a dozen small ways. "I feel really peculiar about food a lot of the time," she says. "Some days I can't eat anything. My hearing has become really acute, and my sense of smell. My mother says I smell things when I'm not even there. Another thing—I've always been a calm person, and now I can become nervous and uptight very easily. I think it's because there is so little happening in my life other than leukemia. I used to be so incredibly busy that I took little things in stride. Now, because there's nothing really happening, anything that does becomes really important. Because I have so much energy still, it *all* goes into that."

Before the Angells attempted their Vermont vacation, Karyn and her parents had talked about the possibility of transferring from Memorial back to Norwalk hospital for the remainder of treatment, to make life easier for everyone. Dee Angell still commuted to New York daily whenever Karyn was hospitalized, and was beginning to worry about neglecting her other children. Dave Angell, whose work schedule continued to take him out of the country frequently, had a harder time getting in to see his daughter, rarely arriving at Memorial before six in the evening, and then not reaching home till nearly ten. If she were at Norwalk, everyone in the family could visit her, for short stays or long, and it would seem less of a big deal all around. That advantage can be so important, in Tim Gee's opinion, that in fact it was he who suggested to the Angells that they consider the change at some point. Karyn's progress had been good, and Dr. Schulman, who had referred the Angells to Dr. Gee in January, knew the protocol as well as anyone. Though he and Memorial are at one end of it, Gee is a believer in cutting the umbilical as soon as it is safe to do so. Since it had become clear that Karyn would be making the break in the fall to go back to school, Gee told the Angells there was no reason not to do it sooner. Sensible though Gee's position seemed to Dee Angell, Karyn and her father were apprehensive. Dave Angell did not want to give up Dr. Gee's expertise, and Karyn was nervous about the skill of the I.V. teams at Norwalk. Her veins were a real problem, and the thought of less than expert insertion, even before Dartmouth, frightened her.

After Dartmouth, none of the Angells wanted to switch hospitals any sooner than was necessary, and the issue was dropped, but in a larger sense, the question of breaking away from Memorial was a metaphor for the tug of war that would continue, probably as long as Karyn was in treatment, between the Angells' instinct to push ahead as if all were well and their new reality. "I remember thinking when Karyn went into remission," her mother said in May, after four months of the disease, "Okay, we've got two years to live a normal life. I knew that even if she came out of remission, they could keep her alive for two years. Of course, I know that if she were to come out of remission, I'd feel differently, but for the moment, I don't feel the pressure to do anything immediately." She shook her head at the strange words it was now possible for her to say, and added, "The human organism is *amazing*."

Except that Karyn answers the door wigless and is the wrong age and too smart to be hanging around the house without something urgent to occupy her time, the Angells' house could still pass as the site of normal life. Her sisters come and go—loudly; friends visit; and most phone conversations are interrupted midway by a click that means another caller is trying to break through. Dee Angell is still trying to get the curtains up in the living room eight months after moving in, and Dave Angell has dismantled his old MG in the garage in order to rebuild it. Life is in all these ways much as it was before Karyn got sick, and yet a tension that is new to this family plays on them all.

On a day when Karyn's counts are sinking predictably toward the floor, a long nap does not restore her, and Dave Angell risks getting snapped at when he suggests that she take another. At the dinner table, her sisters' eyes fly quickly past, rarely landing on Karyn's face, and their voices fill the air with conversation that is both naturally boisterous, and perhaps a bit more, as if meant to convey that there is no need to be somber. A birthday celebration takes on a poignancy that almost no one can bear when Karyn opens a card from her father and reads aloud the rhymed verse that transfers to her the affections and title of his old Volkswagen, *Hubie*, before she has even gone for her driver's license.

When her sisters have left the table one night to finish their homework, Karyn lowers her chin between folded arms on the tabletop and confesses her exhaustion. "I haven't been sleeping well lately," she explains. Her parents are silent, their eyes fixed on her carefully, consciously trying not to overwhelm her with concern. She says that she has been having some weird dreams lately, and in an unusually quiet voice, tells of one in which "someone was putting me down because I had leukemia. I wanted to prove I was as healthy as he was, so I challenged him to do twenty pushups. I dropped to the floor, but I couldn't do a single one," she says, looking up at her mother sadly. Dee Angell hesitates a half second before saying, "And immediately after Karyn told me this dream, she dropped to the floor and did ten pushups." Karyn sighs and says, "Well, I wanted to see if I could."

Her status in the family is so peculiar now, a mix of what it once was and of the special circumstances that keep her among them. Her parents refer to their other three daughters as "the kids," and it is clear that they do not think of Karyn as one. Though she is close to them both, she has not spent this much time with them in years, and it is a bittersweet intimacy at times, because if all were well it would be a thing of the past. Karyn and her father spend many hours together without speaking, as they always have, while she and her mother jabber together like sisters, treating each other with an irreverence they rarely display in public. They feel lucky that their temperaments are so different—Karyn so essentially calm, her mother a chafer at obstacles, always prepared to blast roadblocks from her path, politely, but definitely—

and lucky that they like each other so much. Still, each is eager to get on with her own life. Dee Angell has been planning to get a job since they came back from Paris, and now that Karyn's treatment seems stable, she has begun to look around. Karyn has made a deal with a sailing school in Westport that will let her work in the office on weekends, when bookings are busiest. With any luck, she will be able to fit her remaining treatments in during the week and miss only a weekend or two because of fever.

At the end of May—high from the success of her trip to Wellesley, where she stayed up all night and no one but her close friend had any idea that she was anything but normal—she checks in at Memorial for her third consolidation treatment, another Methotrexate–Ara-C mix. The last time out she had a milder combination, Ara-C and a drug called 6-Thioguanine, and no fever afterward. The Methotrexate mix is rougher and will most likely produce fever, but she is close to schedule at the moment and hopeful of finishing consolidation in time for school, so her mood is good. She is in for less than a week and home by Memorial Day. On the eighth of June, she and her mother appear in clinic full of news about Karyn's first couple of days at the sailing school. Karyn looks as robust as her mother this morning, but a few days later she wakes up with a headache, is driven to Norwalk for a blood test, and is found to have a fever. When Dr. Schulman calls Dr. Gee to confer, Gee says there is no reason Karyn can't stay where she is instead of coming to New York. Lying on a bed at Norwalk, feeling weak and achy, Karyn decides that she would rather stay put than be moved, and thus is the question of whether to switch to Norwalk for treatment unexpectedly settled. There is trouble with her veins—"of course"—but it is tolerable trouble, and in every other respect she and her family are delighted with Norwalk. The timing happens to be excellent, since the fever turns out to consist of two seven-day stretches back to back—one fever runs its course only to be followed immediately by a second. The policy for fever at Norwalk is stricter than at Memorial—a private room automatically, no flowers, no fresh fruits brought in from the outside. Visitors have to wash their hands, but there are more visitors, popping in and out all the time, and that is a great boon. At the end of the first week, Karyn has heard that she will have to stay another, but before she is hooked back up to antibiotics, her father asks if he can take her out for a short drive. They get permission and drive down to Long Island Sound, within sight of the hospital's upper windows. Karyn is back in bed within a couple of hours, but for practical reasons the outing, which would have been permitted but unlikely to take place if she had been at Memorial, gives her and her family the sense that they are not totally at the mercy of the disease.

In early July Karyn and her mother come to New York for an appointment with Dr. Gee that is not quite final but certainly the last that they will have for some time to come, and they carry with them a half-formed expectation that some kind of ceremony, or declaration, will materialize to mark the moment. Somehow it does not. Gee is at pains to emphasize what good shape Karyn is in and the excellence of both Schulman and Paul Hetzel, a former fellow now working at a hospital in Springfield, Massachusetts, to whom he has referred Karyn for treatment when she returns to school. He is equally at pains, it seems to Dee Angell, to avoid a sentimental leave-taking as Karyn departs the Memorial nest. "I kept thinking I wanted to reach up and kiss him on the cheek, or hug him, or something." Dee said afterward, "but I didn't think he would like it."

Walking up the block away from the hospital, Karyn says it feels strange to leave. There are loose ends everywhere—other patients whose stories she may never know the end of, several fellows whose names she may never hear again, and the place itself, from which she had always kept her distance. It is good to leave it behind, possibly forever, barring occasional appointments with Dr. Gee over the next several years, but also very odd, like quitting a campus without graduating. Like Jimmy Polack, she has set her sights for months on the relative freedom that not having to be here means, but it leaves her in no-man's-land a bit ahead of schedule.

August had been her personal deadline for being done with Memorial, for two reasons. First, because she wanted to finish the consolidation phase of treatment before school began, and second, because she believed that if she made it to August, she was home free altogether. When she was diagnosed in January, she says, Schulman told her parents that before the current leukemia treatments were developed patients generally lived no more than eight months. Though she had played very little with the notion of dying, that outdated sentence had stuck in her mind, and she had decided that if she could make it to August, she would be all right. So settled was she on the fact that life would begin over again on September 1 that it was as if nothing special could possibly happen for her before then.

And so August turned out to be a bonus—six months of chemotherapy had left her thinner than she had been in several years, enough of her hair had come in to make her believe that she really would have her own again someday, and midway through the summer she met a boy named Sam Cook, who not only thought she was terrific but was funny and interested in hearing about leukemia. "He's the first person I've told right off about my situation," Karyn said in explaining how they met. "Most people I meet are so afraid of it. *I* was very uncomfortable with cancer before I got it, so I can understand. I was surprised that Sam was willing to get involved. He told me that the night we met he went home and had to figure out whether he liked me because I had leukemia or if he just liked me. And I had to decide whether I liked him or just the return to being normal, which I so desperately needed." They were able to agree in a short time that it was not leukemia that brought them together, yet the fact that they were able to talk about it made all the difference to Karyn.

For Karyn it had been a long time between close friends, and she had never needed one more. And for all her resilience and good humor about being confined, bald, and prescheduled for several years to come, she had suffered some real loss of confidence in her own attractiveness and worth. "I was always very sure of myself before, very popular," she says in late August, hooked up to a computerized I.V. rig in a room at Norwalk, with a white foam board anchoring a needle in her right arm. "Now I feel very *un*sure in social situations, because I don't know how I'm going to act. I feel like a new person, but I haven't gotten used to her yet."

Tan and thin, with a soft-brown cap of hair and her blue eyes pale and clear, Karyn has probably never looked prettier, but it is true that she does not look a great deal like her former self. It is as if five years have passed, not eight months. Her face is no longer a young girl's, no longer so round and open. Everything has registered with her, as Dr. Gee will observe the next time he sees her, but the effect is not to make her look troubled, only rather more substantial. She is lively again, nearing the end of treatment and boosted by a recovery of a social life, but her liveliness plays from a new frame of reference. "Because I'm the kind of person who tries to make do and look on the bright side, it wasn't so obvious how low I was," she says. "But I can remember one night just looking in the mirror and thinking, God, how *ugly*. I felt I was so unattractive, and I think it was because of how it came about."

Hard as it had been, the long stretch of isolation just ending has given her time to think about her life in a new way, and she is not unhappy about that. "I've learned a lot about myself," she says. "When I was a little girl, I used to look at my parents and think, I'm never going to grow up and have a relationship like that—I'll get hit by a car, or something else will happen. And when I was diagnosed, all those fears came back. Mainly it was that I was afraid I wouldn't be able to have a relationship. And so when I first met Sam, I was really urgent about the whole thing, until finally I said to myself, Look, you've got the rest of your life for this. Just to *have* a relationship, however short-lived it turns out to be, helped me get past that."

Having sorted out some of her more fanciful anxieties, she is left with plenty of realistic worries to juggle. There is death, of course, but so far she has sidestepped the subject pretty successfully. And anyway, she says, "I was never as afraid of dying because I had leukemia as I was upset about the deprivation of things I wanted to do." One of those things is a long-standing desire to add a fifth generation to her mother's side of the family, but she will not know for several more years whether the effects of chemotherapy have destroyed her chances of having children. She will be tested when she has finished with maintenance, but until then must live with the question unresolved. She does not pretend equanimity but is trying for it. "I would be really disappointed if I didn't have children," she says. "I always wanted to. But I've thought about it a lot, and I realize that without me, there would be no baby. So if you look at it that way . . ."

Her ability to let in the dark side has grown over the last months, but her resilience has not disappeared, and she switches back and forth between good news and bad, irritation and exuberance, as if, as is the case, she is on similar terms with them both. Pushing her I.V. pole ahead of her into the bathroom, she says, "One thing I really hate is the smell of all this—of the chemo, of the alcohol, of my urine, everything. I just want it to be *over*."

A minute later she is talking about Sam again, mentioning what beautiful veins he has—the sort of observation only a cancer patient would make—and of how they plan to celebrate her safe arrival in the month of September the coming week. There is school to contemplate. She has all her courses worked out, with the schedule arranged to accommodate chemo, and she talks about how there are three kinds of teachers—those who will not be fazed by her condition at all; those who will make a point of telling her not to expect to get away with anything; and those who will readily let her slide. A young woman named Joyce Arena, a former Hodgkin's patient of Schulman's who now works at the hospital, has talked to Karyn about the "secondary gains" of being a cancer patient, what Karyn calls "the business of getting away with things because of having cancer." For someone so conscientious, this possibility has a subversive ring, but, in fact, any perks that she acquires from having leukemia will be nothing in comparison with the effort it will take to stay afloat academically and socially in the coming months.

September arrives, and Karyn and Sam celebrate as planned. She is supposed to be back at Mount Holyoke on September 12 to start classes, but on September 12 she is in the hospital with a fever. "My mood is not the best," she says. "Sam was here last night when I had one of my fits. It was one of my better ones. He loved it." Except when visitors come, she hibernates for the duration. "I try to leave behind as much of myself as I can when I come in," she says. "I just bring in my shell."

Ten days later she arrives at school and starts classes. She has one more consolidation treatment to go, which she could get as an outpatient, driving an hour each day to and from the hospital in Springfield. But after talking to Dr. Hetzel, she decides that she wants to have a catheter installed in her chest, a semipermanent main line through which she can get all her chemo and any transfusions or antibiotics she might need. She consults with her parents, but essentially she sets up the whole thing herself, arranging to have both her treatment and the surgery seen to at Memorial in early October. She leaves school on a Saturday morning, drives first to Westport and then into New York, where she checks into Memorial.

Two days later, the catheter is installed. Two incisions are made, one at the collarbone, where the catheter is anchored in an artery, another above her right breast, from which the end of the catheter emerges—some four or five inches of flexible white tubing that end in a plastic lock, and can be looped and taped flat against Karyn's chest, to be easily hidden under her clothes. A pair of I.V. nurses teach her how to care for it—it needs to be irrigated every day and the bandage changed twice a week to prevent infection. She must beware of air bubbles that could kill her, guard her supply of syringes and tips, and never go off on a trip without taking along her equipment. Karyn memorizes the steps, and lying flat on her back to avoid getting a headache from a spinal that she had received earlier in the day, she painstakingly demonstrates her skill. "Oh, you're so smart," one of the nurses says when she gets it right. "That's because I'm in college," Karyn replies.

Because she has elected to come to Memorial this time, and expects that the catheter will make her life much more pleasant, Karyn experiences little of the depression that overcame her on earlier stays. Yet it is not easy to be here again, and she has to keep telling herself how changed the circumstances are. "As I lie here now, it's like I never left," she says. "Everything else just fades. When I came home the other day, it felt really weird to be there, and when I was at school, *it* had an air of unreality. At school, I kept thinking, Do I really have to get more chemotherapy? It didn't seem possible. And then I got home and I thought, Have I ever been to school? Am I still sick? I couldn't get oriented at all."

It is a feeling that will wax and wane for months to come, with continual change the only thing she can count on. When she returns to school a week after she left, it is to a less than happy situation with a roommate who, it turns out, cannot handle living with someone who has leukemia. Karyn had found the tension unbearable the first ten days after arriving in late September and had determined to change rooms as soon as she could. Her reaction is healthily mixed—she is hurt by the roommate's attitude and annoyed at having to adjust to one more complication in her life. Hearing from a mutual friend that the roommate has expressed the fear that leukemia is catching, Karyn jokes maliciously about switching mattresses before moving to a new room, then announcing the fact a few weeks later and recommending the services of her several doctors. Her new roommate, Cindy Pattison, is terrific and supportive as is the institution of Mount Holyoke itself. Over the winter Karyn sees the school psychiatrist regularly and finds it a big help. "I save all my dumping for her," she says. "I'm very conscious of not wanting to dump my problems on my friends all the time—they think they should be able to help, and sometimes they can't."

Karyn's departure has an effect on her family that none of them would have thought possible before she became sick. "The air is just lighter in this house," her mother says. No matter that everyone wanted desperately to accommodate, to make up to Karyn while she was unnaturally at home for what had happened—it was a terrible strain on them all to live with a problem that they could not fix. "When Karyn is at school, we forget about her being sick," her mother said, "and start to think of her as being completely normal again. Only when she comes home do we call up all the associations of the illness."

It was impossible to avoid the link between Karyn's presence in Westport and her illness, and so holidays proved less easy than in the past. Over Thanksgiving, Karyn and Sam broke up, and over Christmas, approaching the anniversary of her diagnosis, she felt more tension than she had felt in some time. On New Year's Eve, the Angells had a small party, and her mother invited Karyn to join in. "I wanted her to meet my friends," Dee said, "but she said, 'Mom, don't show me off.' And I did want to show her off, it's true. 'Here she is, alive and well.'"

A year after her diagnosis, back at school, she broke down and cried for three nights in a row. Waking up in the morning, she reported to her parents, she would hear voices and think she was back in the hospital. "I felt it, too," Dee said. "That sheer terror that you can't do anything about." Looking for some relief herself, she said she had called Hetzel at Karyn's one-year date. "I said, 'Well, we're out of the woods, aren't we?' wanting him to say, 'That's right, Mrs. Angell,' But he didn't. He said, 'No, we're just a year down the road.'"

And that's how it continues, a day and a week and a month at a time. By March, Karyn was again happy at school and had enough hair on her head to arrive wigless in Grand Central Station on a weekend visit to the city. She had friends she felt comfortable with, and a 3.2 average despite fevers. She swam with her catheter taped securely beneath her bathing suit, drove herself to and from Springfield regularly for treatments, and spent spring vacation driving Hubie to Florida with two friends. In June she started working full time at the sailing school in Westport, managing the office and appearing there day in and day out with her own hair flying loose, curly and beige and very unlike the hair she grew up with. In July she came to New York for a visit and one of Dr. Gee's Monday nights, where she listened to a panicked man a few years older than she talk about coming out of remission. Along with the other patients at the meeting, she confessed fears of relapse—fears that she had not previously articulated to herself—and heard Dr. Gee assure them all that such fears would always be with them. "I go along cruising, feeling fine," she said, "and then the day before treatment, I become a case." Everyone there nodded, and Karyn realized that it had been a long time since she had been someplace where everyone knew just how she felt.

In September 1982 she started school again, switching for her junior year to Trinity College, in Hartford, in lieu of the junior year abroad that she would have attempted if she had not had leukemia. She had chosen the school with some care, aiming for a coed institution with a good academic reputation within easy driving distance of Springfield. A couple of weeks into the first semester she could report that everyone she met had been friendly, though the atmosphere reminded her of high school more than she cared to be reminded. She hadn't realized how competitive girls on a college campus could get when there were boys to compete for. But all that would sort out, she imagined, "as long as I keep the right attitude." Her teachers were good, and her classes looked promising. She told one of her professors of her illness, and the woman replied that a good friend of hers had just died of leukemia. She seemed eager to talk about it, which made Karyn feel good, particularly as she had not yet told any of her schoolmates of her illness and was still contemplating the best moment to break the news. She was going in for a treatment in a couple of days, and, though it would be possible to pass off a one-day reaction as a stomach virus, she would eventually need their help to get through the year. Also, she did not think it was fair to keep it a secret, and so she knew she must tell them soon. Only, it was so sweet for a while not to have anyone know. It made it almost seem as if it were not really so.

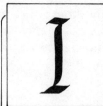I f it is true, as Freud says, that no one can imagine his own death, it is also true that few of us dare to examine the prospect with the sort of interest we bring to other fantasies. One's own death is an event that can hardly be acknowledged, much less believed in ahead of time. In our deepest being, we all expect a reprieve.

Cancer patients are no exception, save perhaps that their need to manufacture hope is more pressing, and that reprieves, if they come, can be dated, and even credited—to a doctor, a drug, nature or a benevolent God. The cancer patient is always measuring time: how long it has been since diagnosis, how many months it has been since treatment began, how much of the statistical survival period has already been exhausted. The patient keeps an eye on the papers, ears alert to the nightly news: one of these days will come the "breakthrough," and then no more chemo, no more radiation, no more disease, no more death.

Talking about his putative relapse one day, Sal Giovia said that he wasn't too worried about coming out of remission in the future, because "even if I did, I'm sure by then they'll have something new." Johanne Johnson, in almost total retreat from the world after her doctor confirms that the last plausible drug available to treat her is not working, still manages to speak of her hope that "they'll think of something." Ray Fink, trying to keep up Celine's spirits—and his own—after two and a half years' continuous treatment for breast cancer, speaks of her fourth course of radiation—aimed at a fresh outbreak of tumors—as "buying time." And Jimmy Polack, no longer toying with the idea of death, but persuaded of a long life of health, says of leukemia, "I know there's a reason, so I know there's a cure."

Such expectations have probably always been instinctive with cancer patients, but the current climate of cancer research makes them irresistible. And when someone as highly placed and regarded as Lewis Thomas, author and chairman emeritus of Memorial Sloan-Kettering declares in print* that he looks for "the end of cancer before this century is over," and further, that "it could begin to fall in place at almost any time, starting next year or even next week," personal expectations of deliverance can no longer be laid to mere wishfulness.

And yet the margins cancer patients live by, and within, are very slim. Surviving five years without recurrence after diagnosis is the generally accepted indicator of cure for most cancers, but none of the eight patients in this book was even diagnosed five years ago, and three of the eight suffered relapses within two years of being diagnosed. For the others, at least two more years must pass without a relapse before the statistical haven of safety is reached. Even then, as they all know, there is no guarantee. Getting cancer, like being born, means drawing an indeterminate sentence.

Indeed, the most dangerous illusion of the cancer patient is not so much that of believing in a cure—because in many instances a cure is possible—as of imagining that without cancer, or post-cancer, immortality is possible. In fact, that illusion remains more compelling to others than it does to cancer patients; it is not possible to have cancer and not consider the fact of one's own death at some point. What is remarkable is how cancer patients live with this intimate awareness of their own mortality, how they push aside ambiguity in order to pursue normal life.

The pursuit is, of course, easiest for those who have no active disease and are finished with treatment. It has been two years since Lou Finkelstein signed off with his surgeon, two and a half since his last chemotherapy treatment. Howard Mindus finished his last cycle of chemotherapy in June 1981 and was restaged and pronounced free of disease the following month. Life comes very close to being as it was for them both, though in Howard's case, the fact of cancer has greatly complicated one of life's most ordi-

---

*The Youngest Science (Viking, 1983).

nary and joyful decisions—whether to have another child. Like every male Hodgkin's patient, Howard was advised before beginning treatment that chemotherapy might render him sterile, or at any rate greatly reduce his sperm count. Accordingly, he made several trips to a sperm bank on Madison Avenue to insure at least the possibility of future progeny. Now, two years after ending treatment, with Howard's expectations of survival virtually identical to those of his never-diagnosed contemporaries, the Minduses' periodic thoughts about having another child are colored by the fact that to do so would almost certainly entail artificial insemination. If they did not have Daniel, now four years old, they might well go ahead, Howard says. But added to all the other considerations of his and Myriam's age and present circumstances, the introduction of technology—and an unguaranteed technology at that—has resulted in a recurrent postponement of the question.

For Jimmy Polack, Sal Giovia, and Karyn Angell, all of whom will have finished treatment by late 1983 or early 1984, roughly three years after they were diagnosed with leukemia, normal life the last few years has been what they have insisted upon in spite of illness. It has taken place in fits and starts, and been regularly punctuated with reminders that life cannot be taken for granted.

Jimmy Polack did go to California after leaving New York in May 1981, but neither he nor his grandfather liked the doctor they had hoped would take over for Dr. Gee in Los Angeles, and when it turned out that Jimmy could not stay with an aunt living in Westwood, his plan to enroll in school there collapsed. He didn't really mind, though, because by then he had had a taste of what it meant to be back in Seattle.

"He wouldn't see anybody for a week," his grandfather reported, "but then all his friends got wind of him being back," and all Jimmy's notions of hiding out until he was ready to be seen bald were forgotten. By early June, he had started maintenance at the Fred Hutchinson Institute, under the care of the doctor who had diagnosed him six months before. Though he was still concerned enough about not losing his hair to request an experimental ice-pack treatment for his scalp ("It looked like a diaper on a baby's ass," he joked, "but I don't care—if it works"), he was also relaxed enough around his friends to have given up wearing hats. And he soon had his first experience as a cancer counselor, when his doctor asked him to talk to another young patient who was refusing treatment. "This guy had ALL for about four months, and he was gonna let Jesus heal him," Jimmy said, "but

274

Jesus was on vacation or something. I told him, 'Don't be stupid, it's your life. Take a little chemo—so what if you lose your hair? It's worth it.'" He laughed. "I didn't tell him I went to a healing service. I mean, I have to be able to talk him into it—I talked myself into it."

In August, he would report that he was "ten pounds lighter and a hundred pounds stronger." He was exercising regularly, working out on a speedbag and getting closer to his old self every day. He could even joke about how a dose of Dactinomycin "made me puke in public in downtown Seattle—right on Pine Street. I'm standing there spilling my guts, and my friend says to me, 'Don't worry, Jim. I threw up here when I was nine years old.'"

He returned to school in September, enrolling in Seattle University and living for a time in one of the dorms. "Life is totally normal," he said that fall, "Better than normal." He described himself as "greedy" for all that he missed while he was sick, and the briefly frenzied existence he pursued at first—a couple of wild trips to California and Nevada with friends, a minor motorcycle accident, a bit of drinking—had both a compensatory quality and a hint of cheating the executioner. "When I got back, I was afraid I couldn't do a lot of things," he said, "So I proved I could." His family watches him anxiously during this time, torn between worry that he will overdo, and relief that he is so much himself again. But they do not press him hard, in recognition of the changes that leukemia has worked in him. "Leukemia set me back six months, sure," Jimmy says at one point, "but I think it sped up my maturity more than a couple of years."

Like Sal, Jimmy has found that going for treatment gets harder and harder all the time, and he complains, long distance, to Dr. Gee that he would like to quit. But he does not, and he makes a deal with Dr. Gee to the effect that if he ever gets ready to quit, the first thing he will do is come back to New York, and give Gee the chance to talk him out of it.

After one semester of college, Jimmy dropped out again, having decided to spend more time working with his grandfather, and to take an accounting course or two at night. His enthusiasm for Acme is real this time out, and he discusses methods of scalding chickens and shipping turkeys with the same sort of technical affection that he once reserved for the disassembly of his various "ve-hicles." In honor of *that* expertise, Morris has placed Jimmy in charge of Acme's small truck fleet, an assignment that pleases them both.

The two men travel together on business now and then, as Morris always hoped they would—to poultry conventions in California and every six months or so to New York, to see suppliers and buyers, and to check in with Dr. Gee, who remains a talisman of sorts for them both and, in a pinch, a trusted mediator. On those trips to New York, Jimmy and his grandfather are like a pair of army veterans returned to tour the front after a year's truce. They walk the midtown streets together, Morris's sports clothes formalized by a string-tie, Jimmy in blue jeans and a jacket that Morris never believes will keep him warm, the two of them bumping shoulders and remarking with delight on all the crazy New Yorkers, the traffic, the overflowing garbage cans. "Jimmy is a good boy," Morris says every hour or so. "That's right, Grampa," Jimmy replies, and slaps the old man gaily on his broad shoulder.

Sal Giovia may have reached his peak of equanimity in the summer of 1982—chastened, hard at work, fit, optimistic, persuaded that life was under control. But he remained susceptible to sweeping transformations of mood that he could neither explain, nor, it seemed, control, and by the fall of that year, he had quit work again and was "hanging out" once more while waiting to start the spring semester at a community college. He was at odds with his parents more often than not, restless, and alternately bored and excited by life. In February 1983, he got an infection and had to spend a week at Memorial as an inpatient, his first hospitalization in almost two years. But, although it depressed him to be back, he knew that his stay did not represent a serious setback; in fact, a year after his suspected relapse, it appeared that it might have been a false alarm. After the time Dr. Gee found Sal's spleen slightly enlarged and then got a dirty marrow reading, he watched him more closely than usual. But subsequent marrows looked good, and when Sal's spleen did not respond to chemotherapy, Gee began to consider its enlargement as possibly due to something other than leukemia. Unless there was a clear change in Sal's condition, then, there was nothing to do medically but continue his treatment, and continue to keep a close watch on him. As for Sal, he remained persuaded that he would die of something pleasurable at a very old age, still a headache—"'cause that's the way I am"—but famous.

Karyn Angell knew that sooner or later she would have to tell her new roommates that she had leukemia, but she did not anticipate its happening quite as it did. In October 1982, a month after starting the new semester, she went for treatment and received a dose of Vincristine, her third or fourth since getting leukemia. A few days later, she woke up with hair on her pillow. This time she did not expect it, and it hit her so hard that she couldn't stand it. She packed up, told her roommates there was a problem at home and drove straight to Westport. "It just isn't fair," she told her parents, who agreed absolutely. And her grandmother, who had taken her shopping for her first wig, now took her out to buy a new one, for the hair that was now falling out was nothing like her old hair or her old wigs. And a week after she had left, she returned to Trinity, where she sat her roommates down and explained herself one more time. As it had done several times already, life started over again. She began to like Trinity better than she had liked it at the start, and in the middle of the semester, she learned of an internship offered by the Leukemia Society in Hartford, which would allow her to work with patients and get college credit for two full courses. Having already decided that she wanted at some point to work professionally with cancer patients, possibly as a psychologist, Karyn applied for the internship and was accepted. Two years earlier, waiting to come into remission, she had answered a question about whether she might consider working with patients when she was finished with her own treatment by saying, "I don't think so. I want to put in my time now and have it behind me." Now she had come full circle, understanding not only that contact with other patients was something she needed to get as well as give, but also—and this was something it would have been impossible to acknowledge at the outset—that you never quite put something like leukemia behind you.

One day, when she had had cancer for about two years, Celine Fink was talking about how it was only natural that people's kindnesses would grow less frequent in the course of time. "I've been sick too long," she said, as if there were a time limit of some kind on compassion. And in a way, she was right, so accustomed are we all to thinking of illness as temporary, reparable, something that can be made to go away or, failing that, that will end quickly. When it does not, we are in some part of ourselves astonished, then made angry. This is not the way life is supposed to turn out. But for Celine, and for Johanne Johnson, having cancer has turned out to be a very untidy experience, a drama with a seemingly interminable terminal act and no prospect of a last-minute reprieve.

In fact, it sometimes seemed as if the two of them had been sentenced to lifetimes of cancer, monthly crises of unpredictable dimensions following one upon another. In the beginning, Celine had read every fresh outbreak of tumors as a potential herald of the end, but as each was treated—cut out, radiated, contained or slowed by chemotherapy, she became warily accepting of the idea that her disease could be managed. In early 1983 Hakes had taken her off Aminoglutethimide, which was no longer working for her, but he put her on another drug, Cytoxan, in its place. She had another round of radiation, continued her monthly visits to Memorial, got around without her walker when she could, used it when she had to, and did her best to remain optimistic. And because breast cancer characteristically moves slowly, she is quite right to go on believing in her chances. Her life is very hard some days, but it is still filled with family and affection and the annoyances and sorrows that are our common lot. And it is still hers.

For Johanne Johnson, that would be true only a little while longer. Following surgery in January 1982, she began a new program of chemotherapy with a drug called dhac-platinum. "There's no comparison to *cis*-platinum," she reported in February, "but it's rougher than I thought it was going to be." Her earliest treatments were given in hospital, and each one effectively put her out of commission for two weeks every month. Marijuana did not ease her nausea, nor did hot baths or Maalox, and in the first six weeks after surgery she lost fourteen pounds. It very soon did not seem worth it. "This time I'm not so gung-ho," she said. "I wonder whether it wouldn't be better to have it over with. I do. I'm entertaining these ideas." Still, mixed in with thoughts of quitting were the jokes. "My body will remember the insults," she said one day. "All of a sudden, it will probably say, 'The hell with you. Let's vacate.'"

She spoke of God's will and of His unknown intentions for her often. "Thy will be done," she said. "But while I say it's in His hands, I keep thinking, what should *I* do?" Trying to sum up her view of how things were going one day, she wagged her index finger at her listener and declared tongue-in-cheek, in tones meant to suggest the voice of the Lord, "See this rock here, Johanne? I'm not going to move it for you. Jump over."

In April her job at Lincoln Hospital was eliminated in a budget cutback, and in order to continue to be able to get medical care Johanne applied for welfare. It was a galling experience. "When I was at Lincoln," she said, "I used to help clients get through all the bureaucracy. Now here it is, my turn." All she wanted was to be eligible for Medicaid, after a lifetime of being self-supporting, but she found she had to pay a very high price in terms of pride and effort to get help. And though she continued to look for part-time work between treatments, she was no longer a very appealing employee. By the fall, the issue was moot. Everything hurt. Her neuropathy was worse than ever, her chest was permanently weighted with pain, and she could neither sleep properly nor walk more than a couple of blocks without stopping to rest on a stoop or a fire hydrant, "Just like the bag ladies and winos." By December, Johanne was down to 106 pounds, the lightest she'd been since her original surgery, almost three years earlier. She continued to complain to Hakes of the pressure in her chest, and in December she was admitted to Memorial once more, where fluid was drained from her lungs.

By spring, although Hakes was now trying Methotrexate, it was clear that Johanne's cancer had advanced beyond containment. And she had begun her retreat from life as well. She did not return to the Bahamas as her cousin Evelyn had, but week by week she withdrew into a limbo state—she was not by her former standards fully alive, but neither had she given up. And her old instinct to try something the doctors could not offer was still there. In April 1983 she sent away to California for a two-month supply of laetrile. It arrived in early May, a totem of the fight still in her as much as an emblem of delusion. "I have to give it a chance," she said. "I've had chemo for three years and it didn't save me. So why not?" Why not, indeed. After all, as she had said once about an earlier choice, "A hundred years from now it will still be my decision."

On June 1, 1983, complaining of extreme discomfort in her chest, Johanne asked to be admitted to Memorial as an emergency patient. Dr. Hakes saw her early the next morning and later remarked that it was the first time she did not have a joke or a light word for him. It was clear that the process of dying that had been under way for months had now speeded up. "I would have said [she had] several weeks," Hakes said. "And they would have been painful."

She had suffered her cancer for more than three and a half years, often in great confusion and agitation, but also bravely and against all reasonable expectation of survival. When she was first hospitalized, she had been advised to forgo surgery and spend her last days getting her "house in order." But she had taken another path. Now she had lived long past the point at which anything could be done for her medically, and perhaps to the very limit of her own will to live as well. As if that were exactly the case, an hour or so after leaving Johanne's bedside, Hakes got word from the floor that she had without warning died. In the absence of an autopsy, which was not performed, Hakes could provide no further detail on the manner of Johanne's dying. Johanne, always eager to point out the limits of conventional medicine, surely would have had something to say about that.

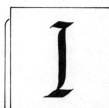I t is probably true that if Terry O'Brien had set herself the problem ahead of time, she might have tried to arrange some better way to die than circumstances and the pace of her unchecked cancer dictated.

If she had understood how quickly her life would unravel at the end, or if she had given up hope sooner than she did, she might have concentrated more on the manner of her death than on fending it off. But it is also true that she had few illusions about enjoying a "good death" and that she understood all too well that no matter how loving a husband she had, no matter how many devoted children were prepared to gather round, she was going to die alone. That's what death meant—an end to human company, a certain and lonely passage into darkness.

Terry O'Brien had believed since childhood that in death she would meet her Maker, but as the moment neared she took less and less consolation from that belief. Not so much because she feared God's punishment—although she did occasionally speak of Hell with the kind of hollow-voiced terror one sees in over-pious children—as because she just wasn't ready to die. Images of heaven could not make up to her for the losses she had begun to experience inch by inch at the end, and it is arguable that however painful it was for her family to watch, the drug-induced derangement that settled over her family was a blessing of sorts, creating the distance necessary to her leave-taking with more clarity than would have been possible otherwise.

Bit by bit, she was simply disappearing before her family's eyes, becoming harder and harder to reach, growing less and less like herself. But there were moments, even at night, when her senility usually was worst, when she could surprise, when she seemed very much there again and impossible to think of as finished with life.

Susie O'Brien remembers her mother being angry a good portion of the last ten days of her life, and occasionally hilariously funny in her fury. "One day," Susie remembers, "she wanted the bed up higher, and Leo and I were there, and we got it up and it got stuck too high, and Leo had to get all the way under the bed to fix it. He got it down, and then she said right away, 'Make it go up again!' And I said, 'Ma, we can't, it'll get stuck.' And she said, 'Oh, sure, *you* go home. *I'll* stay in the hospital in the bed that doesn't work.'"

Susie also remembers that two different hospital chaplains visited her mother during the last couple of weeks (as did a priest from her parish in New Jersey). One of the priests Mrs. O'Brien liked, but the other she thought was an idiot. Susie was there one night when the one her mother didn't like came in. "It was right near the end, when she was being really senile, and the old priest came in that she had joked about before—this little guy who seems like *he's* senile, and he starts to say to her, 'Oh, Theresa, Theresa, I pray for you.' And she looked at him and said, *'You* pray for *me?'* I started to think, Oh my God—and she goes on. *'You? You* are saying prayers for *me?'* I said, 'She doesn't know who you are, Father.' And he starts patting her on the head! He says, 'You're a good girl, Theresa,' and pats her on the head and she's ignoring him. I said, 'Ma, Father's talking to you,' but whenever he'd say 'I'll pray for you,' she'd say *"You* think that *you* can pray for me?' So after he left, I said to her, 'Ma, what's the matter, why didn't you like him?' And she said, 'That man does not deserve to be a priest.' I said, 'Why?' and she said, 'If you don't know, I'm not going to tell you. But that man does not deserve to be a priest. He doesn't do the right thing.'"

On Thursday, June 11, Dr. Golbey speaks of Mrs. O'Brien's case as one that is "as close to being without a solution as anything I've seen in a while." His note of the evening before had concluded, "Poor outlook has been discussed with husband and family," and now he talks of how unhappy he is to see them all going through this, of the limits of hospitals, of the burden that reverts to families, of how ultimately alone they are in dealing with death.

"Dying is very inconvenient for society," Golbey says, conceding that it is not the thing a hospital like Memorial handles best. He says one of the social workers had been in to see Mrs.

O'Brien this week but could not make contact. "If someone had started working with her months ago, we might have more insight into what's going on with her now," he says, but it is both hard to imagine her agreeing to talk to a social worker when she was still well enough to get around and hard to see how it would help her now. Her problem is that she is dying, and she doesn't want to go.

On Friday she sleeps almost continuously. When she is awake, her speech rambles, but there are "lucid moments," according to her chart.

Kak spends the afternoon with her, reminiscing futilely over days at Roxbury Beach, of Te's blond curls and red streak, of how their mother used to set Te's hair with rags and sugar water. Te listens to this indifferently, tuning in and out, interrupting to ask unrelated questions she doesn't seem to really want the answers to. She announces, "The kids aren't coming tomorrow," and when asked why not, answers, "I'll be dead." She looks straight at Kak and says in an uninflected voice, "Well, it's been fun."

On Saturday Ray and several of the children come in, but she is much as she was on Friday. She responds to conversation, but only vaguely. Golbey's note for the day indicates no change in her condition.

On Sunday, Golbey checks on her and finds her much worse. He attempts to make contact but cannot tell whether he succeeds. "Patient deteriorating steadily," his note reads. "Eccychose [bruising] increasing steadily. Body mass [indecipherable] away. She is critically ill and should have whatever she needs for comfort."

On Monday she is worse. "Steady weakening," Golbey's note reads. "Bleak outlook discussed with Mr. O'Brien. I have promised every effort to avoid suffering. Patient should be on critical list."

When Ray O'Brien, Chris and Sean arrive in the afternoon, they are stunned. "She looks like they dropped her off a building," O'Brien says. There are bruises all over her body, the result of her depleted platelets; a sheet has been drawn up over her body, neatly tucked beneath her arms. The lower half of her body is still, as in death, but above the sheet her hands dance without ceasing, fluttering in front of her shut eyes as her head jerks from side to side on the pillow. Her face is hard to read behind the oxygen mask; she is not wearing her glasses, which accentuates the nakedness of her condition. O'Brien quotes Golbey as having said to him earlier in the day that the cancer has in recent hours "overwhelmed her," that it is now a matter of "hours to days."

283

Chris O'Brien stands at the left side of his mother's bed, looking down on her face in silence, his eyes dry and glassy, his face stiff. Sean sits opposite, facing his mother from the right. He leans over the bed from time to time to rub his mother's hand when he can catch it, and somehow maintains an expectant expression.

Their father stands at the foot of the bed, staring at his wife, and then turning away to shake his head, as if incapable of connecting what he sees with the Terry he used to know. Earlier he had said, as if describing the dimensions of the futility he faced, "I've got a million Jesuits praying for her." Watching his wife writhe on the bed now, O'Brien's voice is thick with pain. "I didn't believe it would be like this," he says.

Susie O'Brien was on duty that night, a forty-minute drive from Memorial, and had not planned to come to see her mother until the following night. But she had asked her father to let her know if her mother got worse, and before leaving the hospital he called to tell her. "I asked him if he thought she would know I was there, and he said, 'Probably not.' So I hung up, and I thought about it rationally, and I thought, She's probably not going to know I'm there, and she could be alive tomorrow. We were really busy, and I felt guilty about leaving the other people I worked with, but then I thought, I have to go. Even if she doesn't know I'm there, I have to go."

Leo came with her, both of them wearing their white coats, which enabled them to go right up without being challenged, though it was long past visiting hours when they arrived.

Susie remembers that her mother looked "worse than a lot of corpses I've seen—waxen and emaciated and her mouth open and the blood on her lips." They had been there about fifteen minutes when she died. Susie called for the intern, the young one her mother had liked, who had given her the Narcan that jolted her back to life ten days earlier. The intern came immediately, checked Mrs. O'Brien's blood pressure and pulse and eyes, and pronounced her dead. It was nine-fifteen, a Monday night in June, long before the cold set in.